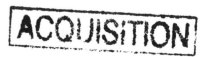

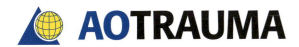

Jesse B Jupiter | Douglas A Campbell | Fiesky Nuñez

Manual of Fracture Management
Wrist

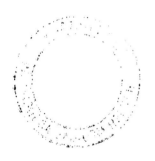

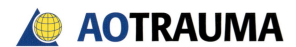

Jesse B Jupiter | Douglas A Campbell | Fiesky Nuñez

Manual of Fracture Management
Wrist

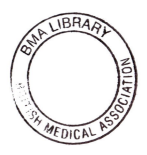

Close to 2,000 illustrations and images and 15 videos

Library of Congress Cataloging-in-Publication Data is available from the publisher.

Hazards

Great care has been taken to maintain the accuracy of the information contained in this publication. However, the publisher, and/or the distributor, and/or the editors, and/or the authors cannot be held responsible for errors or any consequences arising from the use of the information contained in this publication. Contributions published under the name of individual authors are statements and opinions solely of said authors and not of the publisher, and/or the distributor, and/or the AO Group.

The products, procedures, and therapies described in this work are hazardous and are therefore only to be applied by certified and trained medical professionals in environments specially designed for such procedures. No suggested test or procedure should be carried out unless, in the user's professional judgment, its risk is justified. Whoever applies products, procedures, and therapies shown or described in this work will do this at their own risk. Because of rapid advances in the medical sciences, AO recommends that independent verification of diagnosis, therapies, drugs, dosages, and operation methods should be made before any action is taken.

Although all advertising material which may be inserted into the work is expected to conform to ethical (medical) standards, inclusion in this publication does not constitute a guarantee or endorsement by the publisher regarding quality or value of such product or of the claims made of it by its manufacturer.

Legal restrictions

This work was produced by AO Foundation, Switzerland. All rights reserved by AO Foundation. This publication, including all parts thereof, is legally protected by copyright.

Any use, exploitation or commercialization outside the narrow limits set forth by copyright legislation and the restrictions on use laid out below, without the publisher's consent, is illegal and liable to prosecution. This applies in particular to photostat reproduction, copying, scanning or duplication of any kind, translation, preparation of microfilms, electronic data processing, and storage such as making this publication available on Intranet or Internet.

Some of the products, names, instruments, treatments, logos, designs, etc referred to in this publication are also protected by patents and trademarks or by other intellectual property protection laws (eg, "AO", "ASIF", "AO/ASIF", "TRIANGLE/GLOBE Logo" are registered trademarks) even though specific reference to this fact is not always made in the text. Therefore, the appearance of a name, instrument, etc without designation as proprietary is not to be construed as a representation by the publisher that it is in the public domain.

Restrictions on use: The rightful owner of an authorized copy of this work may use it for educational and research purposes only. Single images or illustrations may be copied for research or educational purposes only. The images or illustrations may not be altered in any way and need to carry the following statement of origin "Copyright by AO Foundation, Switzerland".

Check hazards and legal restrictions on www.aofoundation.org/legal

ISBN: 9783132428416
E-book: 9783132428423

1 2 3 4 5 6

Foreword

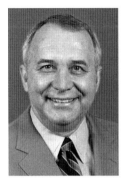

Thomas J Fischer, MD, FAOA, ASSH, AAOS, AOTK
Hand Expert Group
Clinical Associate Professor
Indiana University School of Medicine
Department of Orthopedic Surgery
Section Chief Hand Surgery
Ascension St Vincent, Indianapolis
Indiana Hand to Shoulder Center
8501 Harcourt Rd
Indianapolis, IN 46260
USA

We are now in our 60th year of celebrating the surgeons that came before us and started a unique organization or "working group" the Arbeitsgemeinschaft für Osteosynthesefragen, the AO. The AO had at its core an organizational structure that worked to develop educational programs, documentation of fracture care, research, and instrumentation to make their principles applicable to the variety of fractures.

It was out of this group a text was created, some 30 years ago, called the *Manual of Internal Fixation*. This was the consensus and widely considered technical manual of its time in developing techniques for fracture fixation. It provided a framework for surgeons to approach broken bones and disrupted joints. It provided the integration of thought to perform the documentation, instrumentation, and education of surgeons around the world, thus fulfilling the aims of the organization.

Now several decades and thousands of operations later we find ourselves immersed in a mountain of implants with highly adapted techniques that focus finely on a unique piece of human real estate, the wrist.

Drs Campbell, Jupiter, and Nunez, three lifelong surgeon educators, have tackled this finely focused application of the principles of fracture care and have given us a well-documented and organized text. The text links electronic media with the written word to organize the surgical approaches to primary fracture management and clearly documents the evidence that helps us choose our surgical methods and our surgical implants. But their work does not stop with the primary care of the fracture. The book's hybrid approach to diagrams, case presentations, and evidence-based decision making can also be applied to the described complications and posttraumatic conditions that plague our patients.

In the spirit and innovation that characterized the founders of the AO, these skilled surgeons have approached this task with a passion to perform better and to teach better in a world where online education is the norm. They have used the written text as an anchor and platform to work from and go back to in order to understand the complex repairs of this wonderfully made joint. In reality, the wrist is a series of multiple joints working in harmony to place our hand in space. They have broken down the working components and the common injuries to show us the operative and nonoperative treatment that covers the multitude of internal derangements that can occur.

These surgeons are my valued colleagues and I am honored that they asked me to set the stage for this *Manual of Fracture Management—Wrist*. It is the logical outgrowth of all the learning and development that has taken place since the first development of volar plating for shearing fractures and external fixation with pin fixation for wildly multifragmented fractures. It covers the "lay of the land" quite well and gives us the map we need for lifelong learning in wrist trauma care.

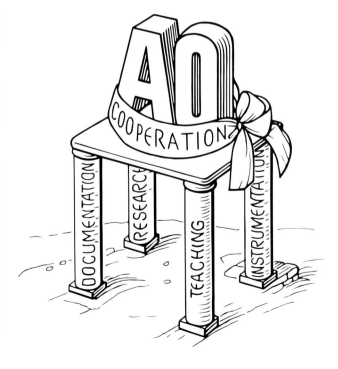

Preface

A considerably greater understanding of traumatic and reconstructive problems about the wrist led us to the decision to revise the initial *AO Manual of Hand and Wrist* into two distinct texts. Following completion and publication of the 2ⁿᵈ edition of the hand fractures volume (now titled *Manual of Fracture Management—Hand*) in 2016, we now offer you the new and expanded *Manual of Fracture Management—Wrist*.

The format of the manual is entirely case based, which has proven to be so successful for both trainees as well as seasoned surgeons in helping to approach and treat both simple and complex injuries. As with the recent hand manual, we have enhanced our clinical case presentations with illustrations taken from the expansive library of the AO Foundation on-line education site, AO Surgery Reference, or used the exceptional skills and resources of the medical illustration and graphic design teams at AO Surgery Reference and the AO Education Institute.

Recognizing the substantial advancements in the understanding of the complex anatomy of the wrist, expanded surgical approaches, and technological improvements in implants specific to a variety of anatomical shapes and injury patterns, this volume covers a wide range of information and is divided into five specific sections. Section one offers the reader ten different surgical approaches to the distal radius, carpus, and distal ulna. Section two examines fractures and fracture dislocations of the carpus including simple and multifragmentary fractures of the scaphoid, nonunions, and even the use of vascular pedicle grafting. The third section focuses on problems of the distal ulna and distal radioulnar joint while the fourth section covers a wide variety of fracture patterns and methods of internal fixation of the distal radius, with

some fascinating clinical cases involving severe multifragmentation and deformity. The final section provides the reader with illustrated cases of various reconstructive problems including nonunion and malunions of the distal radius as well as posttraumatic conditions of the radiocarpal and intercarpal joints.

This wrist manual also reflects the experience and expertise of many teaching faculty that have taught in AO Foundation hand and wrist courses, over many years, and throughout the world. Their concepts as well as clinical examples have assisted and influenced the editors throughout its production. We wish to especially acknowledge the following surgeons for their contributions: Drs Diego Fernandez, Renato Fricker, Fiesky Nuñez Jr, Zhong yu Li, Thomas Fischer, and Juan Del Pino, all of whom contributed unique treatments of specific problems that are illustrated within the manual.

As we first identified in our originally published *AO Manual of Hand and Wrist*, and again emphasized with the recent *Manual of Fracture Management—Hand*, this wrist publication primarily encompasses several examples of operative treatment. It should not be construed to be the only way nor even necessarily the best way to approach the individual problems presented. Likewise it is not intended to be an exhaustive text on the subject. Still, we hope you will find many hours of learning and pleasure in this text in return for the many hours we and others have dedicated in providing this book to you.

Jesse B Jupiter
Douglas A Campbell
Fiesky Nuñez

Acknowledgments

We are well aware that it would not be possible to produce and publish the *Manual of Fracture Management—Wrist*, nor any of the fine AO Foundation book publications you see today, without the dedication and assistance of a large number of contributors. The comradery shown by fellow AO members to share resources, images, and cases, and the hours of education work previously undertaken by wrist surgeon colleagues, plus ad hoc involvement of our own clinical staff means that there truly is a long list of people to thank.

But while there have been countless people involved in some way in the development of this book, we would like to especially mention the following individuals, committees, and groups:

- Members of the AOTrauma Education Commission, for providing the opportunity to develop both this work and the partner publication the *Manual of Fracture Management— Hand*
- Urs Rüetschi and Robin Greene, from the AO Education Institute, for providing access to the resources and AOEI staff required to bring this publication to fruition
- Renato Fricker, for his contributions both as an editor of the *Manual of Fracture Management—Hand* and as an author of this work
- Diego Fernandez and Ladislav Nagy for their previous contributions to hand and wrist education at AO Foundation and contributions and assistance with this publication
- Prof Tom Fischer for kindly providing his Foreword
- Carl Lau, Manager Publishing, and Michael Gleeson, Project Manager for both hand and wrist publications, plus the entire team of graphic design and medical illustration staff and consultants that helped bring hand drawn sketches and verbal ideas into reality
- Lars Veum, Manager AO Surgery Reference, and the teams of current and former project managers, surgeon authors and editors, and illustrators for their editorial and illustration work developing the AO Surgery Reference carpal and distal radius modules
- Fiona Henderson and Andreas Schabert from AO Foundation's publishing partner Thieme
- And last but not least to our partners and family for their continuing and never-ending support for our involvement with the AO Foundation's world-class books, courses, and online education activities and events.

Contributors

Editors

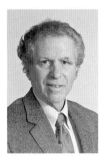

Jesse B Jupiter, MD
Hansjorg Wyss/AO Professor of Orthopaedic Surgery
Harvard Medical School
Massachusetts General Hospital
Yawkey Center, Suite 2100
55 Fruit Street
Boston MA 02114
USA

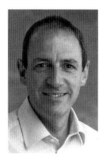

Douglas A Campbell, ChM, FRCS Ed, FRCS(Orth),
FFSEM(UK)
Consultant Hand and Wrist Surgeon
Leeds General Infirmary
Great George St
Leeds LS1 3EX
United Kingdom

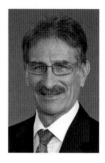

Fiesky A Nuñez Sr, MD
Associate Professor
Department of Orthopaedic Surgery
Wake Forest School of Medicine
Medical Center Boulevard
Winston-Salem NC 27157-1010
USA

Authors

Douglas A Campbell, ChM, FRCS Ed, FRCS(Orth),
FFSEM(UK)
Consultant Hand and Wrist Surgeon
Leeds General Infirmary
Great George St
Leeds LS1 3EX
United Kingdom

Diego L Fernández, MD
Professor of Orthopaedic Surgery
University of Bern
Orthopedic Surgeon
Consultant, Hand and Upper Extremity Surgery
Ch. de la Côte du Bas 12
CH-1588 Cudrefin
Switzerland

Thomas J Fischer, MD, FAOA, ASSH, AAOS, AOTK
Hand Expert Group
Clinical Associate Professor
Indiana University School of Medicine
Department of Orthopedic Surgery
Section Chief Hand Surgery
Ascension St Vincent, Indianapolis
Indiana Hand to Shoulder Center
8501 Harcourt Rd
Indianapolis, IN 46260
USA

Renato Fricker, MD

Member AOTauma Europe, Swiss and American
Societies for Hand Surgery, German speaking Working
Group for Surgery of the Hand
Specialist in Hand Surgery FMH
Senior Consultant Hand, Wrist, Elbow Surgery
Orthopedic and Trauma Surgeons
Hirslanden Clinic Birshof
Reinacherstrasse 28
CH4142 Münchenstein
Switzerland

Juan González del Pino, MD, PhD

Member Spanish Society for Hand Surgery
Member Spanish Society for Orthopaedic Surgery
Former member AOTK Hand Expert Group
Former Editor-in-Chief Spanish Journal of
Orthopaedic Surgery
Former President Spanish Society for Microsurgery
Founder and Head
The Institute of the Hand
Nuestra Señora del Rosario Hospital
80 Castelló St
28006 Madrid
Spain

Jesse B Jupiter, MD

Hansjorg Wyss/AO Professor of Orthopaedic Surgery
Harvard Medical School
Massachusetts General Hospital
Yawkey Center, Suite 2100
55 Fruit Street
Boston MA 02114
USA

Zhongyu Li, MD, PhD, FAOA, FAAOS, ASSH, ASPN

ABOS Board Certified in Orthopaedic Surgery and
Hand Surgery
Professor
Department of Orthopaedic Surgery
Department of Vascular and Endovascular Surgery
Wake Forest School of Medicine
Medical Center Boulevard
Winston-Salem NC 27157-1070
USA

Fiesky A Nuñez Jr, MD, PhD

Hand Surgeon
Bon Secours Mercy Health
Piedmont Orthopedic Associates
35 International Drive
Greenville, SC 29615
USA

Fiesky A Nuñez Sr, MD

Associate Professor
Department of Orthopaedic Surgery
Wake Forest School of Medicine
Medical Center Boulevard
Winston-Salem NC 27157-1010
USA

Abbreviations

APL	abductor pollicis longus
CH	capitate head
CMC	carpometacarpal
DCP	dynamic compression plate
DRUJ	distal radioulnar joint
ECRB	extensor carpi radialis brevis
ECRL	extensor carpi radialis longus
ECU	extensor carpi ulnaris
EDC	extensor digitorum communis
EDM	extensor digiti minimi
EIP	extensor indicis proprius
EPB	extensor pollicis brevis
EPL	extensor pollicis longus
FCR	flexor carpi radialis
FCU	flexor carpi ulnaris
FPL	flexor pollicis longus
LC-DCP	limited contact dynamic compression plate
LCP	locking compression plate
PIP	proximal interphalangeal
SL	scapholunate
SLAC	scapholunate advanced collapse
SNAC	scaphoid nonunion advanced collapse
TFCC	triangular fibrocartilage complex
TFC	triangular fibrocartilage disc
VA	variable angle
VCP	volar column plate

Online book content

Using a QR code scanner on a mobile device, readers will be able to access the approach and demonstration videos featured in this book. The QR code on this page will also bring you to additional online educational content related to this book.

Front matter

Part I
Surgical approach

Part II
Cases

Appendix

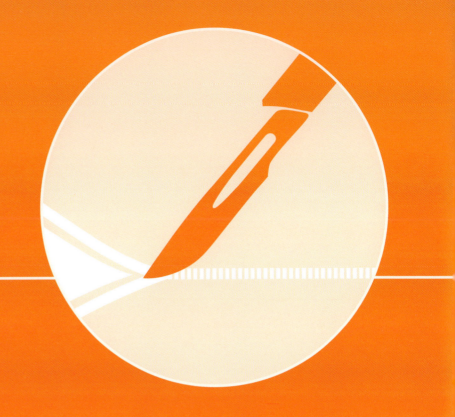

Part I
Surgical approach

1

Approaches

1.1 Palmar approach to the scaphoid

1 Surgical approach

Fig 1.1-1 Injuries involving the scaphoid can be treated using a palmar approach.

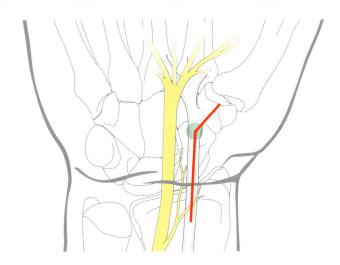

2 Indications

Fig 1.1-2a–b Fractures of the scaphoid are typically described by the location of the fracture, as proximal pole (in the proximal third), scaphoid waist (in the central third), or distal pole (in the distal third). The palmar approach to the scaphoid is indicated for displaced fractures in the central or distal thirds (**a**). It is also indicated for the treatment of scaphoid fracture non-unions (**b**).

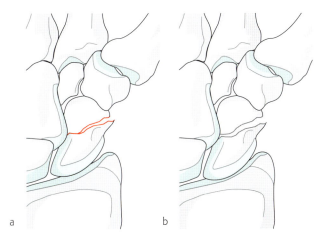

a   b

2 Indications (cont)

Fig 1.1-3 The palmar approach also gives access to those irreducible displaced scaphoid waist (central third) fractures that cannot be reduced and fixed by percutaneous techniques.

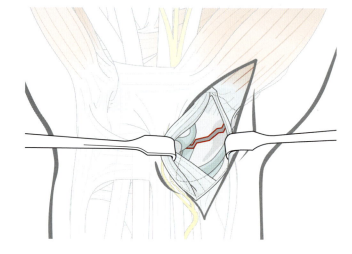

Fracture pattern

Fig 1.1-4a–c Most scaphoid waist fractures are transverse (**a**); however, some can be oblique either in the horizontal (**b**) or vertical plane (**c**).

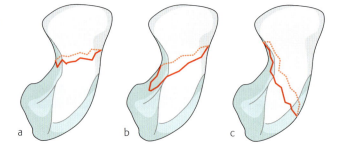

3 Surgical anatomy

Carpal bones

Fig 1.1-5   The bones of the wrist comprise the carpus or carpal bones at the proximal end of the hand, and the radial and ulnar bones at the distal end of the arm. The carpus is made up of eight carpal bones, which include the hamate, capitate, trapezoid, and trapezium in the distal carpal row, and the pisiform, triquetrum, lunate, and scaphoid in the proximal carpal row.

A complex series of soft-tissue structures stabilize the carpal bones and their connection to each other and to the radius and ulna. The scaphoid, however, is by far the most commonly injured carpal bone.

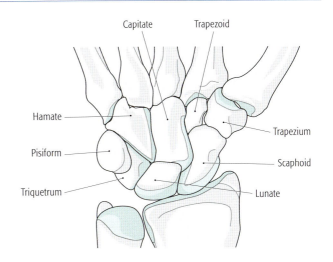

Soft tissues

Fig 1.1-6a–b   On the palmar side of the wrist, the following structures can also be found:
1. Motor branch of the median nerve
2. Palmar cutaneous branch of the median nerve
3. Median nerve
4. Pronator quadratus muscle
5. Flexor digitorum profundus tendons
6. Flexor digitorum superficialis tendons
7. Flexor carpi radialis (FCR) tendon
8. Radial artery.

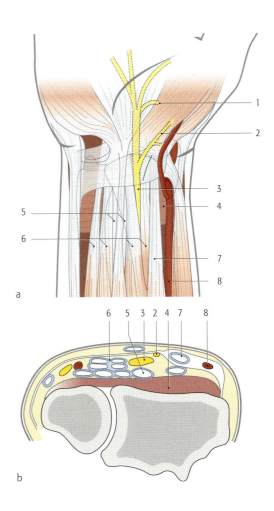

4 Skin incision

Angled skin incision

Fig 1.1-7 Important anatomical landmarks for the angled palmar skin incision are:
- The scaphoid tubercle
- The FCR tendon.

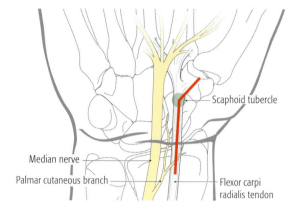

Scaphoid tubercle

Median nerve

Palmar cutaneous branch

Flexor carpi radialis tendon

Fig 1.1-8 The incision line can be marked on the skin in line with the FCR tendon, starting at the scaphoid tubercle and running proximally for about 2 cm. Distal to the scaphoid tubercle, the incision angles toward the base of the thumb over the scaphotrapezial joint. Be aware of the proximity of this incision to the palmar cutaneous branch of the median nerve (as shown in **Fig 1.1-7**) and be sure to avoid injuring it.

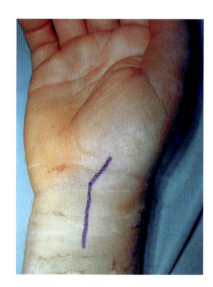

4 Skin incision (cont)

Zigzag incision

Fig 1.1-9 Alternatively, a zigzag palmar incision can be constructed using the same landmarks.

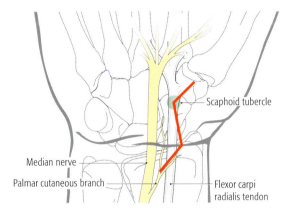

Ligate the superficial palmar branch of the radial artery

Fig 1.1-10 The superficial palmar branch of the radial artery passes toward the palm, running close to the scaphoid tubercle. If necessary, it can be ligated and divided.

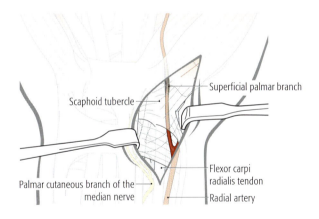

Open the flexor carpi radialis sheath

Fig 1.1-11 The FCR sheath is opened as far distally as possible and the tendon retracted toward the ulnar side.

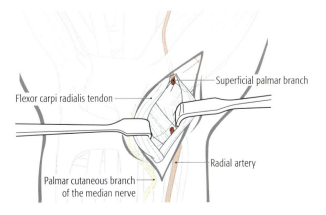

9

4   Skin incision (cont)

Expose the wrist capsule

Fig 1.1-12   The capsule is then incised obliquely from the tubercle distally toward the palmar rim of the radius proximally. This incision also involves the radioscaphocapitate and long radiolunate ligaments. As determined by the fracture configuration, preserve as much of the palmar ligament complex as possible as it helps to contain the proximal pole and prevents palmar tilt of the scaphoid.

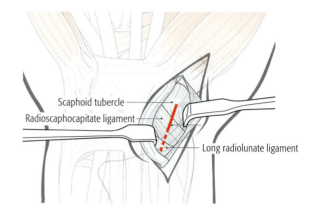

Z-shaped capsular incision

Fig 1.1-13   Alternatively, to preserve the palmar liga-ments, a Z-shaped incision can be made in the joint capsule.

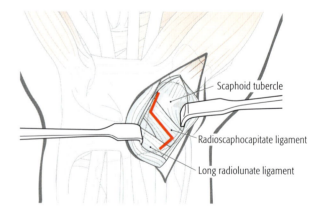

Expose the scaphoid

Fig 1.1-14   Retract the divided radioscaphocapitate ligament to expose the scaphoid.

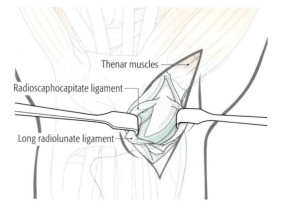

4 Skin incision (cont)

Fig 1.1-15 If it is necessary to expose the proximal part of the scaphoid, divide the long radiolunate ligament proximally as far as the palmar rim of the radius.

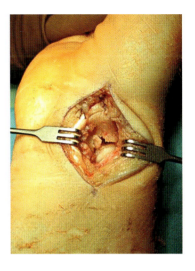

Expose the scaphotrapezial joint

Fig 1.1-16 The scaphotrapezial joint must be exposed to allow optimal positioning of a screw. The incision is deepened distally, dividing the origin of the thenar muscles in line with their fibers.

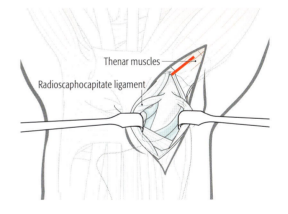

Fig 1.1-17 The scaphotrapezial joint is identified, the scaphotrapezial ligament divided in the line of its fibers, and the joint capsule opened.

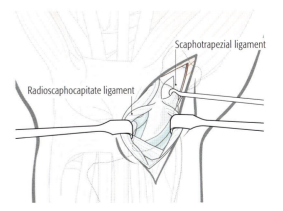

11

5 Wound closure

Fig 1.1-18 The divided palmar ligaments (radioscaphocapitate and long radiolunate) must be repaired with fine interrupted sutures to prevent secondary carpal instability. Approximate the soft tissues over the scaphotrapezial joint. Test the integrity of the soft-tissue repair by passive wrist motion. Finally, the FCR tendon sheath is repaired and covered with subcutaneous tissue.

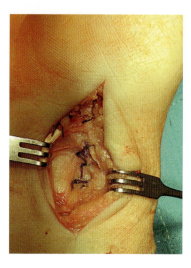

Video

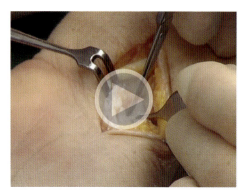

Video 1.1-1 This video demonstrates the palmar approach to the carpals.

1.2 Dorsal approach to the scaphoid

1 Surgical approach

Fig 1.2-1 Injuries involving the scaphoid can be treated using a dorsal approach.

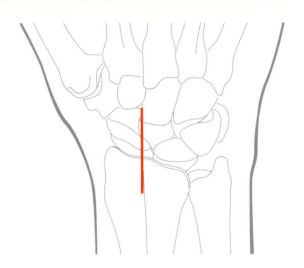

2 Indications

Fig 1.2-2a–b The dorsal approach to the scaphoid is indicated for all acute displaced and nondisplaced fractures of the proximal pole (proximal third) (**a**). It is also indicated for the bone grafting of proximal pole nonunions (**b**).

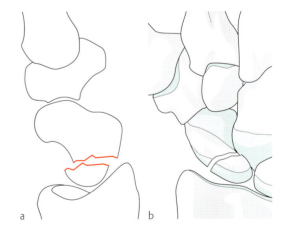

3 Surgical anatomy

Extensor compartments

Fig 1.2-3 There are five extensor compartments on the dorsum of the radiocarpal region and one extensor compartment at the ulnocarpal region. These compartments or tunnels contain the extensor tendons.

The first compartment contains the abductor pollicis longus (APL) and extensor pollicis brevis (EPB) tendons. The second compartment contains the extensors carpi radialis longus (ECRL) and brevis (ECRB). The third compartment contains the extensor pollicis longus (EPL) tendon. The fourth compartment contains the extensor indicis proprius (EIP) and the extensor digitorum communis (EDC). The fifth compartment contains the extensor digiti minimi (EDM). Finally, the sixth compartment hosts the extensor carpi ulnaris (ECU).

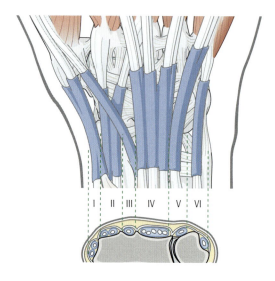

Fig 1.2-4 The superficial radial nerve (1) and the dorsal branch of the ulnar nerve (2) lie in the subcutaneous tissues superficial to the extensor compartments and are vulnerable to injury during surgical approach.

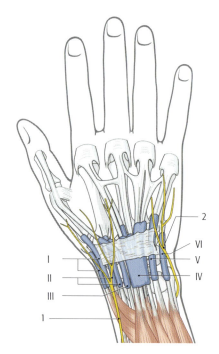

Fig 1.2-5a–b   Make a straight dorsal skin incision starting over Lister tubercle (the bony prominence located at the distal end of the radius) and extend the incision for about 4 cm distally.

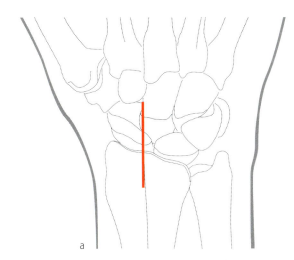

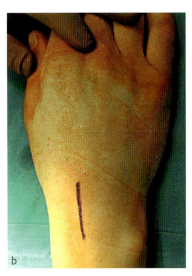

4 Skin incision (cont)

Identify the radial nerve

Fig 1.2-6 Ensure to preserve any parts of the superficial branch of the radial nerve, which runs in the radial skin flap of the wound.

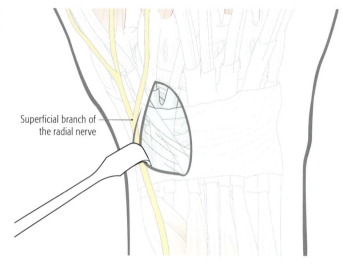

Superficial branch of the radial nerve

Incise the retinaculum

Fig 1.2-7 Incise the distal part of the extensor retinaculum over the EPL tendon, leaving the proximal part intact.

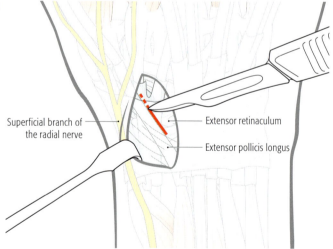

Superficial branch of the radial nerve

Extensor retinaculum

Extensor pollicis longus

4　Skin incision (cont)

Fig 1.2-8　Open the distal part of the third extensor compartment.

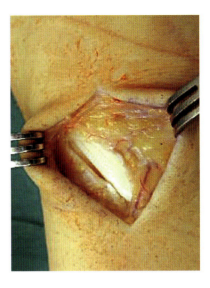

Retraction of the tendons

Fig 1.2-9　The EPL tendon is then retracted radially together with the tendons of the second extensor compartment (the ECRB and the ECRL).

The tendons of the fourth extensor compartment are retracted in an ulnar direction.

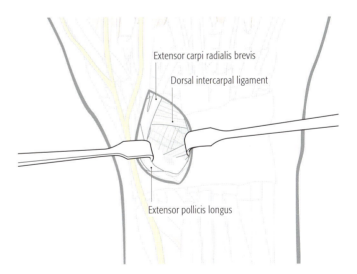

Extensor carpi radialis brevis

Dorsal intercarpal ligament

Extensor pollicis longus

4   Skin incision (cont)

Opening the capsule

Fig 1.2-10   Make a longitudinal or inverted T-shaped incision, starting at the dorsal rim of the distal radius, and extending to the dorsal radiocarpal ligament.

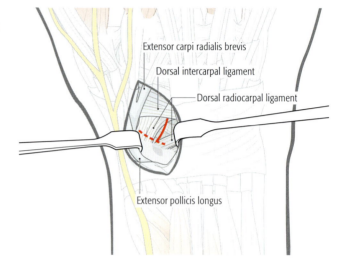

Extensor carpi radialis brevis

Dorsal intercarpal ligament

Dorsal radiocarpal ligament

Extensor pollicis longus

Fig 1.2-11   Take care to preserve the vessels to the dorsal ridge of the scaphoid. The capsule should not be stripped from this area.

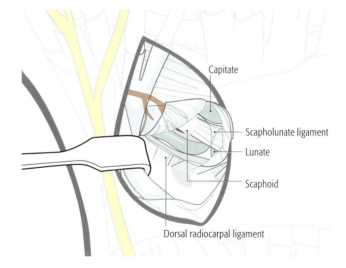

Capitate

Scapholunate ligament

Lunate

Scaphoid

Dorsal radiocarpal ligament

4 Skin incision (cont)

Expose the scaphoid

Fig 1.2-12 To expose the proximal pole of the scaphoid, it is necessary to flex the wrist. The scaphoid now comes into view. And the scapholunate ligament can be identified.

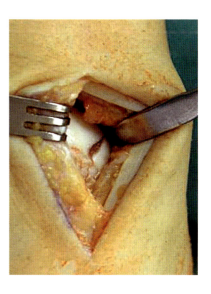

5 Wound closure

Fig 1.2-13 Close the capsule with interrupted sutures.

It is not necessary to repair the third extensor compartment because the proximal part remains intact.

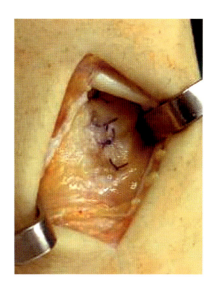

5 Wound closure (cont)

Video

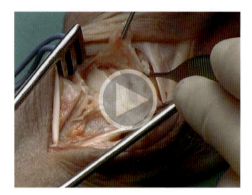

Video 1.2-1 This video demonstrates the dorsal approach to the carpals.

1.3 Combined approach to the lunate and perilunate injuries

Fig 1.3-1   Injuries involving the lunate or its surrounding structures can be treated using a combined dorsal and palmar approach.

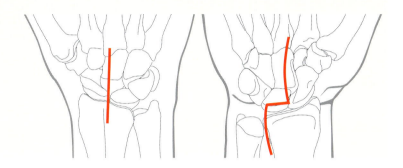

Fig 1.3-2a–c   The combined approach (using both dorsal and palmar incisions) is often indicated for lunate and perilunate injuries.

A lunate dislocation exists when the lunate (**a**) loses contact with the lunate fossa of the distal radius (**b**).

However, a perilunate injury exists when an adjoining carpal bone is damaged or dislocated but the lunate itself remains in contact with the lunate fossa of the distal radius (**c**).

In most cases involving the combined approach, the dorsal approach is made first. However, start with a palmar approach in cases of palmar dislocation of the lunate or in the rarer palmar luxation of other carpal bones.

Note that a combined approach for these injuries is not always necessary. The dorsal aspect of the scapholunate ligament is the stronger, so the dorsal approach is indicated to repair it and to reduce any scapholunate dissociation (ligament injuries). It is also indicated to reduce and stabilize other perilunate fracture dislocations.

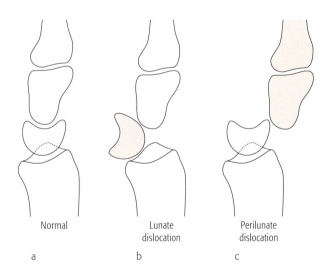

Normal	Lunate dislocation	Perilunate dislocation
a	b	c

---

3 Surgical anatomy

Extensor compartments

Fig 1.3-3   There are five extensor compartments in the dorsoradial region and one extensor compartment at the dorsoulnar region.

The second compartment contains the extensor carpi radialis longus and brevis. The third compartment contains the extensor pollicis longus (EPL) tendon. The fourth compartment contains the extensor indicis proprius and the extensor digitorum communis. Perilunate injuries can be approached through the second, third, and fourth compartments.

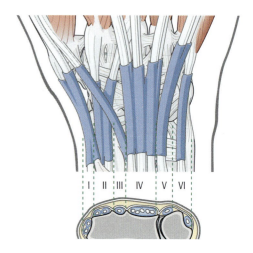

Soft tissues

Fig 1.3-4a–b   On the palmar side of the wrist, the following structures can also be found:
1. Motor branch of the median nerve
2. Palmar cutaneous branch of the median nerve
3. Median nerve
4. Pronator quadratus muscle
5. Flexor digitorum profundus tendons
6. Flexor digitorum superficialis tendons
7. Flexor carpi radialis (FCR) tendon
8. Radial artery.

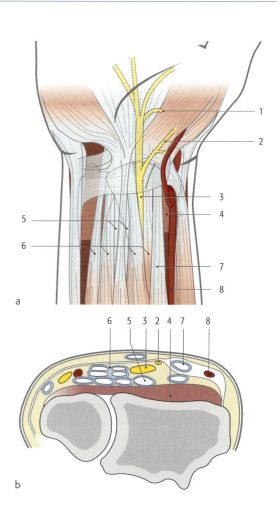

4 Dorsal skin incision

Straight skin incision

Fig 1.3-5 Make a straight skin incision beginning proximally and ulnar to Lister tubercle and ending distally at the level of the third carpometacarpal joint. The incision should be about 8 cm long. The incision can be extended proximally or distally if necessary.

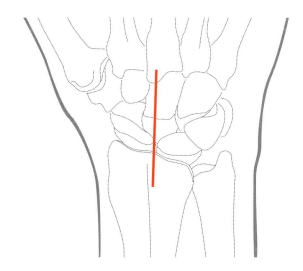

Elevate the skin flap

Fig 1.3-6 Preserve the large longitudinal veins and ligate and divide the crossing branches to achieve exposure.

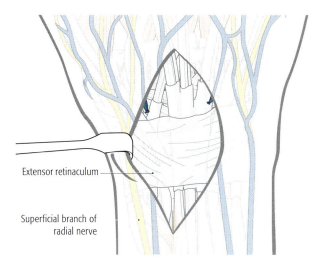

Extensor retinaculum

Superficial branch of
radial nerve

4   Dorsal skin incision (cont)

Fig 1.3-7   Elevate the skin flaps, complete with subcutaneous tissue, from the extensor retinaculum. The superficial branch of the radial nerve should be identified and elevated with the skin flap.

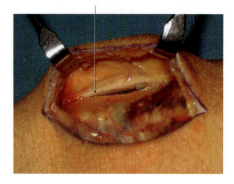

Superficial branch of the radial nerve

Open the third compartment

Fig 1.3-8   Incise the extensor retinaculum over the EPL tendon, opening the third extensor compartment.

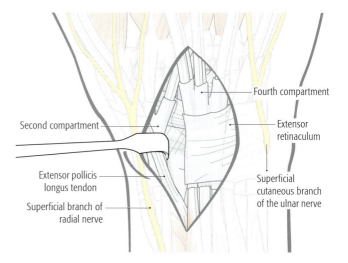

Second compartment

Extensor pollicis longus tendon

Superficial branch of radial nerve

Fourth compartment

Extensor retinaculum

Superficial cutaneous branch of the ulnar nerve

Fig 1.3-9   The EPL tendon is released and retracted radially, together with the extensor tendons of the second compartment.

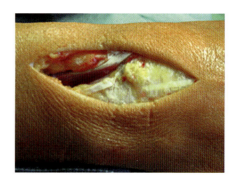

4 Dorsal skin incision (cont)

Open the fourth compartment

Fig 1.3-10 Retract the extensor tendons of the fourth compartment in an ulnar direction to expose the wrist capsule.

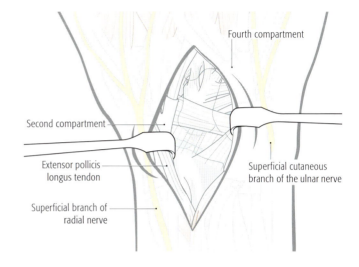

Fourth compartment

Second compartment

Extensor pollicis longus tendon

Superficial branch of radial nerve

Superficial cutaneous branch of the ulnar nerve

Radially based capsular incision

Fig 1.3-11 To gain a complete view of the carpus, a radially based capsular ligamentous flap is elevated. The capsulotomy incision starts radially deep to the floor of the second extensor compartment.

Leave a fringe of 2–3 mm of the capsular attachment at the dorsal rim of the radius for subsequent suture repair.

The incision occurs as follows:
1. The incision continues in an ulnar direction along the dorsal rim of the radius
2. It then turns distally in line with the fibers of the radiolunotriquetral (dorsal radiocarpal) ligament
3. At the triquetrum it turns radially in line with the fibers of the dorsal intercarpal ligament.

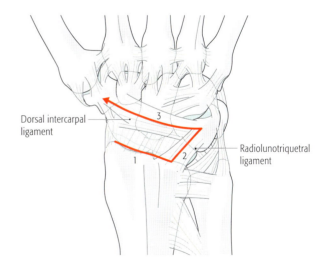

Dorsal intercarpal ligament

Radiolunotriquetral ligament

4 Dorsal skin incision (cont)

Protect the distal radioulnar joint

Fig 1.3-12 Be careful not to cut the dorsal radioulnar ligament or the triangular fibrocartilage of the distal radioulnar joint, which must be protected.

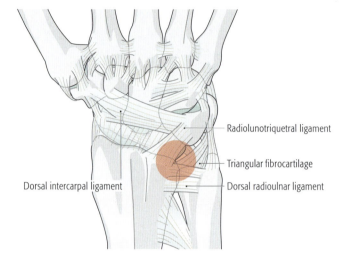

Radiolunotriquetral ligament

Triangular fibrocartilage

Dorsal radioulnar ligament

Dorsal intercarpal ligament

Elevate the capsular flap

Fig 1.3-13 The capsular flap is elevated by sharp dissection in an ulnar to radial direction.

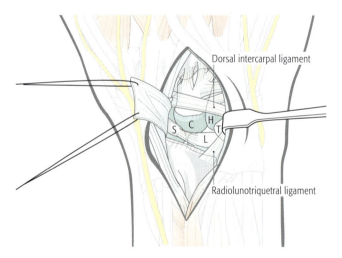

Dorsal intercarpal ligament

Radiolunotriquetral ligament

Fig 1.3-14 The proximal carpal row with its intrinsic ligaments and the midcarpal joint are exposed.

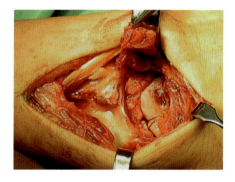

5 Palmar skin incision

Fig 1.3-15   After the dorsal approach, with temporary fixation on the dorsal side, the palmar approach is performed if necessary.

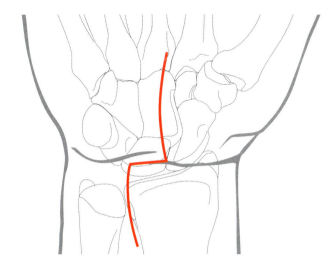

Extended carpal tunnel incision

Fig 1.3-16   The incision begins in the palm, at the level of the distal edge of the flexor retinaculum, in line with the third metacarpal. It continues proximally in the intereminence crease to the level of the transverse flexor crease of the wrist.

At this point, the incision angles 90 degrees in an ulnar direction for 2 cm in the line of the wrist flexor crease. It then turns proximally as a slightly curved longitudinal extension as far as necessary.

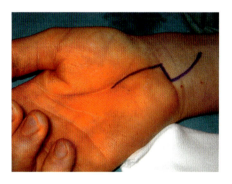

---

5   Palmar skin incision (cont)

Elevate the skin flaps

Fig 1.3-17   Elevate the skin flaps by sharp dissection, firstly from the surface of the palmar aponeurosis distally, then from the antebrachial fascia proximally, on the ulnar side of the palmaris longus tendon. This protects the palmar cutaneous branch of the median nerve, which passes to the radial side of the palmaris longus tendon.

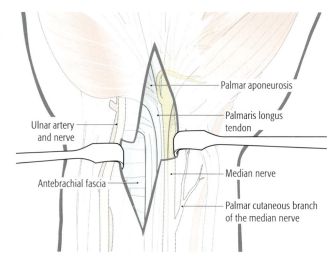

Open the carpal tunnel

Fig 1.3-18   Identify the median nerve, which lies radial and deep to the palmaris longus tendon. Insert a blunt instrument into the carpal tunnel between the median nerve and the flexor retinaculum. Now divide the flexor retinaculum longitudinally over the blunt instrument, which protects the median nerve. The retinaculum should be divided to the ulnar side of the median nerve to protect its motor branch to the thenar muscles.

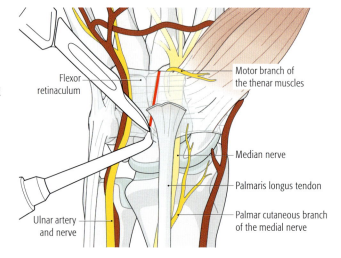

5 Palmar skin incision (cont)

Retract the flexor tendons

Fig 1.3-19 To expose the palmar carpal ligaments, retract all the flexor tendons radially.

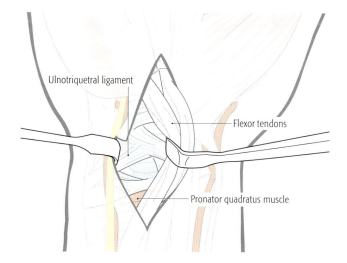

Ulnotriquetral ligament

Flexor tendons

Pronator quadratus muscle

Fig 1.3-20 Only the ulnar nerve and artery remain on the ulnar side.

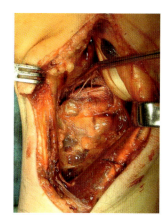

5   Palmar skin incision (cont)

Option: approach to the radial palmar capsule

Fig 1.3-21   Sometimes the median nerve must be carefully retracted radially together with the tendon of the flexor pollicis longus. The flexor tendons of the fingers are retracted in an ulnar direction, thereby exposing the radial side of the palmar capsule.

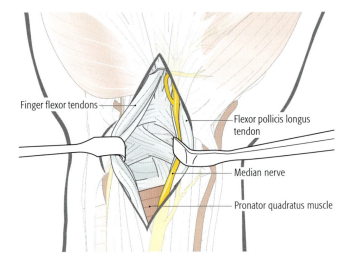

Finger flexor tendons

Flexor pollicis longus tendon

Median nerve

Pronator quadratus muscle

6   Wound closure

Close the capsular incision

Fig 1.3-22   On the dorsal side, repair the radially based flap with interrupted sutures.

To avoid the risk of ischemic rupture of the EPL, it is recommended that it be left above the extensor retinaculum in the subcutaneous tissue.

If an incision is also made on the palmar side, the skin is closed in the standard fashion.

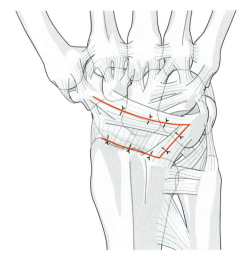

1.4   Radiopalmar approach to the thumb base

1   Surgical approach

Fig 1.4-1   Injuries involving the base of the thumb can be treated using a radiopalmar approach.

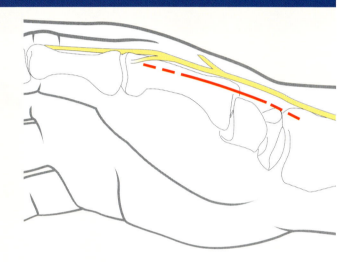

2   Indications

Fig 1.4-2   This approach is indicated for fractures of the trapezium as well as for intraarticular fractures of the first carpometacarpal joint, such as Bennett or Rolando fractures. It is also indicated for basal metacarpal fractures.

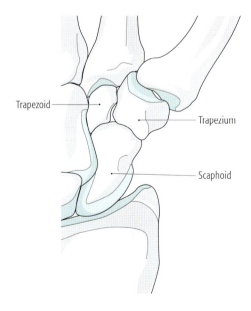

Trapezoid

Trapezium

Scaphoid

3 Surgical anatomy

Fig 1.4-3a–b The joint surfaces of the trapezium and thumb metacarpal resemble two reciprocally interlocking saddles. This articular geometry, the ligamentous support system, and the thumb muscles all work in synergy to enable opposition of the thumb to the fingers.

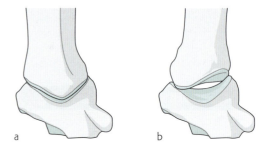

a   b

Fig 1.4-4 The strong palmar oblique ligament is essential as a stabilizing unit of the base of the thumb metacarpal; it inserts into the articular margin of the palmar beak on the ulnar aspect of the first metacarpal base. On the radial side of the metacarpal base is the insertion of the abductor pollicis longus (APL) tendon. The adductor pollicis exerts a force that pulls the thumb in a palmar and ulnar direction.

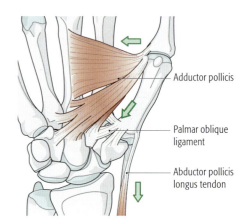

Adductor pollicis

Palmar oblique ligament

Abductor pollicis longus tendon

4 Skin incision

Two different skin incisions can be used:
- The straight radiopalmar incision
- The curved incision, described by Wagner.

Fig 1.4-5 The straight incision is made in the dorsoradial aspect of the thenar eminence at the transition between the dorsal and palmar skin. It starts about 1 cm distal to the tip of the radial styloid and extends distally for 4–5 cm.

The superficial branch of the radial nerve divides into several branches in this area. Identify and protect these branches to avoid troublesome neuroma formation. The radial artery crosses the proximal limit of the incision in an oblique direction and must also be identified, protected, and preserved.

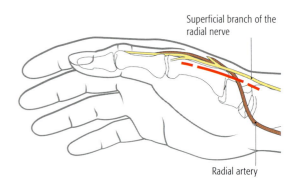

Superficial branch of the radial nerve

Radial artery

4 Skin incision (cont)

Fig 1.4-6 The Wagner incision follows the thenar eminence in a gentle curve toward its palmar aspect. The disadvantage of this incision is the risk of scar formation across the wrist crease and lesions of nerve branches.

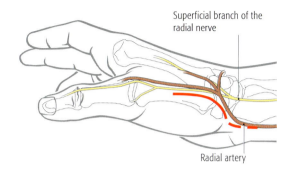

Superficial branch of the radial nerve

Radial artery

Elevate the flap

Fig 1.4-7 Elevate the flaps of skin and subcutaneous tissue by blunt dissection, identifying and protecting the divisions of the superficial branch of the radial nerve and the APL tendon. Gentle retraction with elastic vessel loops aids the exposure.

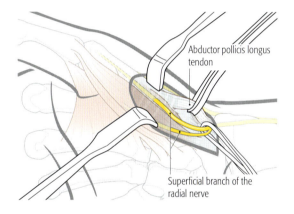

Abductor pollicis longus tendon

Superficial branch of the radial nerve

Fig 1.4-8 However, the excessive retraction of the flaps can impair vascularity of the tissues.

Abductor pollicis longus tendon

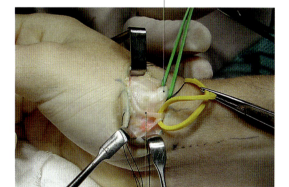

Superficial branch of the radial nerve

4 Skin incision (cont)

Detach the thenar muscles

Fig 1.4-9 After retracting these structures, the thenar muscles come into view. They are then detached from their origins at the base of the first metacarpal and reflected in a palmar direction.

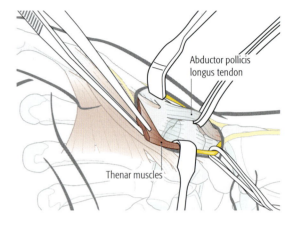

Abductor pollicis longus tendon

Thenar muscles

Fig 1.4-10 Preserving a small part of the insertion will later help with reattachment of the thenar muscles.

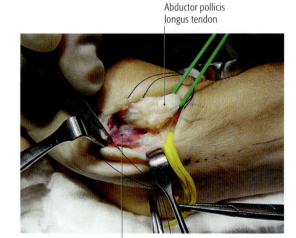

Abductor pollicis longus tendon

Thenar muscles

Capsulotomy

Fig 1.4-11 Perform a transverse or longitudinal capsulotomy to expose the joint.

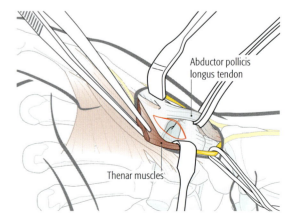

Abductor pollicis longus tendon

Thenar muscles

4   Skin incision (cont)

Inspect the joint

Fig 1.4-12   Inspect the joint by rotating the thumb into pronation and supination, while exerting longitudinal traction. This maneuver also helps to assess the fracture geometry and to reduce Bennett fractures.

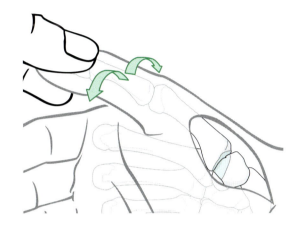

5   Wound closure

Fig 1.4-13   Close the capsule with interrupted sutures. Reattach the thenar muscles to the base of the first metacarpal using interrupted sutures.

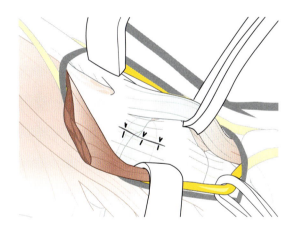

5   Wound closure (cont)

Video

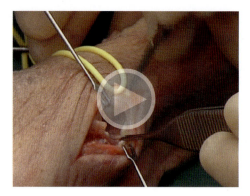

Video 1.4-1   This video demonstrates the radiopalmar approach to the thumb base.

1.5 Dorsoradial approach to the distal radius

1 Surgical approach

Fig 1.5-1 Injuries involving the radial styloid can be treated using a dorsoradial approach.

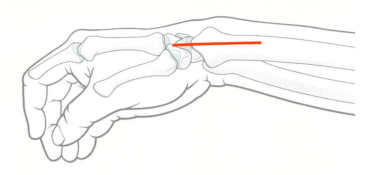

2 Indications

Fig 1.5-2 Depending on the specific fracture pattern, a dorsal approach between the various extensor compartments I-VI is chosen.

In injuries involving the radial styloid, an approach between the first and second extensor compartments (A) is indicated.

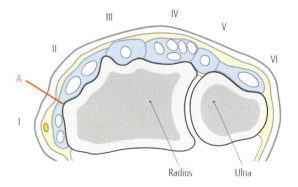

3 Surgical anatomy

Anatomical snuffbox

Fig 1.5-3 The extensor pollicis longus and the extensor pollicis brevis are the landmarks for the anatomical snuffbox, with the tip of the radial styloid forming the floor.

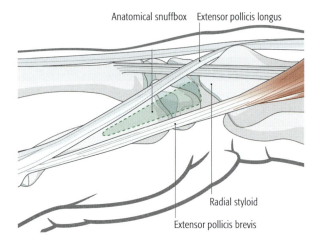

Anatomical snuffbox Extensor pollicis longus

Radial styloid

Extensor pollicis brevis

Fig 1.5-4 Important structures around the anatomical snuffbox include the superficial branches of the radial nerve, which should be carefully protected during any fixation procedure. The radial artery crosses the floor of the anatomical snuffbox and should also be protected.

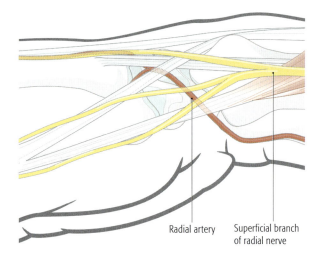

Radial artery Superficial branch of radial nerve

4   Skin incision

Fig 1.5-5   A straight incision is made over the anatomical snuffbox and extended distally and proximally, to the necessary extent, as illustrated. The two resultant skin/subcutaneous flaps are raised by blunt dissection from the underlying extensor retinaculum.

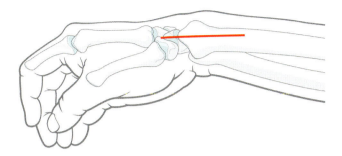

Exposure

Fig 1.5-6   The superficial cutaneous branches of the radial nerve are identified and protected. The radial styloid is approached between the first and second compartments and then exposed by sharp dissection.

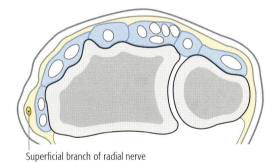

Superficial branch of radial nerve

4   Skin incision (cont)

Fig 1.5-7   The first and second compartments can be elevated as necessary.

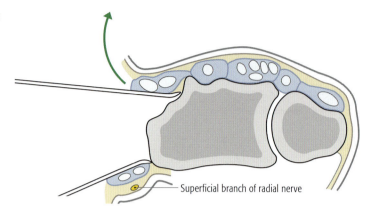

Superficial branch of radial nerve

5   Wound closure

The skin is closed in a standard fashion.

1.6 Modified Henry palmar approach to the distal radius

1 Surgical approach

Fig 1.6-1 Injuries involving the distal radius can be treated using a modified Henry palmar approach.

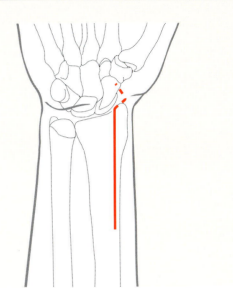

2 Indications

Fig 1.6-2 The modified Henry approach is suitable for most fractures of the distal radius.

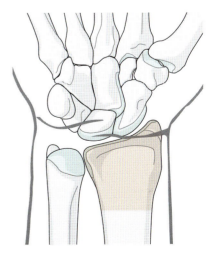

Soft tissues

Fig 1.6-3a–b   On the palmar side of the wrist, the following structures can be found:
1. Motor branch of the median nerve
2. Palmar cutaneous branch of the median nerve
3. Median nerve
4. Pronator quadratus muscle
5. Flexor digitorum profundus tendons
6. Flexor digitorum superficialis tendons
7. Flexor carpi radialis (FCR) tendon
8. Radial artery.

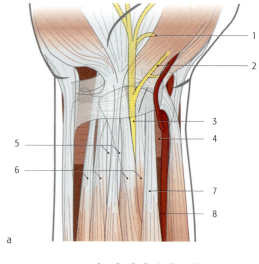

a

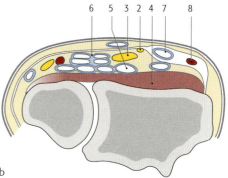

b

3   Surgical anatomy (cont)

Bony anatomy

Fig 1.6-4a–b   In addition to the surrounding soft tissues, the distal radius contains a number of bony protrusions:
1. Ulnar styloid
2. Ulnar head
3. Sigmoid notch
4. Lunate facet
5. Lister tubercle
6. Scaphoid facet
7. Radial styloid
8. Watershed line.

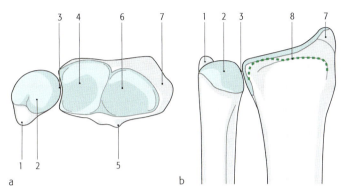

Watershed line

Fig 1.6-5   The watershed line represents the margin between the structures that may be elevated proximally and the capsule of the wrist joint, which should be respected.

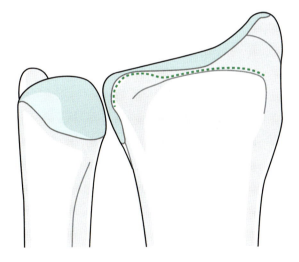

4   Planning the incision

Fig 1.6-6   The modified Henry approach uses the plane between the FCR tendon and the radial artery. The classic Henry approach goes between the brachioradialis and the radial artery, that is, radial to the radial artery; however, the modified Henry approach is ulnar to the radial artery. The FCR tendon is palpated before making the skin incision to the radial side.

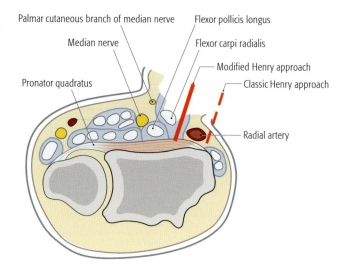

Palmar cutaneous branch of median nerve — Flexor pollicis longus

Median nerve — Flexor carpi radialis

— Modified Henry approach

Pronator quadratus — Classic Henry approach

— Radial artery

Fig 1.6-7   A distal extension of the incision in a zigzag fashion across the wrist flexion crease will allow mobilization of the FCR tendon for a more extensile approach.

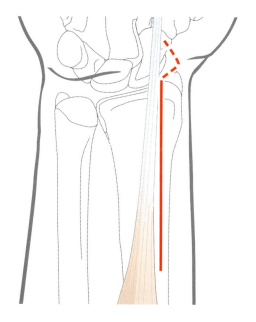

Pitfall

The radial artery and the palmar cutaneous branch of the median nerve are at risk during this approach.

5   Skin incision

Fig 1.6-8   Make the skin incision along the radial border of the FCR tendon. The sheath is opened and the tendon retracted toward the ulnar side. Deepen the incision between the flexor pollicis longus (FPL) tendon and the radial artery.

Care must be taken to avoid damaging the radial artery on the radial side and the palmar cutaneous branch of the median nerve on the ulnar side.

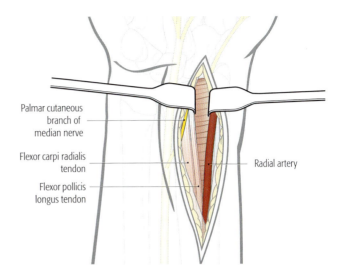

Fig 1.6-9   The FPL muscle belly is swept away toward the ulna. This increases the space and exposes the pronator quadratus muscle.

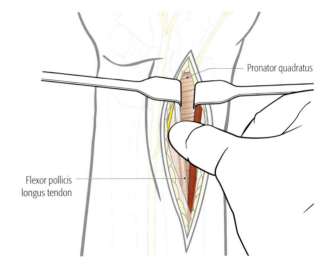

5   Skin incision (cont)

Pearl

Fig 1.6-10   The pronator quadratus muscle should be elevated using an L-shaped incision. The horizontal limb is placed at the watershed line. This lies a few millimeters proximal to the joint line; the position of the joint line can be determined by a hypodermic needle placed in the joint.

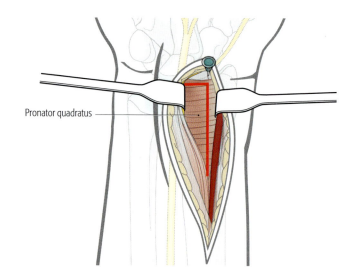

Pronator quadratus

Exposing the distal radius

Fig 1.6-11   The pronator quadratus muscle is incised on its radial border, exposing the distal radius. It is stripped off the distal radius together with the periosteum.

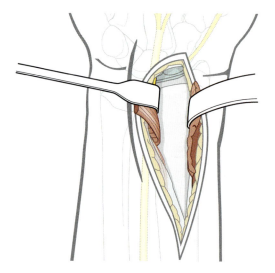

6 Wound closure

Fig 1.6-12 The pronator quadratus should be placed over the plate. Every attempt should be made to reattach the horizontal limb of the pronator quadratus elevation to the capsule. If possible, it should be reattached to its radial insertion.

The tendon sheath may be closed, but care must be taken to avoid catching the cutaneous branch of the median nerve. The skin is then closed.

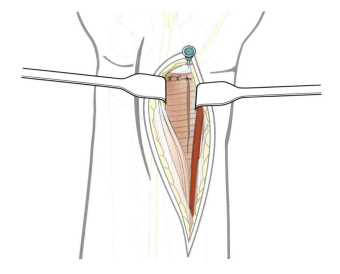

Video

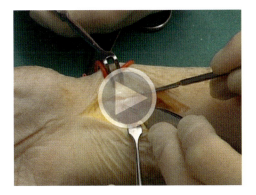

Video 1.6-1 This video demonstrates the palmar approach to the distal radius.

1.7 Ulnar palmar approach to the distal radius

1 Surgical approach

Fig 1.7-1 Injuries involving the distal radius can be treated using an ulnar palmar approach.

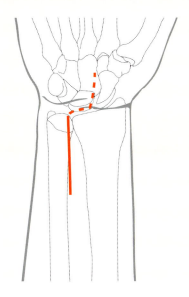

2 Indications

Fig 1.7-2a–b An ulnar palmar approach is preferred to expose the palmar lunate facet. The ulnar palmar approach also facilitates exposure of the sigmoid notch, the palmar wrist capsule, the distal radioulnar joint, and the distal ulna (**a**). It is less suitable for the radial part of the distal radius.

For more complex fractures, an ulnar palmar extensile approach may be used.

If it is desired to decompress the carpal tunnel, this can be performed either through an ulnar palmar extensile approach or two separate approaches (**b**).

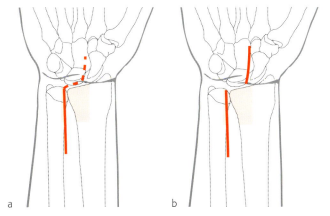

a   b

3 Surgical anatomy

Details on the anatomy involved in this approach can be found in the surgical anatomy topic in chapter 1.6 Modified Henry palmar approach to the distal radius.

4 Planning the incision

Fig 1.7-3 The ulnar palmar approach uses the plane between the ulnar artery and nerve on one side and the flexor tendons on the other side.

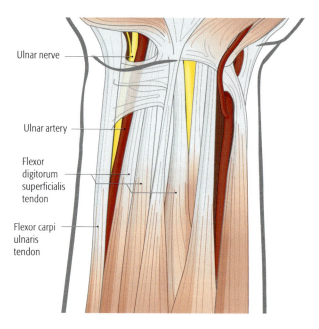

Ulnar nerve

Ulnar artery

Flexor digitorum superficialis tendon

Flexor carpi ulnaris tendon

5 Skin incision

Fig 1.7-4a–b The incision starts at the wrist crease and runs proximally parallel to the ulna (**a**). It can be extended along the wrist crease and distally into the palm. The interval is developed between the ulnar artery and the flexor tendons (**b**).

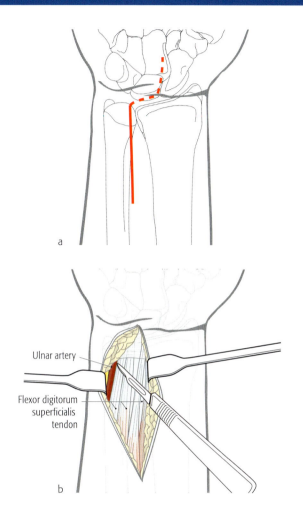

Dissection

Fig 1.7-5 The flexor tendons and median nerve are retracted toward the radial side to provide excellent exposure of the pronator quadratus.

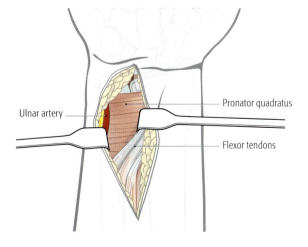

5 Skin incision (cont)

Fig 1.7-6 The pronator quadratus is incised as much as necessary.

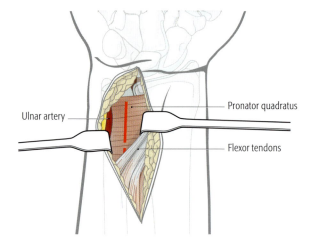

Fig 1.7-7 Expose the ulnar side of the distal radius by elevating the incised portion of the pronator quadratus.

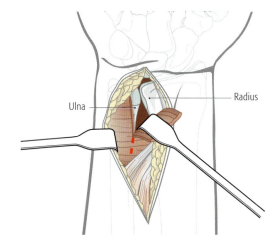

5   Skin incision (cont)

Extension of ulnar palmar approach

Fig 1.7-8   The ulnar palmar approach can be extended distally. This allows decompression of the carpal tunnel and gives good access to the radiocarpal structures in high-energy injuries.

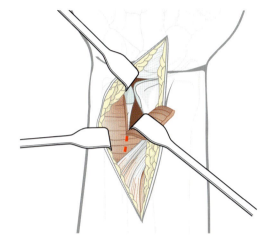

6   Wound closure

The skin is closed in the standard fashion.

1.8 Dorsal approach to the distal radius

1 Surgical approach

Fig 1.8-1 Injuries involving multifragmentary articular fractures, or both the radial and intermediate columns of the distal forearm, can be approached through a single dorsal skin incision with multiple approaches through the extensor compartments.

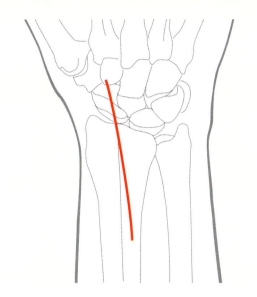

2 Indications

Principle of columns

Fig 1.8-2 The distal forearm can be thought of in terms of three columns. The ulna forms one column (the ulnar column) while the radius can be separated into two (the intermediate column and the radial column).

The radial column includes the radial styloid and scaphoid fossa while the intermediate column includes the lunate fossa and the sigmoid notch, which is part of the distal radioulnar joint (DRUJ). The ulnar column comprises the distal ulna with the triangular fibrocartilage complex (TFCC).

Distally at the wrist joint, the radial column articulates with the scaphoid while the intermediate column articulates with the lunate. The ulnar column terminates distally at the TFCC.

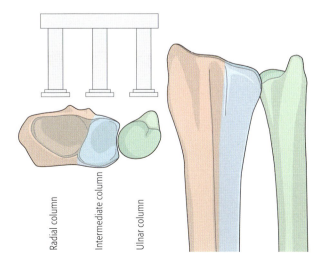

2 Indications (cont)

This 3-column concept helps in describing the location of wrist injuries and is a helpful biomechanical model for understanding the pathomechanics of wrist fractures.

Fig 1.8-3 Depending on the specific fracture pattern, a dorsal approach between the various extensor compartments I-VI is chosen.

In injuries requiring a dorsal approach to the distal radius, approaches (marked as A, B, or C) between the various extensor compartments are indicated:
A: Approach to the radial column
B: Approach to the intermediate column
C: Approach to the intermediate column for the dorsal lunate facet and distal radioulnar joint.

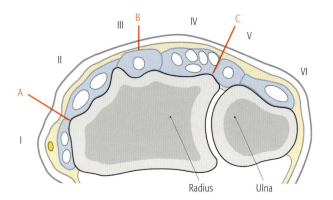

3 Surgical anatomy

Extensor compartments

Fig 1.8-4 There are five extensor compartments in the dorsoradial region (I-V) and one extensor compartment in the dorsoulnar region (VI).

In a dorsal approach to the distal radius, numerous compartments may be involved.

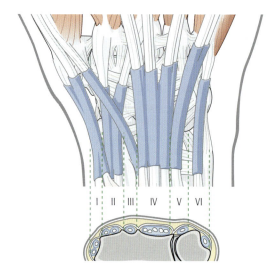

4   Skin incision

Fig 1.8-5   The radial and intermediate columns can be approached separately using a single dorsal skin incision.

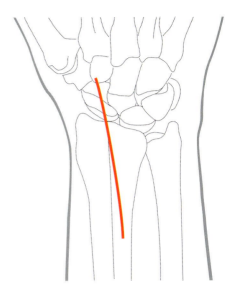

5   Approach to the radial column

Two incision options

Fig 1.8-6   Depending on the fracture configuration, various retinacular incisions are possible to deal with radial column fractures. Either of the following options can be chosen:
1. Approach to the radial column between the first and second extensor compartments
2. Approach to the radial column under the second extensor compartment.

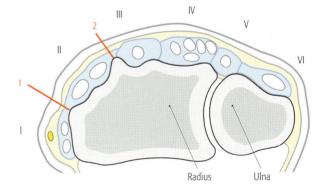

Option 1: between first and second compartments

Fig 1.8-7 The approach in option 1 allows plate positioning on the radial side of the radial column when it is not necessary to expose the articular surface. The radial column is approached with a subcutaneous dissection toward the radial side.

After exposing the extensor pollicis longus (EPL), a second approach is made through the retinaculum between the first and second extensor compartments.

Identify the sensory branch of the radial nerve, which lies in the subcutaneous flap above the first compartment and must be protected.

If it is difficult to obtain satisfactory reduction of a radial styloid fracture, it can be helpful to release the brachioradialis tendon.

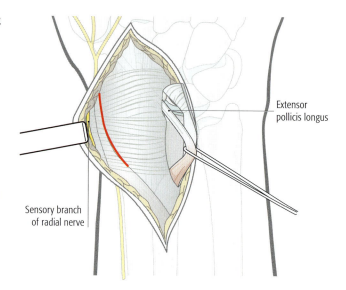

Extensor pollicis longus

Sensory branch of radial nerve

Incision through first compartment

Fig 1.8-8 The first extensor compartment is incised at the level of the musculotendinous transition and is released up to the tip of the radial styloid. The tendons of the first compartment are released and mobilized.

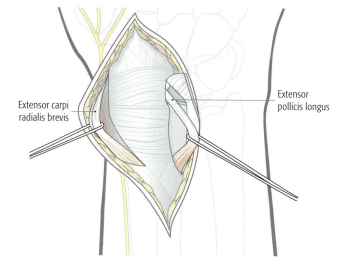

Extensor carpi radialis brevis

Extensor pollicis longus

5 Approach to the radial column (cont)

Subperiosteal elevation of second compartment

Fig 1.8-9 The second compartment is elevated subperiosteally, leaving the compartment itself intact. The radial column is now exposed.

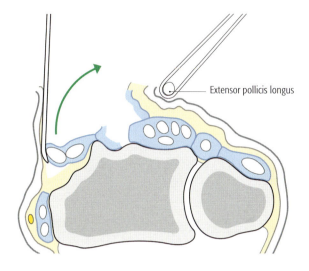

Extensor pollicis longus

Option 2: elevation under the second extensor compartment

Fig 1.8-10 In this approach, Lister tubercle is identified on the radial side and the second compartment is partially elevated. The EPL tendon can be retracted to the ulnar side.

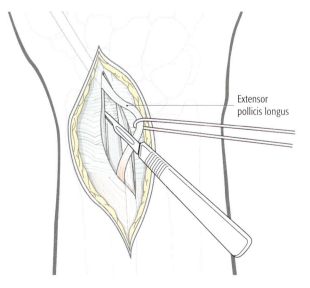

Extensor pollicis longus

5 Approach to the radial column (cont)

Elevation of second compartment

Fig 1.8-11   The second compartment and its contents are elevated from the distal radius by sharp dissection.

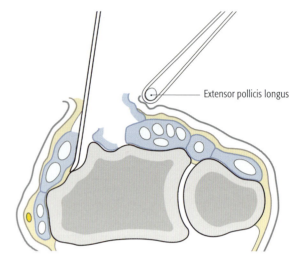

Extensor pollicis longus

Fig 1.8-12   The ECRB tendon is retracted from the floor of the compartment. This allows access to the radiocarpal articular surface on the radial column.

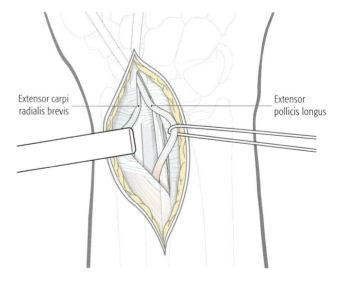

Extensor carpi radialis brevis

Extensor pollicis longus

6 Approach to the intermediate column

Incision of the retinaculum

Fig 1.8-13   In the approach to the intermediate column (B), the third compartment is opened in line with the EPL tendon. When opening the extensor compartment, be careful not to cut the tendon.

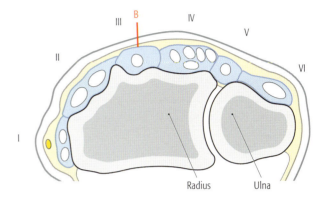

Fig 1.8-14   The incision is extended proximally in line with the EPL. Distally, open the extensor retinaculum as far as needed. It is recommended to preserve the distal part so that the tendon still glides toward the thumb. Alternatively, the compartment can be opened distally and the tendon elevated and retracted radially.

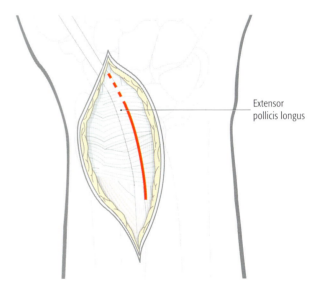

6 Approach to the intermediate column (cont)

Mobilization of extensor pollicis longus tendon

Fig 1.8-15 The EPL tendon is freed and a vessel loop is passed around it.

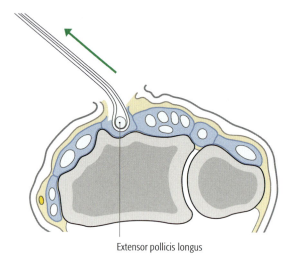

Extensor pollicis longus

Subperiosteal elevation of the fourth compartment

Fig 1.8-16 The fourth compartment is elevated subperiosteally, leaving the compartment itself intact. The intermediate column is now exposed.

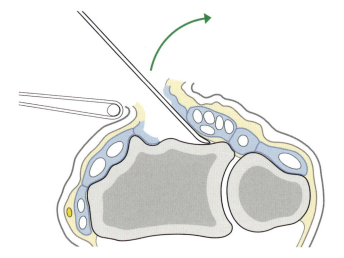

6 Approach to the intermediate column (cont)

Option: arthrotomy

Fig 1.8-17 Once the compartments have been elevated and the distal radius exposed, the capsule can be opened to expose the articular surface. A plate can be applied to the radial column through this approach. The EPL and ECRB tendons can be retracted in either direction, as dictated by the fracture configuration.

The capsular incision should be big enough to see the lunate facet and a part of the scaphoid facet in cases of distal radial articular compression or carpal bone injury.

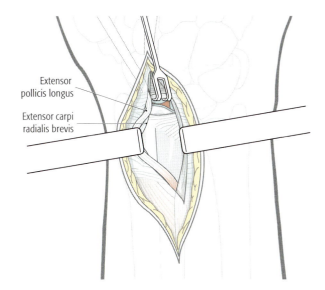

Extensor pollicis longus

Extensor carpi radialis brevis

7 Approach to the intermediate column for the dorsal lunate facet and distal radioulnar joint

Fig 1.8-18 An approach between the fourth and fifth extensor compartments (C) is also possible.

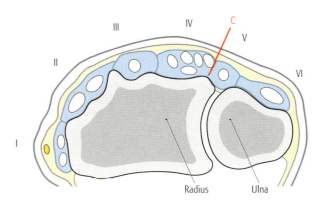

Radius

Ulna

7   Approach to the intermediate column for the dorsal lunate facet and distal radioulnar joint (cont)

Fig 1.8-19   This will allow clear access to the ulnar side of the intermediate column to treat lunate facet and DRUJ injuries.

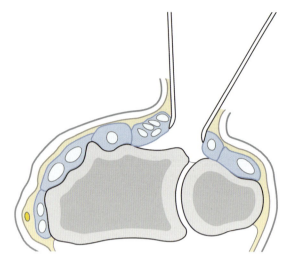

8   Wound closure

A range of wound closures exist for the various dorsal approaches to the distal radius. These are described in further detail in Part II Cases.

Video

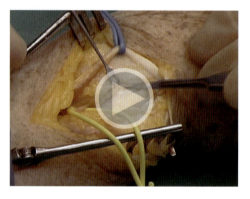

Video 1.8-1   This video demonstrates the dorsal approach to the distal radius.

1.9 Extended dorsal approach to the distal radius

1 Surgical approach

Fig 1.9-1 Injuries involving the distal radius can be treated using an extended dorsal approach.

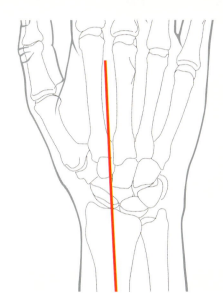

2 Indications

Fig 1.9-2 The extended dorsal approach can be used for wrist fusions or for joint bridging (spanning) plate fixation of multifragmentary intraarticular distal radial fractures.

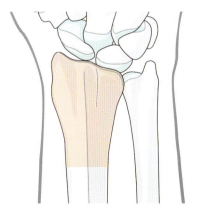

3 Surgical anatomy

Extensor compartments

Fig 1.9-3 There are five extensor compartments in the dorsoradial region (I-V) and one extensor compartment in the dorsoulnar region (VI).

In an extended dorsal approach to the distal radius, numerous compartments may be involved.

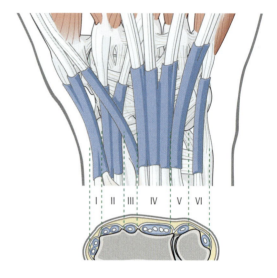

4 Planning the incision

Fig 1.9-4 When mobilizing the skin flaps, make sure not to injure the superficial radial nerve.

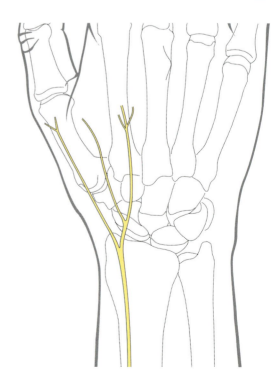

5 Skin incision

Incision options

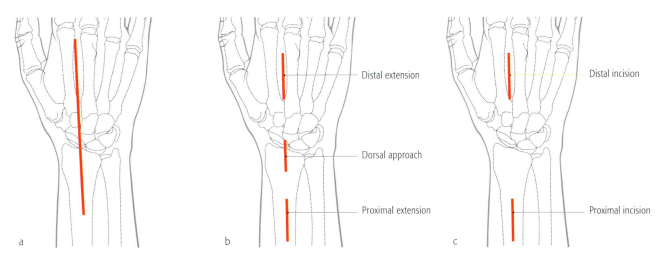

a

b

Distal extension

Dorsal approach

Proximal extension

c

Distal incision

Proximal incision

Fig 1.9-5a–c Depending on the fracture configuration or disorder, various incisions are possible. The following options can be chosen:
1. Longitudinal skin incision (**a**)
2. Standard dorsal incision with an additional extended proximal or extended distal incision or both (**b**)
3. Proximal and distal incisions only (**c**).

Option 1: longitudinal skin incision

Fig 1.9-6 A longitudinal skin incision is made along a line over Lister tubercle to the interspace between the second and third metacarpal.

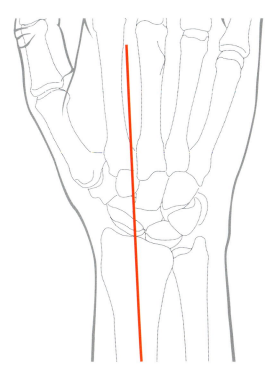

Incision of retinaculum

Fig 1.9-7 The third compartment is opened in line with the extensor pollicis longus (EPL). When opening the extensor compartment, be careful not to cut the tendon.
The incision is extended proximally in line with the EPL tendon. Distally, the extensor retinaculum is fully opened.

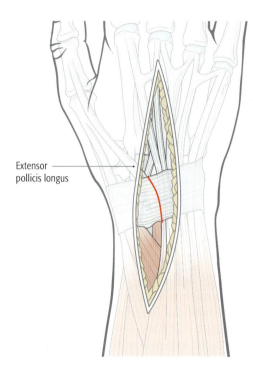

Extensor
pollicis longus

Mobilize the extensor pollicis longus

Fig 1.9-8 The EPL tendon is freed and a vessel loop is passed around it. The tendon is retracted toward the radial side.

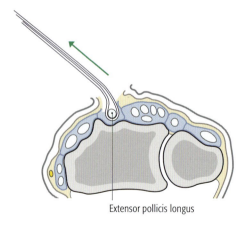

Extensor pollicis longus

5   Skin incision (cont)

Subperiosteal elevation of the fourth compartment

Fig 1.9-9   The fourth compartment is elevated subperiosteally, leaving the compartment itself intact. The intermediate column is now exposed. The tendons of the fourth extensor compartment are retracted to the ulnar side. If necessary, the tendons of the second extensor compartment are mobilized to the radial side.

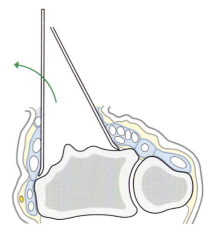

Fig 1.9-10   The periosteum is incised on the dorsal side of the third metacarpal and the interosseous muscles elevated subperiostally, if necessary.

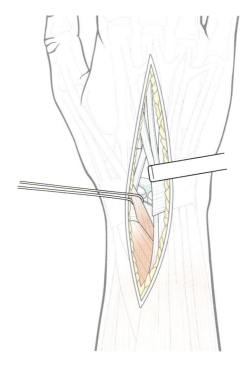

5 Skin incision (cont)

Option 2: dorsal incision with additional proximal or distal incisions

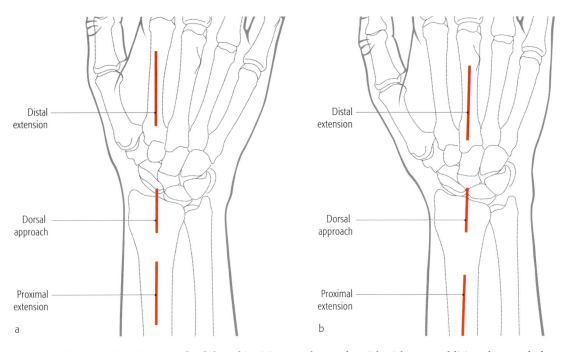

Fig 1.9-11a–b In option 2, a standard dorsal incision can be made with either an additional extended proximal or extended distal incision or both. However, it is first necessary to determine which metacarpal aligns best when the fracture is reduced. Note that a minimum of three screws should be placed in the metacarpal. The method for determining which metacarpal to use is as follows:
1. Provisionally reduce the fracture
2. Place the plate onto the dorsal surface of the wrist
3. Use the image intensifier, to make small adjustments in radioulnar deviation allowing the optimal plate location to be determined over either the second or third metacarpal
4. Make the incisions.

5 Skin incision (cont)

Mark incision lines through the plate holes

Fig 1.9-12 Using this approach, it is helpful to mark all incisions at the beginning through the plate holes. Draw a 3 cm straight first skin incision line over the chosen metacarpal. A second incision line of 2 cm is drawn over Lister tubercle. The third and final straight incision line of 3 cm is drawn over the radial shaft holes.

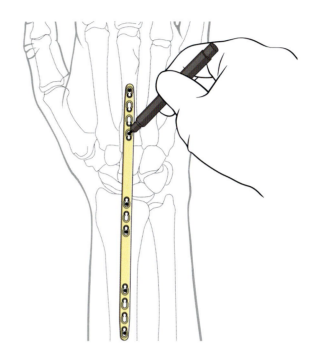

Make the distal incision

Fig 1.9-13 A 3 cm incision is made at the base of the selected metacarpal and continued over the shaft. The metacarpal is exposed while the extensor tendons are retracted and protected.

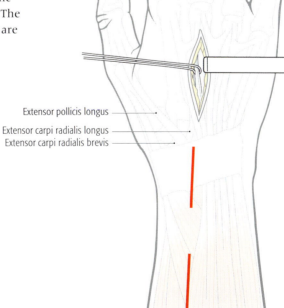

Extensor pollicis longus

Extensor carpi radialis longus
Extensor carpi radialis brevis

5 Skin incision (cont)

Make the dorsal incision and mobilize the extensor pollicis longus

Fig 1.9-14a–b The middle incision is recommended to avoid any damage to the EPL (**a**). Palpate Lister tubercle and make a 2 cm longitudinal incision directly over the bony landmark. Fully release the EPL and retract it toward either the radial or ulnar side depending on the fracture configuration (**b**). Mobilizing the EPL facilitates plate insertion, fracture reduction, and stabilization of the articular surface, as well as the application of bone graft for filling voids (if necessary). This incision also allows sliding of the plate under the second compartment tendons to avoid impinging them under the plate.

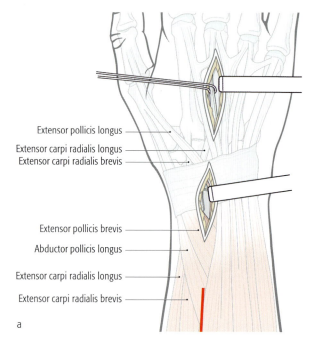

Extensor pollicis longus
Extensor carpi radialis longus
Extensor carpi radialis brevis

Extensor pollicis brevis
Abductor pollicis longus

Extensor carpi radialis longus

Extensor carpi radialis brevis

a

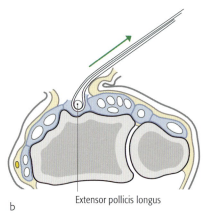

Extensor pollicis longus

b

5   Skin incision (cont)

Make the proximal incision

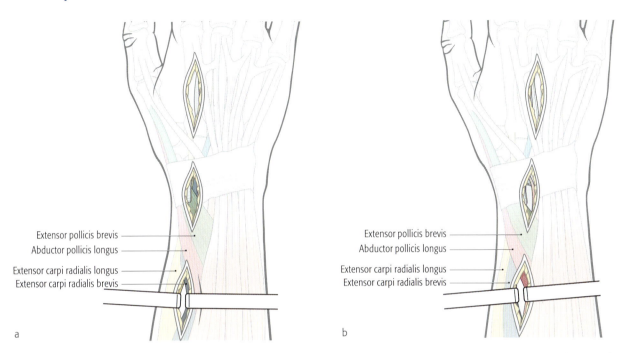

Extensor pollicis brevis
Abductor pollicis longus
Extensor carpi radialis longus
Extensor carpi radialis brevis

Extensor pollicis brevis
Abductor pollicis longus
Extensor carpi radialis longus
Extensor carpi radialis brevis

a

b

Fig 1.9-15a–b   Using the image intensifier for guidance, an incision measuring approximately 3 cm is made over the dorsal aspect of the radius just proximal to the muscle bellies of the abductor pollicis longus (APL) and the extensor pollicis brevis (EPB) tendons, in line with the extensor carpi radialis longus (ECRL) and brevis (ECRB) tendons.

The exact location of the incision may depend on whether the plate will attach distally at the second or third metacarpal. For a second-metacarpal fixation by blunt dissection, the interval between the ECRL and ECRB is developed and the diaphysis of the radius is exposed (**a**).

For a third-metacarpal fixation by blunt dissection, the interval between the first compartment (containing the APL and EPB tendons) and second compartment (ECRL and ECRB tendons) is developed and the diaphysis of the radius is exposed (**b**). Retract the first compartment muscles ulnarly and the second compartment radially.

5   Skin incision (cont)

Option 3: proximal and distal incisions

Fig 1.9-16   As an alternative, the approach can be made using just proximal and distal incisions.

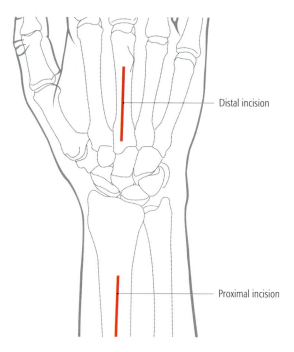

Distal incision

Proximal incision

Fig 1.9-17   This is done by marking the skin at the level of the proximal and distal screw holes of the plate and making 3–4 cm incisions.

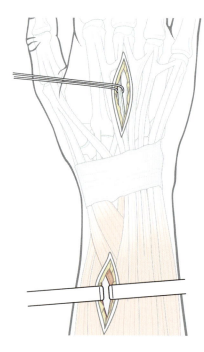

6 Wound closure

The skin is closed in a standard fashion.

1.10 Ulnar approach to the distal ulna

1 Surgical approach

Fig 1.10-1 Injuries involving the distal ulna can be treated using an ulnar approach.

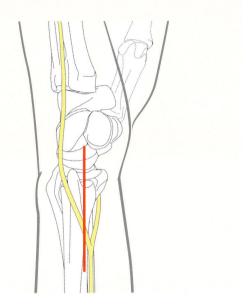

2 Indications

Fig 1.10-2 The ulnar approach is indicated for all fractures of the distal ulna.

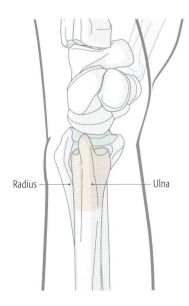

Radius ———•————— Ulna

3   Skin incision

Fig 1.10-3   The ulnar shaft and the fracture gap between the ulnar styloid and the distal metaphysis are usually easily palpated.

A straight longitudinal incision is made over the distal ulna between the tendons of the extensor and flexor carpi ulnaris.

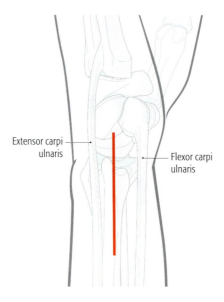

Extensor carpi
ulnaris

Flexor carpi
ulnaris

Dissection

Fig 1.10-4   The dorsal branch of the ulnar nerve should be able to be seen. Care should be taken to avoid injury to this nerve. The fracture site is then exposed, if necessary, releasing the ulnar attachment of the extensor retinaculum.

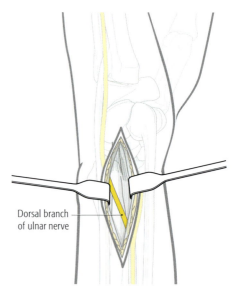

Dorsal branch
of ulnar nerve

3 Skin incision (cont)

Fig 1.10-5a–b Supination of the forearm results in the ulnar styloid lying dorsally. This exposes the distal ulna without interference from the extensor carpi ulnaris (**a**). Pronation of the forearm exposes the ulnar styloid in the center of the approach (**b**).

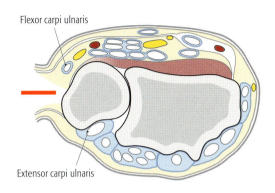

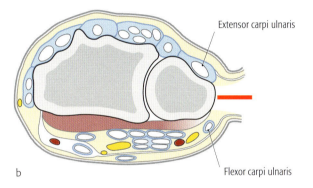

a

b

4 Wound closure

The extensor retinaculum is repaired as necessary, and the wound is closed in layers.

Video

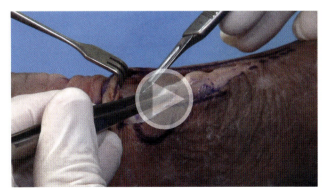

Video 1.10-1 This video demonstrates the ulnar approach to the distal ulna.

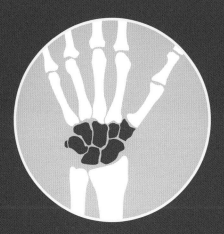

Part II
Cases

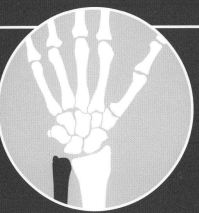

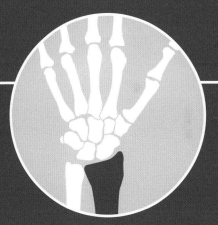

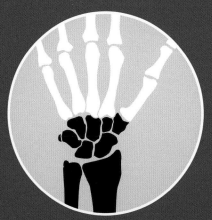

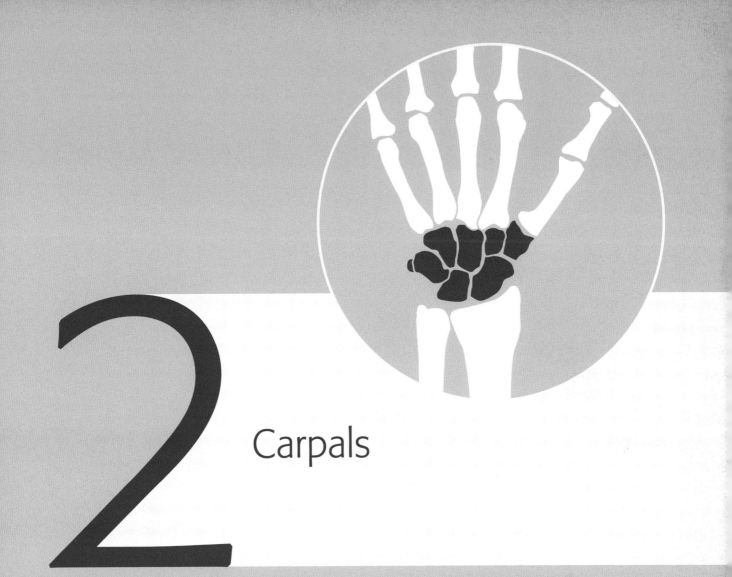

2

Carpals

2.1 Scaphoid—nondisplaced fracture treated percutaneously with a headless compression screw

1 Case description

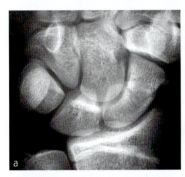
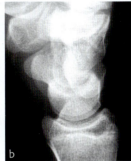

Fig 2.1-1a–b A 26-year-old man fell onto his outstretched right hand during a club soccer game noting immediate acute pain. An examination revealed pain in the anatomical snuff box of his wrist. The AP and lateral x-rays revealed a fracture line across the waist of the scaphoid, however, carpal alignment appeared normal.

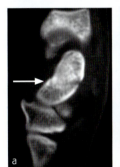
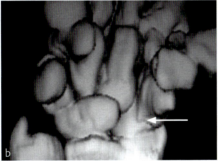
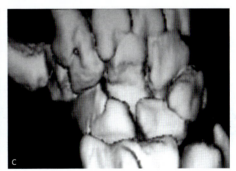

Fig 2.1-2a–c The 2-D and 3-D CT scans identified the fracture as having minimal displacement but going through both cortices of the scaphoid in the frontal and sagittal planes (arrows).

2 Indications

Nondisplaced scaphoid fractures

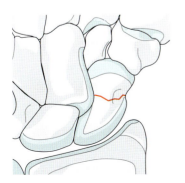

Fig 2.1-3 Percutaneous (minimally invasive) fixation is largely indicated for nondisplaced or minimally displaced fractures of the waist of the scaphoid.

85

2 Indications (cont)

Internal fixation vs nonoperative treatment

In general, internal fixation of fractures is thought to provide effective bone healing in at least the same if not less time than nonoperative treatment, but that the period of immobilization is shortened. Percutaneous treatment brings the advantages of avoiding a wide surgical approach, preserving the palmar ligament complex and local vascularity, and avoiding the extended immobilization required for healing after a wider open exposure.

Readers of this publication are immediately reminded that in some instances of wrist injury, nonoperative treatment is a viable alternative. However, the detailed cases provided throughout this book outline situations where, for those patients, surgical techniques were deemed the more appropriate treatment option.

Imaging

With nondisplaced and minimally displaced scaphoid fractures, conventional x-rays often do not adequately demonstrate the complete fracture configuration. As shown in the case description of this patient, CT scans were therefore performed and are strongly recommended if a percutaneous procedure is planned.

Anatomical considerations

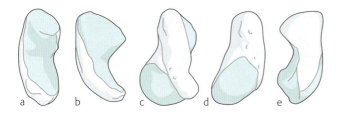

Fig 2.1-4a–e With all scaphoid fractures, the anatomy and vascularity of the scaphoid need to be considered. Close to 80% of the surface of the scaphoid is covered with articular cartilage, which greatly limits the points of entry for fixation devices. An additional constraint is the curved morphology of the scaphoid. This means that it can be difficult to pass a wire or fixation device along the true long axis of the bone, yet this is the implant location that provides the greatest stability and compression. Occasionally, access to the correct distal entry point for a device can only be gained by a limited excision of the overhanging edge of the trapezium.

Vascularity

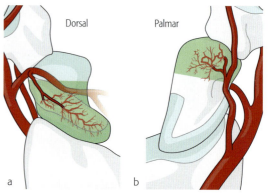

Fig 2.1-5a–b The blood supply of the scaphoid is derived from two sources. The main source is a group of blood vessels entering the dorsal surface of the distal pole (**a**). This is the largest contribution to the vascularity of the scaphoid as the dorsal group supplies the proximal two thirds of the bone. However, the proximal pole relies on a retrograde blood flow, a fact that makes this part of the scaphoid more prone to suffer avascular bone necrosis and a consequent nonunion.

A second group of vessels enters the palmar aspect of the distal pole (**b**). These vessels contribute largely to the vascularity of the distal third.

3 Preoperative planning

Equipment

- Headless compression screw set 2.4 or 3.0
- 1.1 mm K-wires, 150 mm length
- Hypodermic needle
- Osteotome
- Image intensifier

Fig 2.1-6 Before starting the procedure, re-examine the fracture pattern under an image intensifier. Be sure that the fracture is suitable for a percutaneous technique and that no secondary displacement has occurred. Position the patient supine and place the forearm on the hand table. By abducting the patient's shoulder it is possible for the surgeon and the assistant to sit on either side of the hand table. A nonsterile pneumatic tourniquet is used. Prophylactic antibiotics are optional.

Patient preparation and positioning

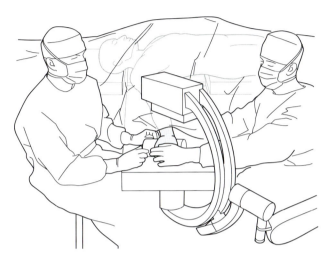

4 Surgical approach

Approach

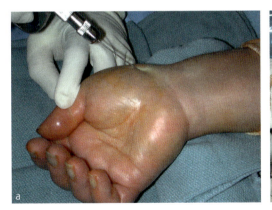
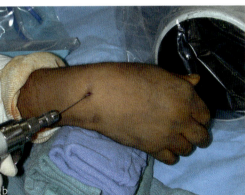

Fig 2.1-7a–b Two approaches exist for percutaneous screw fixation, entering either palmarly (**a**) or dorsally (**b**) to reach the scaphoid from either the distal or proximal pole. For the patient in this chapter, the palmar approach was used, entering through the distal pole of the scaphoid.

4   Surgical approach (cont)

Hyperextend the wrist

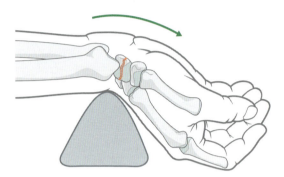

Fig 2.1-8   To assist in the approach, place a rolled towel or bolster under the wrist and hyperextend it. The use of the support helps access the correct entry point for a guide wire.

Mark the skin

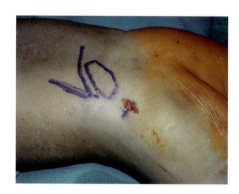

Fig 2.1-9   It can be helpful to mark on the skin the position of the scaphoid, the palmar rim of the distal radius, and the level of the scaphotrapezial joint.

Skin incision

A stab incision of 5–10 mm is made distally to the scaphotrapezial joint. Deepen the incision through the subcutaneous tissues by blunt dissection then incise the capsule of the scaphotrapezial joint. The distal pole of the scaphoid is now accessible for insertion of a K-wire, which will be used as a guide wire.

5   Reduction

Determine insertion point for the guide wire

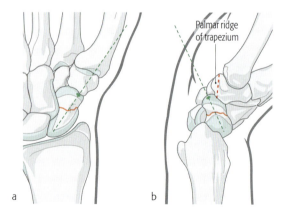

Palmar ridge of trapezium

a   b

Fig 2.1-10a–b   The correct entry point for the guide wire is the center of the distal pole of the scaphoid. However, to get proper access, it may be necessary to remove the palmar ridge of the trapezium with an osteotome or a bone nibbler/rongeur. This reveals the distal pole of the scaphoid and allows the path of the guide wire to be made more centrally within the bone.

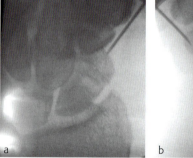

a   b

Fig 2.1-11a–b   Use a hypodermic needle to determine the insertion point radiologically before inserting the guide wire.

5 Reduction (cont)

Insert the guide wire

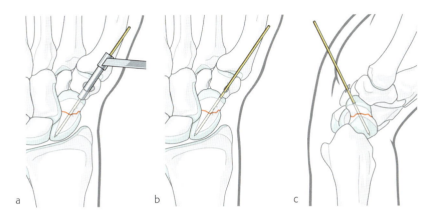

a   b   c

Fig 2.1-12a–c   The guide wire should be inserted through a drill guide (**a**). If no drill guide is available, use a protective sleeve. The position of the wire should be as perpendicular as possible to the fracture line (**b–c**). In oblique fractures, this principle may have to be compromised. Do not penetrate beyond the proximal cortex of the scaphoid.

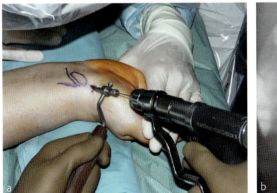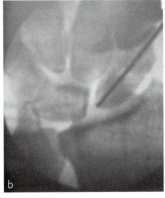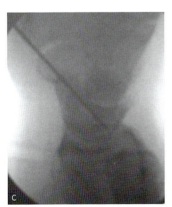

a   b   c

Fig 2.1-13a–c   The guide wire was inserted at the confirmed entry point.

6   Fixation

Measure screw length

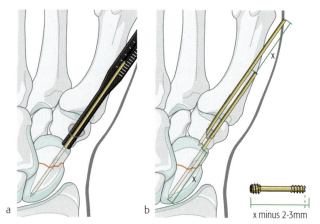

Drilling

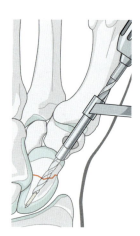

Fig 2.1-14a–b   Two methods can be employed for measuring the desired length of the headless screw. Insert the dedicated measuring device over the guide wire, through the drill guide, which must be firmly positioned on the tubercle for a reliable measurement (**a**). Alternatively, if the dedicated measuring device is not available, take another guide wire of the same length and place its tip onto the bone at the insertion point (**b**). The difference between the protruding ends of the two wires indicates the length of the drill hole for the screw. Subtract 2–3 mm to determine the screw length.

Fig 2.1-15   Use only the dedicated drill bit. A power drill will exert less force on the fragments than manual drilling and will reduce the risk of displacing the fragments. A small power drill with slow rotation is the preferred choice. Use saline solution to cool the drill bit in order to minimize thermal injury. Check the position of the tip of the drill bit under image intensification.

Select the screw

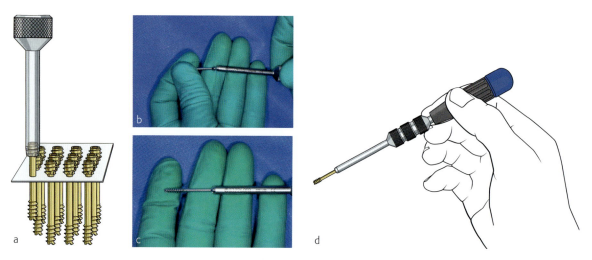

Fig 2.1-16a–d   Select the appropriately sized cannulated (ie, hollow) headless compression screw (**a–c**). The selected screw is inserted into the internal thread of the compression sleeve (**d**).

6   Fixation (cont)

Insert the screw

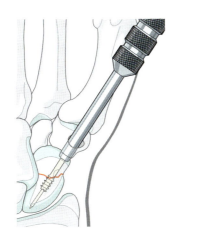

Fig 2.1-17   The screw and compression sleeve are inserted over the guide wire.

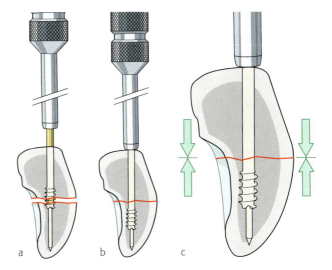

Fig 2.1-18a–c   The screw is tightened until sufficient compression is achieved.

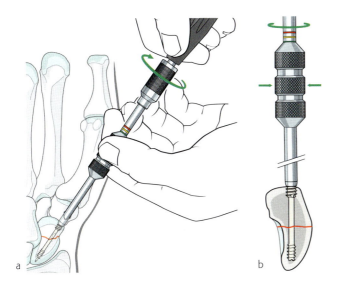

Fig 2.1-19a–b   The cannulated screwdriver is inserted. The compression sleeve is held still, using the thumb and index finger to firmly hold the compression sleeve, as the screwdriver turns the screw and advances it out of the compression sleeve and into the bone. Compression is maintained by the compression sleeve during this action.

6 Fixation (cont)

Advance and countersink the screw

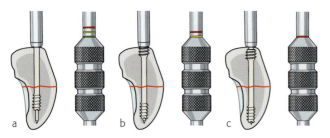

Fig 2.1-20a–c The screwdriver has three colored markings that are visible at the edge of the compression sleeve. The green mark indicates the screw is still fully retained within the compression sleeve (**a**). The yellow mark indicates the screw has been advanced level with the surface of the bone (**b**). The red mark indicates the screw has been countersunk 2 mm under the bone surface (**c**). Countersink the screw by turning the screwdriver shaft while simultaneously holding the compression sleeve stationary.

Ensure correct screw and thread length

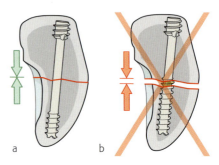

Fig 2.1-21a–b It is vital that the threaded section of the tip of the screw passes completely beyond the fracture plane if interfragmentary compression is to be achieved. Also ensure that the screw is not too long nor overtightened as it could protrude beyond the cortical surface and lose compression, or endanger the soft tissues, especially tendons and neurovascular structures.

Complete the fixation

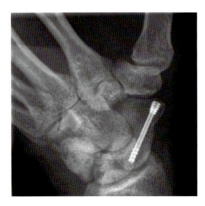

Fig 2.1-22 Before final tightening, remove the guide wire. Make sure that the threads at the near end of the screw are fully buried in the bone at the insertion site. Check the final position of the screw and scaphoid stability using image intensification or x-rays.

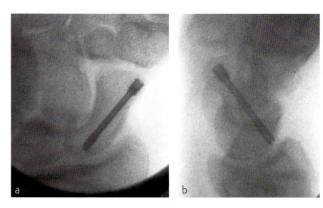

Fig 2.1-23a–b Intraoperative images of the patient show the placement of the headless screw in line with the longitudinal axis of the scaphoid with the screw crossing the fracture line.

7 Rehabilitation

Aftercare

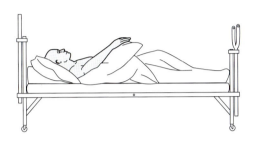

Fig 2.1-24 While the patient is in bed, use pillows to keep the hand elevated above the level of the heart to reduce swelling.

Immobilization

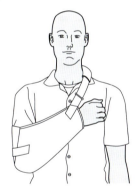

Fig 2.1-25 Rest the wrist with a well-padded below-elbow splint for 48–72 hours. For ambulating patients, dispense with the splint and apply an elastic bandage. If necessary, put the arm in a sling and elevate to above the heart.

Follow-up

See the patient after 2–5 days to change the dressing. After 10 days, remove the sutures and confirm with x-rays that no secondary displacement has occurred.

Functional exercises

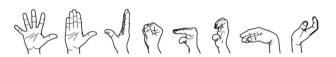

Fig 2.1-26 Following surgery, begin active controlled range of motion exercises. Active motion exercises and later resistance exercises should be initiated based upon the surgeon's decision as to time after surgery and patient compliance. Load-bearing activities are usually delayed until radiological evidence of bone healing. The importance of mobilization must be emphasized to the patient and rehabilitation should be supervised by a physical therapist.

8 Outcome

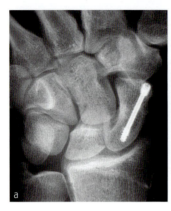
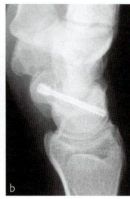

Fig 2.1-27a–b At the 1-year follow-up, the AP and lateral x-rays indicated excellent healing.

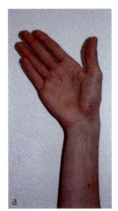
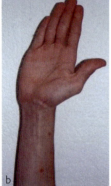
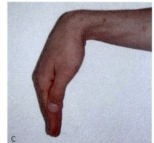
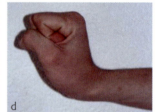

Fig 2.1-28a–d There was full clinical motion and return of normal strength.

Video

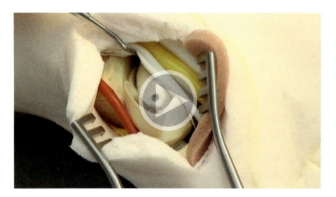

Video 2.1-1 This video demonstrates a scaphoid fracture procedure treated with percutaneous fixation with a 3.0 mm headless compression screw.

2.2 Scaphoid–displaced fracture treated with a headless compression screw

1 Case description

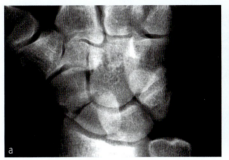 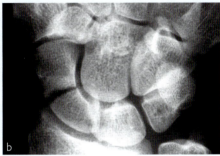

Fig 2.2-1a–b A 38-year-old construction worker injured his dominant left wrist when he fell from a 3 m platform at work. The initial x-rays confirmed an unstable displaced fracture of the waist of the scaphoid.

2 Indications

Displaced scaphoid fractures

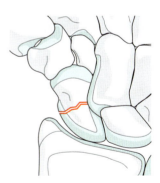

Fig 2.2-2 Acute scaphoid fractures are considered to be displaced when there is a 1 mm gap between the fragments on any single view. Displacement in an acute fracture increases the risks of nonunion if the injury is managed nonoperatively in a cast. Consequently, consideration must be given to reduction and stabilization by internal fixation.

Anatomical and vascularity considerations

The scaphoid's unique anatomy and vascularity must also be considered. Refer to the indications topic in chapter 2.1 Scaphoid—nondisplaced fracture treated percutaneously with a percutaneous screw for more information.

Choice of implant

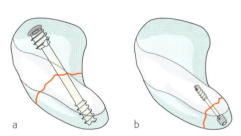

Fig 2.2-3a–b A 2.4 mm or 3.0 mm implant using retrograde insertion (distal entry point) is indicated for scaphoid waist fractures or when the proximal fragment is larger than 10 mm (**a**). For smaller proximal fragments, the use of an antegrade insertion (proximal entry point) with single or multiple mini headless bone screws (1.5 mm) is advisable (**b**). As this patient had a scaphoid waist fracture, a palmar retrograde insertion was required.

Imaging

Obtaining a full series of scaphoid x-rays of the affected and normal contralateral side is necessary for surgical planning.

95

3   Preoperative planning

Equipment

- Headless compression screw set 2.4 or 3.0
- 1.1 mm K-wires
- Osteotome
- Image intensifier

Patient preparation and positioning

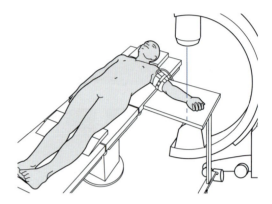

Fig 2.2-4   Position the patient supine and place the forearm on the hand table. Supinate the forearm. A nonsterile pneumatic tourniquet is used. Prophylactic antibiotics are optional.

4   Surgical approach

Approach

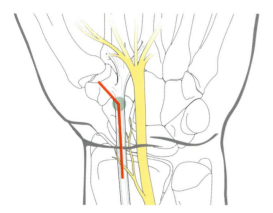

Fig 2.2-5   In cases where reduction cannot be achieved closed, a direct open approach is necessary. The surgical approach used for this patient was a palmar approach involving a radial longitudinal angled skin incision (see chapter 1.1 Palmar approach to the scaphoid).

Hyperextend the wrist

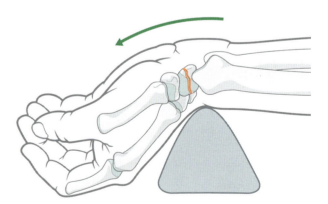

Fig 2.2-6   To assist in the approach, place a rolled towel or bolster under the wrist and hyperextend it. The use of the support helps access the correct entry point for a guide wire. This position also helps to reduce the scaphoid fragments.

5 Reduction

Determine insertion point for the guide wire

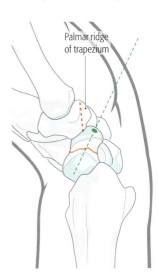

Palmar ridge
of trapezium

Fig 2.2-7 The correct entry point for the guide wire is the center of the distal pole of the scaphoid. However, to get proper access, it may be necessary to remove the palmar ridge of the trapezium with an osteotome or a bone nibbler/rongeur. This reveals the distal pole of the scaphoid and allows the path of the guide wire to be made more centrally within the bone.

Insert the guide wire

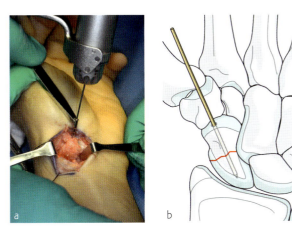

Fig 2.2-8a–b The guide wire should be inserted through a drill guide (**a**). If no drill guide is available, use a protective sleeve. The position of the wire should be as perpendicular as possible to the fracture line (**b**). In oblique fractures, this principle may have to be compromised. Do not penetrate beyond the proximal cortex of the scaphoid.

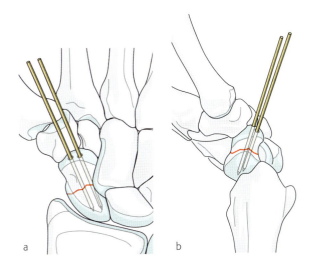

Fig 2.2-9a–b A second K-wire is useful to prevent rotation of the fragments as compression is achieved. The second K-wire should be removed before final tightening of the screw. Image intensification in at least two planes is used to confirm accurate advancement of the guide wire in the scaphoid axis and perpendicular to the fracture plane. Reduction can often be achieved by compression alone as the cannulated screw is carefully inserted.

6 Fixation

Measure screw length

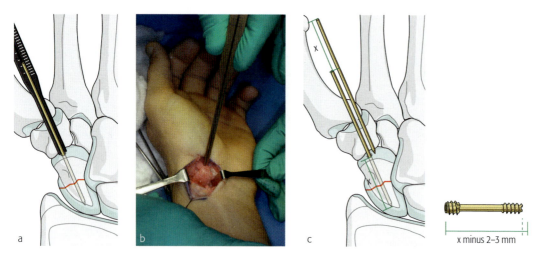

a   b   c

x minus 2–3 mm

Fig 2.2-10a–c Two methods can be employed for measuring the desired length of the headless screw. Insert the dedicated measuring device over the guide wire, through the drill guide, which must be firmly positioned on the tubercle for a reliable measurement (**a**) (as shown on the patient) (**b**). Alternatively, if the dedicated measuring device is not available, take another guide wire of the same length and place its tip onto the bone at the insertion point (**c**). The difference between the protruding ends of the two wires indicates the length of the drill hole for the screw. Subtract 2–3 mm to determine the screw length.

Drilling

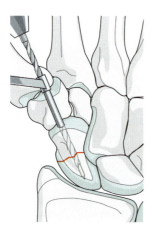

Fig 2.2-11 Use only the dedicated drill bit. A power drill will exert less force on the fragments than manual drilling and will reduce the risk of displacing the fragments. A small power drill with slow rotation is the preferred choice. Use saline solution to cool the drill bit in order to minimize thermal injury. Check the position of the tip of the drill bit under image intensification.

Select the screw

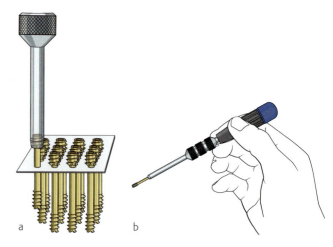

a   b

Fig 2.2-12a–b Select the appropriately sized cannulated headless compression screw (**a**). The selected screw is inserted into the internal thread of the compression sleeve (**b**).

6 Fixation (cont)

Insert the screw

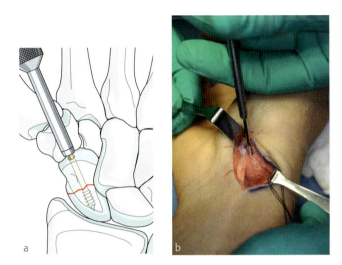

Fig 2.2-13a–b The screw and compression sleeve are inserted over the guide wire.

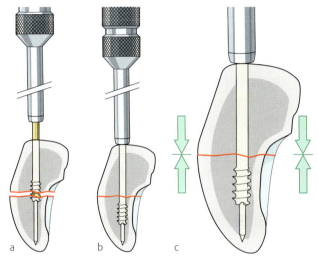

Fig 2.2-14a–c The screw is tightened until sufficient compression is achieved.

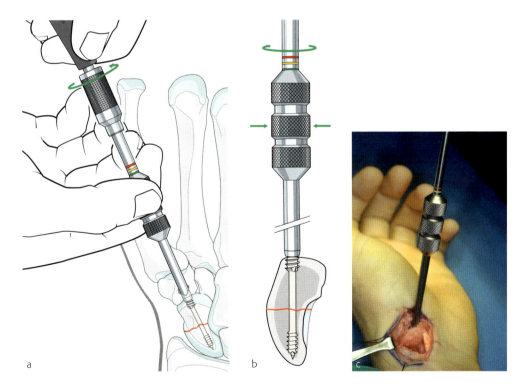

Fig 2.2-15a–c The cannulated screwdriver is inserted. The compression sleeve is held still, using the thumb and index finger to firmly hold the compression sleeve, as the screwdriver turns the screw and advances it out of the compression sleeve and into the bone. Compression is maintained by the compression sleeve during this action.

6 Fixation (cont)

Advance and countersink the screw

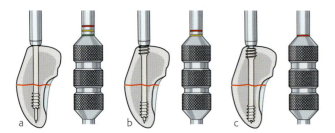

Fig 2.2-16a–c The screwdriver has three colored markings that are visible at the edge of the compression sleeve. The green mark indicates the screw is still fully retained within the compression sleeve (**a**). The yellow mark indicates the screw has been advanced level with the surface of the bone (**b**). The red mark indicates the screw has been countersunk 2 mm under the bone surface (**c**). Countersink the screw by turning the screwdriver shaft while simultaneously holding the compression sleeve stationary.

Ensure correct screw and thread length

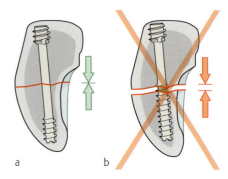

Fig 2.2-17a–b It is vital that the threaded section of the tip of the screw passes completely beyond the fracture plane if interfragmentary compression is to be achieved. Also ensure that the screw is not too long nor overtightened as it could protrude beyond the cortical surface and lose compression, or endanger the soft tissues, especially tendons and neurovascular structures.

Complete the fixation

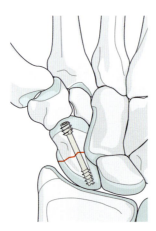

Fig 2.2-18 Before final tightening, remove the guide wire. Make sure that the threads at the near end of the screw are fully buried in the bone at the insertion site. Check the final position of the screw and scaphoid stability using image intensification or x-rays.

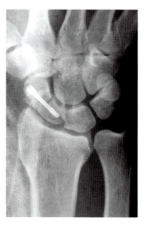

Fig 2.2-19 The intraoperative x-ray confirmed correct positioning of the implant together with reduction of the unstable fracture.

7 Rehabilitation

Aftercare

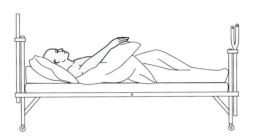

Fig 2.2-20 While the patient is in bed, use pillows to keep the hand elevated above the level of the heart to reduce swelling.

Immobilization

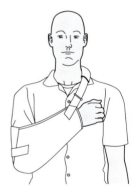

Fig 2.2-21 The type and duration of postoperative immobilization depends on a number of factors including the quality of the internal fixation as well as patient activity and reliability. It may be necessary to rest the wrist for several weeks in a plaster or removable splint. During that time, the patient is encouraged to remove the splint for short periods to allow gentle wrist motion.

Follow-up

See the patient after 2–5 days to change the dressing. After 10 days, remove the sutures and confirm with x-rays that no secondary displacement has occurred.

Functional exercises

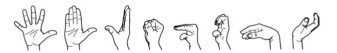

Fig 2.2-22 Following surgery, begin active controlled range of motion exercises. Active motion exercises and later resistance exercises should be initiated based upon the surgeon's decision as to time after surgery and patient compliance. Load-bearing activities are usually delayed until radiological evidence of bone healing. The importance of mobilization must be emphasized to the patient and rehabilitation should be supervised by a physical therapist.

8   Outcome

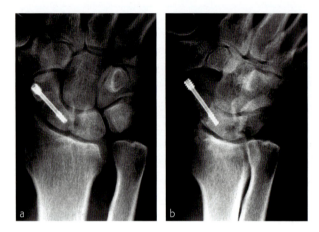

Fig 2.2-23a–b   At the 14-month follow-up, the x-rays confirmed healing.

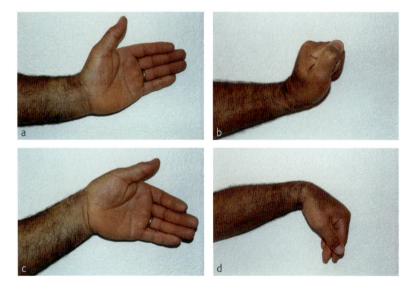

Fig 2.2-24a–d   The patient had achieved a full range of motion.

2.3 Scaphoid—multifragmentary fracture treated with a headless compression screw and lag screw

1 Case description

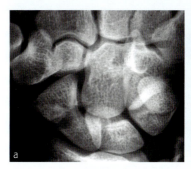
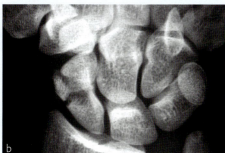

Fig 2.3-1a–b A 29-year-old teacher was involved in a high-speed collision on his motorcycle. He injured his right dominant wrist. The x-rays confirmed a displaced multifragmentary fracture of the scaphoid.

2 Indications

Multifragmentary scaphoid fractures

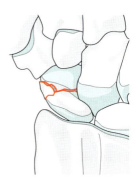

Fig 2.3-2 Acute displaced and multifragmentary scaphoid fractures are often the result of high-energy impact. They are unstable fractures and there is a strong possibility of later displacement even if they do not appear displaced on primary presentation. These injuries are at a high risk of nonunion if the injury is managed nonoperatively in a cast. Consequently, consideration must be given to open reduction and stabilization by internal fixation.

A systematic approach to the stabilization of each of the large fragments may be required. When the fragments are too small for individual stabilization, consideration should be given to excision of these fragments and replacement by primary bone graft.

Choice of implant

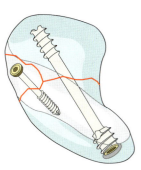

Fig 2.3-3 In multifragmentary fractures, a 2.4 mm or 3.0 mm implant is indicated for stabilization of the large fragments. For the smaller additional fragments, the use of mini headless bone screws or small cortical lag screws is advisable. K-wires are always an option if the introduction of an implant proves difficult. For this patient, a combination of a headless compression screw and a lag screw was required.

2 Indications (cont)

Anatomical and vascularity considerations

The scaphoid's unique anatomy and vascularity must also be considered. Refer to the indications topic in chapter 2.1 Scaphoid—nondisplaced fracture treated percutaneously with a headless compression screw for more information.

Imaging

Obtaining a full series of scaphoid x-rays of the affected and normal contralateral side is necessary for surgical planning.

3 Preoperative planning

Equipment

- Headless compression screw set 2.4 or 3.0
- Modular screw set 1.5 or 2.0
- 1.1 mm K-wires
- Pointed reduction forceps
- Osteotome
- Image intensifier

Patient preparation and positioning

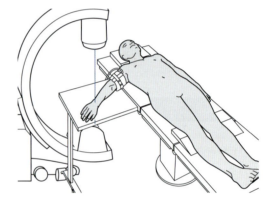

Fig 2.3-4 Position the patient supine and place the forearm on the hand table. In multifragmentary fractures, a dorsal antegrade or palmar retrograde approach can be used, depending on fracture configuration. Pronate the forearm on the hand table for a dorsal approach. In unusual circumstances, a combined dorsal and palmar approach may be required. A nonsterile pneumatic tourniquet is used. Prophylactic antibiotics are optional.

Approach

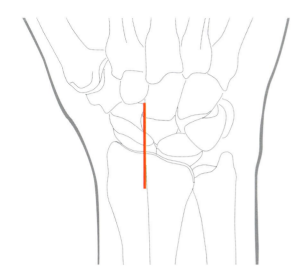

Fig 2.3-5   The surgical approach used was a dorsal approach due to the particular fracture configuration (see chapter 1.2 Dorsal approach to the scaphoid).

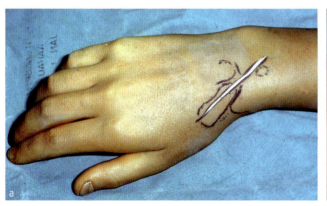

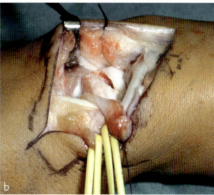

Fig 2.3-6a–b   For this patient, a longitudinal dorsoradial skin incision was made, starting over the distal radius, and extending toward the base of the thumb passing around the dorsal aspect of the scaphoid.

5 Reduction

Direct reduction

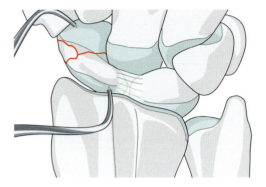

Fig 2.3-7 With multifragmentary scaphoid fractures, it is often difficult to achieve closed reduction. If open reduction is required, reduce the fracture with small pointed reduction forceps.

Insert K-wires

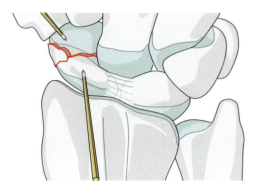

Fig 2.3-8 If the fracture cannot be reduced with the forceps, insert a K-wire into each fragment and use the wires as joysticks to manipulate the fragments.

Determine insertion point for the guide wire

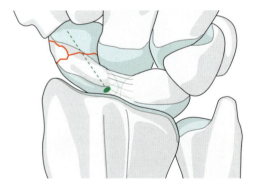

Fig 2.3-9 The correct entry point for the guide wire is in the center of the proximal pole, directly adjacent to the scapholunate ligament insertion.

Insert the guide wire

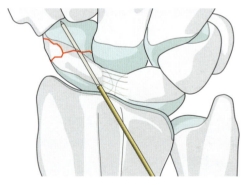

Fig 2.3-10 The guide wire is inserted in the axis of the shaft of the first metacarpal, in radial abduction. During the introduction of the guide wire, the wrist should be in flexion otherwise the entry point cannot be reached. Do not penetrate the scaphotrapezial joint with the guide wire. In multifragmentary fractures, the guide wire also helps to maintain the reduction.

Image intensification in at least two planes is required to confirm accurate advancement of the guide wire in the scaphoid axis and to make sure that there is no rotational deformity.

6   Fixation

Insert lag screw

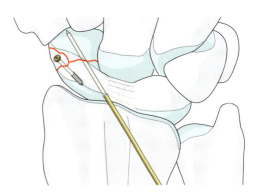

Fig 2.3-11   Multifragmentary fractures involving the proximal half of the scaphoid cannot be fixed with a headless screw alone. Additional K-wires, or as in this case an additional lag screw, should be considered.

A 1.5 mm lag screw is first placed into the scaphoid to make the 3-part fracture into 2 parts. The comminuted fragment is directly secured to the body of the scaphoid.

Use of lag screws

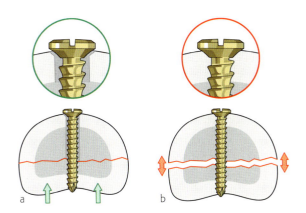

Fig 2.3-12a–b   Be sure to insert the screw as a lag screw, with a gliding hole in the near cortex, and a threaded hole in the far cortex (**a**). Inserting a screw across a fracture plane that is threaded in both cortices (position screw) will hold the fragments apart and apply no interfragmentary compression (**b**).

Countersinking

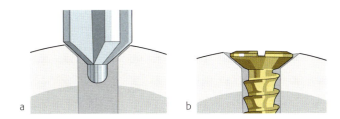

Fig 2.3-13a–b   Also ensure to countersink the screw to reduce the risk of soft-tissue irritation, so that the screw head has maximal contact area with the bone.

6   Fixation (cont)

Measure screw length

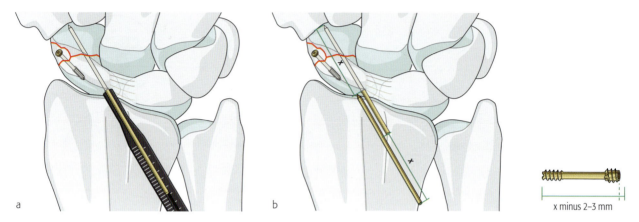

a   b   x minus 2–3 mm

Fig 2.3-14a–b   Two methods can be employed for measuring the desired length of the headless screw. Insert the dedicated measuring device over the guide wire, through the drill guide, which must be firmly positioned on the tubercle for a reliable measurement (**a**). Alternatively, if the dedicated measuring device is not available, take another guide wire of the same length and place its tip onto the bone at the insertion point (**b**). The difference between the protruding ends of the two wires indicates the length of the drill hole for the screw. Subtract 2–3 mm to determine the screw length.

Drilling

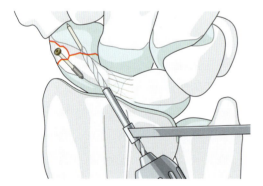

Fig 2.3-15   Use only the dedicated drill bit. A power drill will exert less force on the fragments than manual drilling and will reduce the risk of displacing the fragments. A small power drill with slow rotation is the preferred choice. Use saline solution to cool the drill bit in order to minimize thermal injury. Check the position of the tip of the drill bit under image intensification.

6   Fixation (cont)

Select and insert the screw

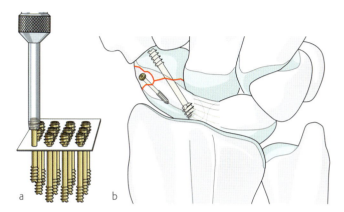

Fig 2.3-16a–b   Select the appropriately sized cannulated headless compression screw. Insert the screw over the guide wire. However, as this is a multifragmentary fracture, strong compression/overcompression with the screw is not recommended because of the possibility of collapse of the fracture. Instead of a compression screw, a position screw is recommended in this situation, although by virtue of the differential pitch of the threads on the screw, there will be some compression regardless. One of the advantages of these headless screws is that they can be inserted without the compression sleeve, helping to avoid the possible complication of unstable fracture collapse.

Ensure correct screw and thread length

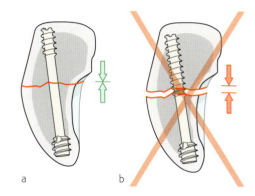

Fig 2.3-17a–b   It is vital that the threaded section of the tip of the screw passes completely beyond the fracture plane if interfragmentary compression is to be achieved. Also ensure that the screw is not too long nor overtightened as it could protrude beyond the cortical surface and lose compression, or endanger the soft tissues, especially tendons and neurovascular structures.

Advance the screw

The proximal end of the screw should be advanced until it is buried beneath the subchondral bone.

Complete the fixation

Before final tightening, remove the guide wire. Make sure that the threads at the near end of the screw are fully buried in the bone at the insertion site. Check the final position of the screw and scaphoid stability using image intensification or x-rays.

7 Rehabilitation

Aftercare, follow-up, and functional exercises

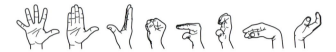

Fig 2.3-18   The patient should receive the standard postoperative rest, injury elevation, follow-up, removal of stitches, and immobilization as required. Following surgery, begin active controlled range of motion exercises. For further information, see the rehabilitation topic in chapter 2.2 Scaphoid—displaced fracture treated with a headless compression screw.

8 Outcome

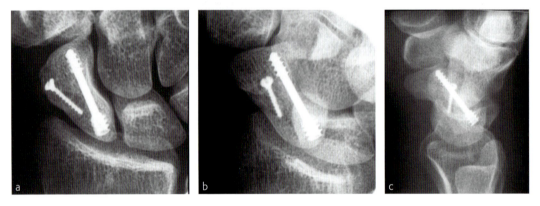

Fig 2.3-19a–c   At the 2-year follow-up, PA, oblique, and lateral x-rays confirmed full healing.

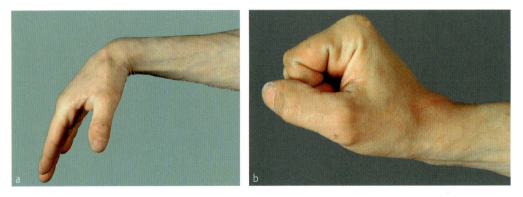

Fig 2.3-20a–b   The patient had nearly full range of wrist extension and flexion.

2.4 Scaphoid, proximal pole—fracture treated with a headless compression screw

1 Case description

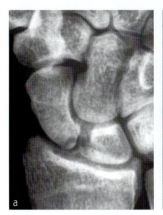 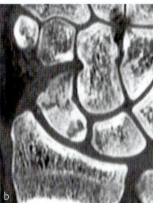 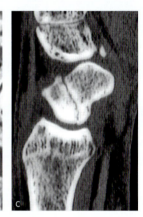

Fig 2.4-1a–c A 20-year-old university student was seen in the emergency department following a fall onto his outstretched right hand. The man suffered wrist pain, which was elicited by the flexion of the wrist, during palpation over the snuffbox, and when axial compression was applied to the thumb. The initial PA x-ray showed a tiny fracture of the proximal pole of the scaphoid. Additional CT scans were performed in the true longitudinal axis of the scaphoid in the coronal and sagittal plane, which also indicated the proximal pole fracture. The sagittal view showed that the fragment was not as small as was suspected with the x-ray.

2 Indications

Proximal pole fractures

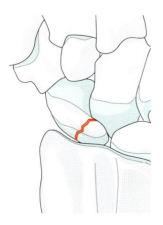

Fig 2.4-2 Scaphoid fractures are the most common carpal fractures and approximately 10–20% of these involve the proximal pole. The proximal pole relies largely on a retrograde blood flow, so the bone relies on distal to proximal intraosseous blood supply for healing. This makes proximal pole fractures highly prone to avascular bone necrosis, delayed union, and nonunion. Nonoperative treatment requires a prolonged period of immobilization of 3–6 months. Therefore, operative treatment via a dorsal approach should be considered.

Choice of implant

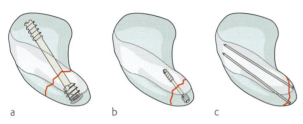

a   b   c

Fig 2.4-3a–c   For proximal pole fractures, if the proximal fragment is large enough, a 2.4 mm or 3.0 mm implant using antegrade insertion is advisable (**a**). For smaller proximal fragments, single or multiple mini headless bone screws (1.5 mm) can be used (**b**). For very small fragments (flakes), K-wires may be a better option (**c**). For this patient, a headless compression screw using an antegrade insertion was required.

Anatomical and vascularity considerations

The scaphoid's unique anatomy and vascularity are critically important in cases involving the proximal pole. Refer to the indications topic in chapter 2.1 Scaphoid—nondisplaced fracture treated percutaneously with a headless compression screw for more information.

Imaging

Obtaining a full series of scaphoid x-rays of the affected and normal contralateral side is necessary for surgical planning. Additional CT scans in the true longitudinal axis of the scaphoid are helpful to identify deformity.

3   Preoperative planning

Equipment

- Headless compression screw set 2.4 or 3.0
- 1.1 mm K-wires
- Pointed reduction forceps
- Image intensifier

Patient preparation and positioning

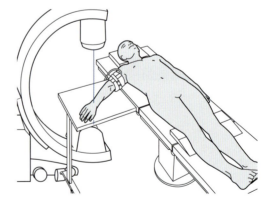

Fig 2.4-4   Position the patient supine and place the forearm on a hand table. Pronate the forearm. A nonsterile pneumatic tourniquet is used. Prophylactic antibiotics are optional.

4 Surgical approach

Approach

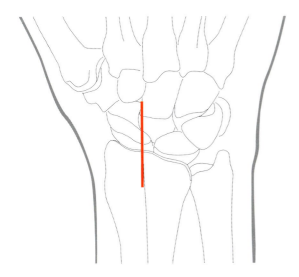

Fig 2.4-5 The surgical approach used was a dorsal approach (see chapter 1.2 Dorsal approach to the scaphoid).

5 Reduction

Direct reduction

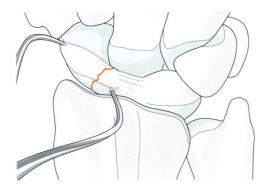

Fig 2.4-6 Use small pointed reduction forceps to reduce the fracture.

Determine insertion point for the guide wire

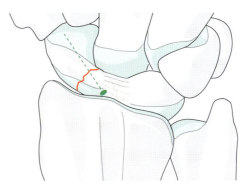

Fig 2.4-7 The correct entry point for the guide wire is in the center of the proximal pole, directly adjacent to the scapholunate ligament insertion.

5   Reduction (cont)

Insert the guide wire

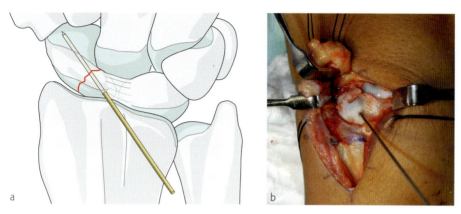

Fig 2.4-8a–b   The guide wire is inserted in the axis of the shaft of the first metacarpal, in radial abduction (**a**). During the introduction of the guide wire, the wrist should be in flexion otherwise the entry point cannot be reached. Do not penetrate the scapho-trapezial joint with the guide wire. The guide wire was carefully inserted across the patient's fracture (**b**).

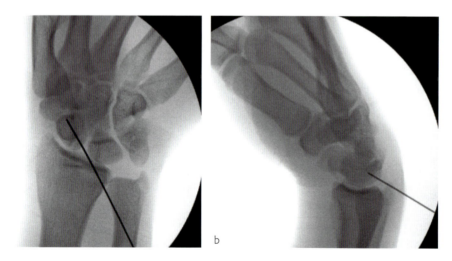

Fig 2.4-9a–b   Image intensification in at least two planes was used to confirm accurate advancement of the guide wire in the scaphoid axis and perpendicular to the fracture plane.

6 Fixation

Measure screw length

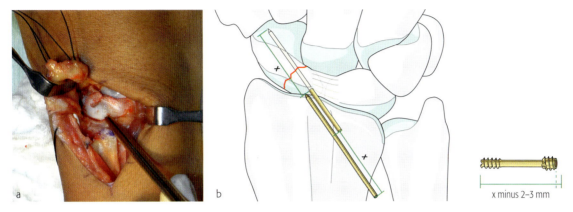

Fig 2.4-10a–b Two methods can be employed for measuring the desired length of the headless screw. Insert the dedicated measuring device over the guide wire, through the drill guide, which must be firmly positioned on the tubercle for a reliable measurement (as shown on the patient) (**a**). Alternatively, if the dedicated measuring device is not available, take another guide wire of the same length and place its tip onto the bone at the insertion point (**b**). The difference between the protruding ends of the two wires indicates the length of the drill hole for the screw. Subtract 2–3 mm to determine the screw length.

Drilling

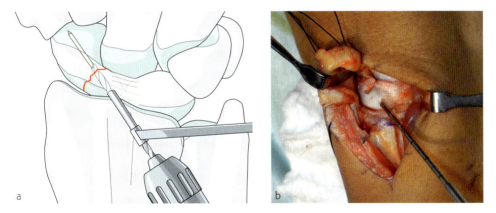

Fig 2.4-11a–b Use only the dedicated drill bit. A power drill will exert less force on the fragments than manual drilling and will reduce the risk of displacing the fragments. A small power drill with slow rotation is the preferred choice (**a**). Use saline solution to cool the drill bit in order to minimize thermal injury. Check the position of the tip of the drill bit under image intensification. Intraoperative image of drilling into the affected scaphoid (**b**).

6 Fixation (cont)

Select the screw

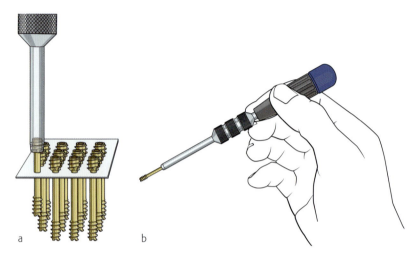

a   b

Fig 2.4-12a–b Select the appropriately sized cannulated headless compression screw. The selected screw is inserted into the internal thread of the compression sleeve.

Insert the screw

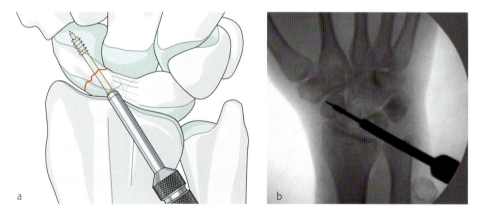

a   b

Fig 2.4-13a–b The screw and compression sleeve are inserted over the guide wire (**a**), as shown in the intraoperative image (**b**).

6   Fixation (cont)

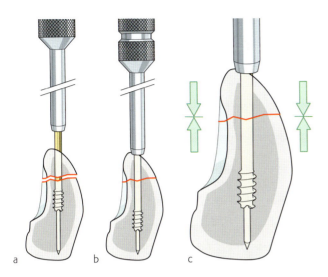

Fig 2.4-14a–c The screw is tightened until sufficient compression is achieved.

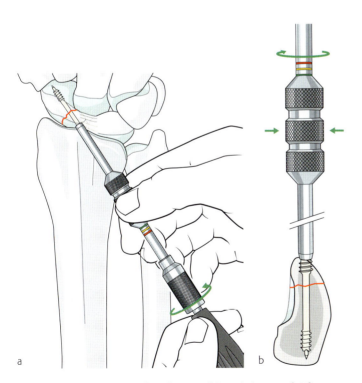

Fig 2.4-15a–b The cannulated screwdriver is inserted. The compression sleeve is held still, using the thumb and index finger to firmly hold the compression sleeve, as the screwdriver turns the screw and advances it out of the compression sleeve and into the bone. Compression is maintained by the compression sleeve during this action.

6   Fixation (cont)

Advance and countersink the screw

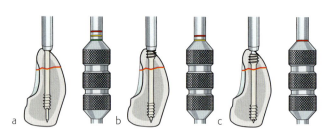

Fig 2.4-16a–c   The screwdriver has three colored markings that are visible at the edge of the compression sleeve. The green mark indicates the screw is still fully retained within the compression sleeve (**a**). The yellow mark indicates the screw has been advanced level with the surface of the bone (**b**). The red mark indicates the screw has been countersunk 2 mm under the bone surface (**c**). Countersink the screw by turning the screwdriver shaft while simultaneously holding the compression sleeve stationary.

Ensure correct screw and thread length

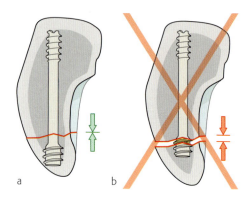

Fig 2.4-17a–b   It is vital that the threaded section of the tip of the screw passes completely beyond the fracture plane if interfragmentary compression is to be achieved. Also ensure that the screw is not too long nor overtightened as it could protrude beyond the cortical surface and lose compression, or endanger the soft tissues, especially tendons and neurovascular structures.

Complete the fixation

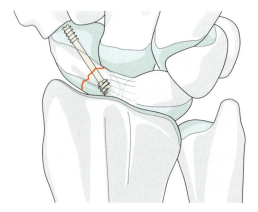

Fig 2.4-18   Before final tightening, remove the guide wire. Make sure that the threads at the near end of the screw are fully buried in the bone at the insertion site. Check the final position of the screw and scaphoid stability using image intensification or x-rays.

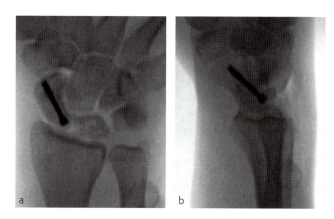

Fig 2.4-19a–b   Intraoperative images showed there was correct positioning of the screw.

7 Rehabilitation

Aftercare, follow-up, and functional exercises

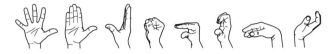

Fig 2.4-20 The patient should receive the standard postoperative rest, injury elevation, follow-up, removal of stitches, and immobilization as required. Following surgery, begin active controlled range of motion exercises. For further information, see the rehabilitation topic in chapter 2.2 Scaphoid—displaced fracture treated with a headless compression screw.

8 Outcome

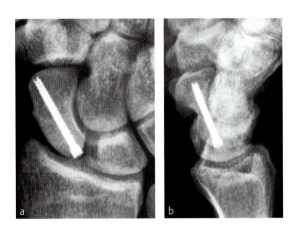

Fig 2.4-21a–b At the 6-month follow-up following the initial trauma, the PA and lateral x-rays showed complete healing of the fracture.

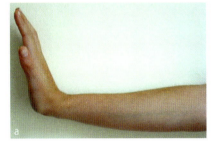

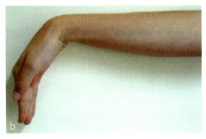

Fig 2.4-22a–b There was restored range of motion and an excellent functional outcome.

9 Alternative technique: case description

Using an additional guide wire

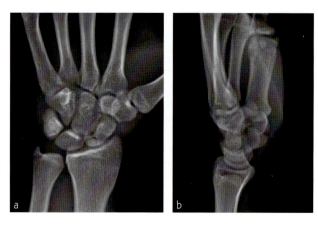

Fig 2.4-23a–b The torque forces of the screw on dense bone in young patients are high that an additional guide wire may be required. This was so for a 17-year-old female school student sustaining a fracture to the proximal pole of her scaphoid after a fall over her outstretched hand during sporting activities.

10 Alternative technique: reduction and fixation

Insert the guide wires

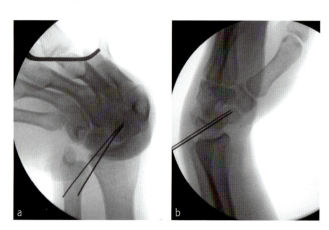

Fig 2.4-24a–b In order to avoid undesirable rotation of the distal fragment of the scaphoid during screw tightening, instead of one guide wire, two parallel guides were used. Image intensification in at least two planes is recommended to confirm the accurate location of both guide wires in the scaphoid.

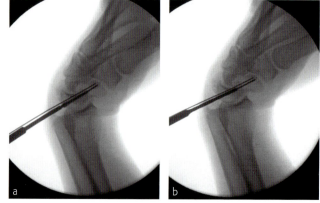

Fig 2.4-25a–b Once the location of the guides has been checked, drilling is performed, followed by the insertion of the screw. In cases of multifragmentation from the proximal third to the scaphoid waist, the additional guide can be left in place to reinforce the fixation.

10 Alternative technique: reduction and fixation (cont)

Outcome

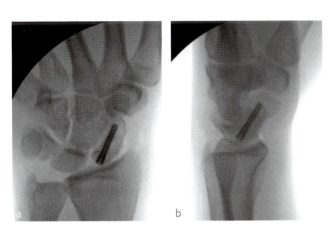

Fig 2.4-26a–b Confirm the position of the screw using image intensification. Note that a fully threaded screw was actually used in this case, however, the principles and techniques remain the same.

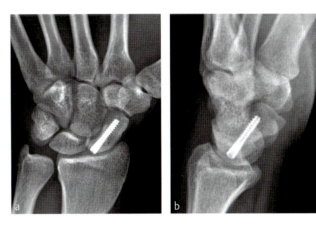

Fig 2.4-27a–b The x-rays showed complete fracture healing 1 year after the initial trauma.

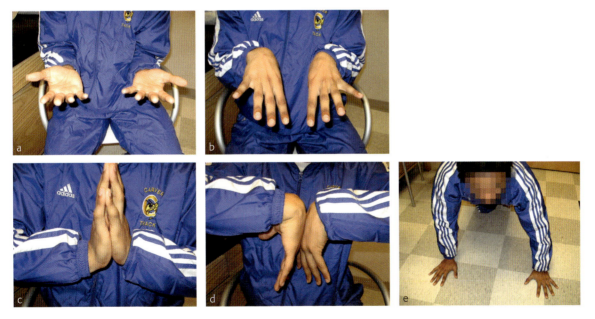

Fig 2.4-28a–e Importantly for this young aspiring athlete, there was an excellent functional outcome.

2.5 Scaphoid, proximal pole—nonunion treated with a headless compression screw and bone graft

1 Case description

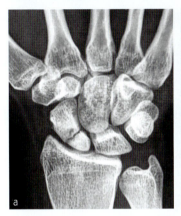
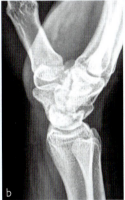

Fig 2.5-1a–b A 21-year-old male student presented with wrist pain, swelling, and limitation of motion having had a fall onto an outstretched right hand some time earlier. The reduced range of motion involved flexion of 15 degrees, extension of 40 degrees, with pronation and supination normal. Pain was elicited by flexion of the wrist, during palpation over the snuffbox, and when axial compression was applied to the thumb. The PA and lateral x-rays demonstrated a well-defined nonunion.

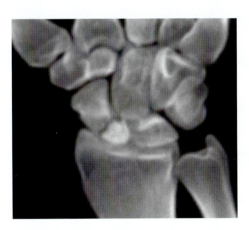

Fig 2.5-2 The images also demonstrated sclerosis (hardening) of the proximal pole of the scaphoid, suggesting avascularity, but there were no major changes to the shape of the bone and no substantial bone resorption was evident.

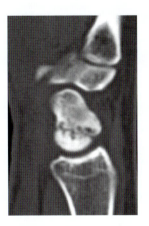

Fig 2.5-3 The CT scan showed a nonunion with a dense proximal pole. The CT scans were performed in the true longitudinal axis of the scaphoid and indicated nonunion with multiple cysts located proximal to the dorsal apex ridge, with minor dorsal displacement of the distal portion of the scaphoid. No collapse was evident and the intrascaphoid angle was 35 degrees.

2 Indications

Proximal pole nonunion

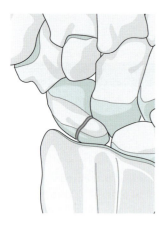

Fig 2.5-4 There are various reasons why a fracture can fail to heal, such as late diagnosis, inadequate immobilization, or severity of trauma. Scaphoid fractures suffer a high rate of nonunion and the poor vascularity of the scaphoid is often to blame (refer to the indications topic in chapter 2.1 Scaphoid—nondisplaced fracture treated percutaneously with a headless compression screw). There are other factors that can also influence the rate of scaphoid union, such as the tremendous forces of flexion and extension that act over this bone, and the fact that approximately 80% of the scaphoid surface is covered with cartilage and bathed in synovial fluid, resulting in bone healing by direct healing without callus formation.

Proximal pole fractures rely largely on a distal to proximal intraosseous blood flow and are therefore especially prone to delayed union and nonunion. A nonunion will result in osteoarthritis of the wrist (also known as arthritis). Nonoperative treatment of acute proximal pole fractures requires a prolonged period of immobilization (3–6 months), therefore operative treatment is recommended at an early stage.

Goals of surgical treatment of a scaphoid nonunion

The following are the main goals for the surgical treatment of scaphoid nonunions:
- To restore anatomy (morphology and scaphoid length)
- To obtain healing
- To stop progression of carpal instability
- To reduce progression of osteoarthritis.

Imaging

Obtaining a full series of scaphoid x-rays of the affected and normal contralateral side is necessary for surgical planning. Also, CT scans in the true longitudinal axis of the scaphoid are helpful in order to identify deformity.

Choice of implant

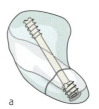
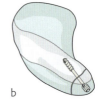
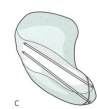

a   b   c

Fig 2.5-5a–c For proximal pole nonunions, if the proximal fragment is large enough, a 2.4 mm or 3.0 mm implant using antegrade insertion is advisable (**a**). For smaller proximal fragments, single or multiple mini headless bone screws (1.5 mm) can be used (**b**). For very small fragments (flakes), K-wires may be a better option (**c**). For this patient, a headless compression screw combined with bone grafting was required.

Equipment

- Headless compression screw set 2.4 or 3.0
- 1.1 mm K-wires
- Pointed reduction forceps
- Autogenous bone graft equipment
- Image intensifier

Patient preparation and positioning

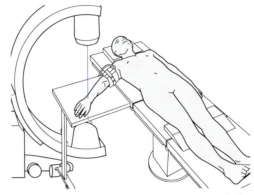

Fig 2.5-6   Position the patient supine and place the forearm on a hand table. Pronate the forearm. A nonsterile pneumatic tourniquet is used. Prophylactic antibiotics are optional.

Approach

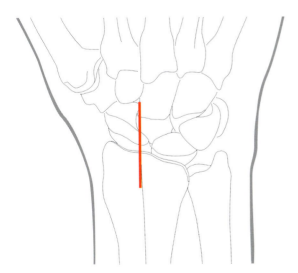

Fig 2.5-7   The surgical approach used was a dorsal approach (see chapter 1.2 Dorsal approach to the scaphoid).

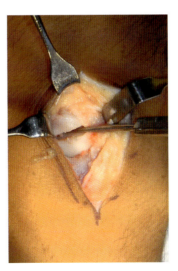

Fig 2.5-8   Through a small dorsal approach and dorsal capsulotomy, the nonunion was identified. Minimal bone resorption and minimal fracture sclerosis were noted. The fibrous tissue interposed in the nonunion area was removed using a small curette until healthy bone was found on both sides. Care was taken to ensure the external shape of the scaphoid was not changed significantly to maintain normal carpal kinematics.

5 Reduction

Direct reduction

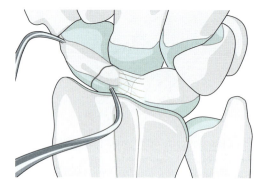

Fig 2.5-9 Use small pointed reduction forceps to reduce the nonunion.

Bone graft

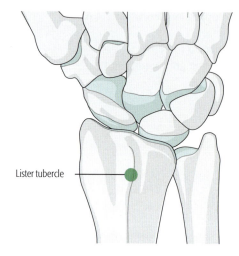

Lister tubercle

Fig 2.5-10 Harvest the graft material from the distal radius. A good and safe place is proximal and slightly radial to Lister tubercle.

Harvesting

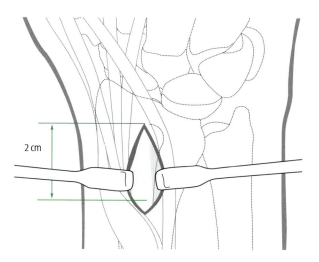

2 cm

Fig 2.5-11 Make a 2 cm longitudinal incision proximal to Lister tubercle. Retract the tendons of the second compartment radially, and the extensor pollicis longus in an ulnar direction.

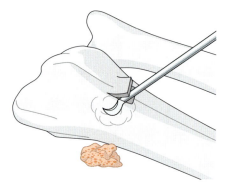

Fig 2.5-12 Use a chisel to cut three sides of a small square. Lift the dorsal radial cortex as a flap. After harvesting cancellous bone, replace the "lid", and suture the periosteum and the skin incision. Use a pusher instrument to impact the bone graft.

5 Reduction (cont)

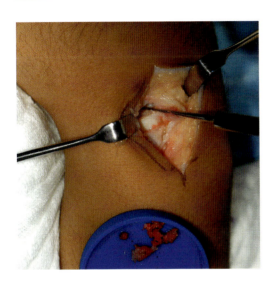

Fig 2.5-13 Cancellous bone graft taken from the distal radius was interposed in the nonunion area.

Determine insertion point for the guide wire

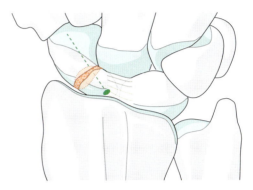

Fig 2.5-14 The correct entry point for the guide wire is in the center of the proximal pole, directly adjacent to the scapholunate ligament insertion.

Insert the guide wire

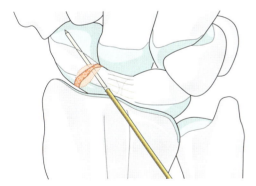

Fig 2.5-15 The guide wire is inserted in the axis of the shaft of the first metacarpal, in radial abduction. During the introduction of the guide wire, the wrist should be in flexion otherwise the entry point cannot be reached. Do not penetrate the scaphotrapezial joint with the guide wire.

Image intensification in at least two planes should be used to confirm accurate advancement of the guide wire in the scaphoid axis and perpendicular to the nonunion.

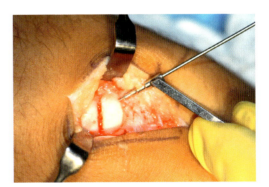

Fig 2.5-16 Vascularity was evaluated and found to be adequate through direct observation of the bleeding spots on the proximal pole. While monitoring with the image intensifier, the guide wire was advanced through the drill guide from proximal to distal into the bone until the tip was anchored in the far cortex.

6 Fixation

Scaphoid fixation

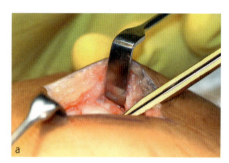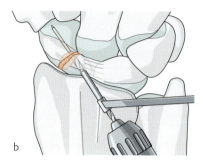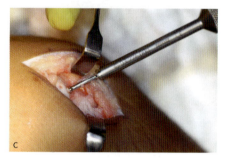

Fig 2.5-17a–c After measuring and drilling, the headless compression screw was settled on the compression sleeve, placed through the drill guide, and carefully tightened until compression of the nonunion was achieved. Forceful tightening was avoided as this could cause stripping of the shaft thread. Predrilling made it substantially easier to insert the screw into dense bone.

The fixation procedure follows the usual steps of measuring screw length, drilling, selecting the screw, inserting the screw, and advancing and countersinking the screw. For further information on these steps see chapter 2.4 Scaphoid, proximal pole—fracture treated with a headless compression screw.

Ensure correct screw and thread length

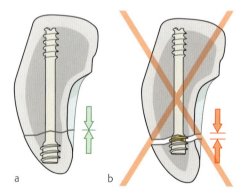

Fig 2.5-18a–b It is vital that the threaded section of the tip of the screw passes completely beyond the fracture plane if interfragmentary compression is to be achieved. Also ensure that the screw is not too long nor overtightened as it could protrude beyond the cortical surface and lose compression, or endanger the soft tissues, especially tendons and neurovascular structures.

Complete the fixation

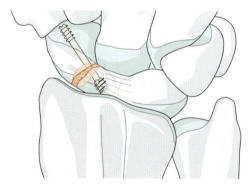

Fig 2.5-19 Before final tightening, remove the guide wire. Make sure that the threads at the near end of the screw are fully buried in the bone at the insertion site. Check the final position of the screw and scaphoid stability using image intensification or x-rays.

6 Fixation (cont)

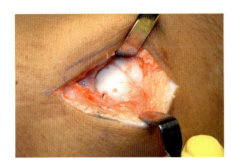

Fig 2.5-20 Through direct vision, it was confirmed that perfect reduction was achieved and that the screw had been sunk beneath the articular cartilage.

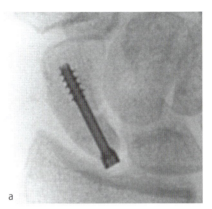

a

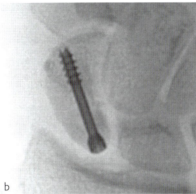

b

Fig 2.5-21a–b With the help of the image intensifier the correct location of the screw was confirmed.

7 Rehabilitation

Aftercare, follow-up, and functional exercises

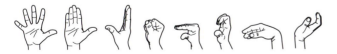

Fig 2.5-22 The patient should receive the standard postoperative rest, injury elevation, follow-up, removal of stitches, and immobilization as required. Following surgery, begin active controlled range of motion exercises. For further information, see the rehabilitation topic in chapter 2.2 Scaphoid—displaced fracture treated with a headless compression screw.

8 Outcome

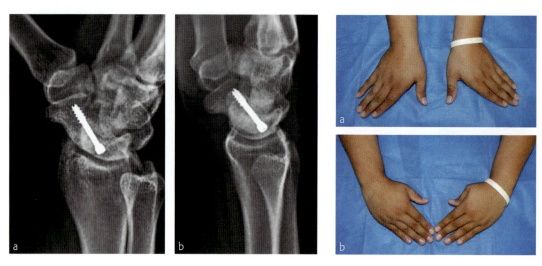

Fig 2.5-23a–b At the 6-month follow-up the postoperative x-rays showed there had been complete healing.

Fig 2.5-24a–b There was also excellent ulnar and radial deviation.

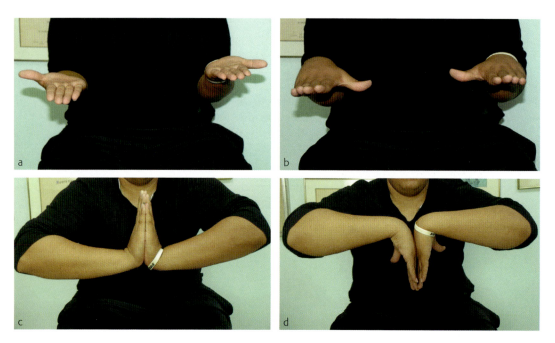

Fig 2.5-25a–d At this stage, excellent range of motion was also shown.

2.6 Scaphoid, waist—nonunion with deformity treated with a headless compression screw and bone graft

1 Case description

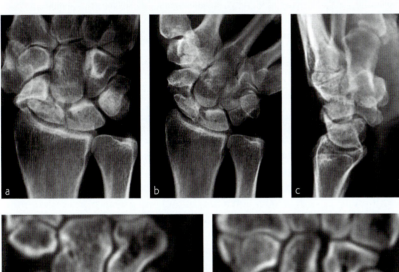

Fig 2.6-1a–c A 47-year-old store manager presented with a symptomatic nonunion of the scaphoid of his right hand following an earlier injury. He presented with pain, limited range of motion, and a weak grip. The PA, PA in ulnar deviation, and lateral x-rays revealed a well-defined nonunion with deformity of the scaphoid.

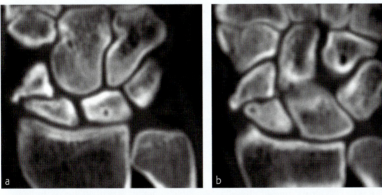

Fig 2.6-2a–b The 2-D CT scans clearly defined the nonunion but without radiographic evidence of osteoarthritis.

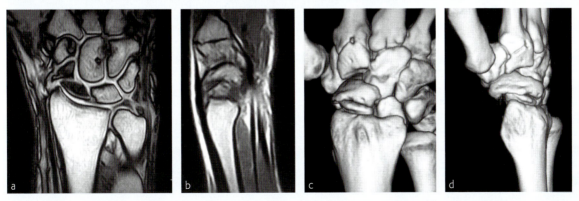

Fig 2.6-3a–d While the MRIs showed preserved cartilage within the radioscaphoid joint, the 3-D CT scan showed a "humpback" deformity pattern of the scaphoid.

2 Indications

Scaphoid waist nonunion

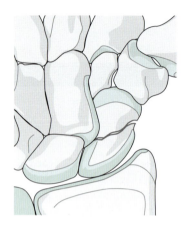

Fig 2.6-4 For a variety of reasons, scaphoid fractures suffer a high rate of nonunion, and a nonunion of a scaphoid waist fracture presents a well-recognized risk of developing intercarpal arthritis. With scaphoid waist nonunions, the goal is often not only to gain union but also to restore the normal functional anatomy of the scaphoid, which may have become deformed. Additionally, it is important to correctly restore the scaphoid's relationship to the adjacent lunate carpal bone.

Nonunion and the humpback deformity

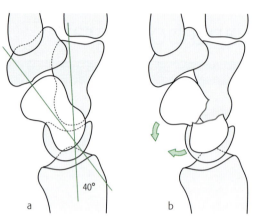

Fig 2.6-5a–b In fractures of the waist of the scaphoid, the distal half tends to rotate into flexion in relation to the proximal half, the lunate, and the triquetrum, which all lie in extension. This can result in a rotational and angular deformity and a nonunion known as humpback deformity. Furthermore, due to the forces exerted over the scaphoid in its palmar aspect, it suffers bone loss with consequent shortening. These changes to the bone often induce carpal collapse.

Scaphoid nonunion advanced collapse

Due to the changes of load over the radiocarpal joint, deformities of the scaphoid can also be responsible for causing osteoarthritis, which can produce what is known as scaphoid nonunion advanced collapse (SNAC). If osteoarthritis develops, only salvage reconstruction procedures can be offered.

Goals of surgical treatment of a scaphoid nonunion

The following are the main goals for the surgical treatment of scaphoid nonunions:
- To restore anatomy (morphology and scaphoid length)
- To obtain healing
- To stop progression of carpal instability
- To reduce progression of osteoarthritis.

Carpal collapse correction

Where there are indications of carpal collapse as a result of scaphoid deformity, an osteotomy or corticocancellous bone graft may be required to fill the defect. This will help to induce healing and to prevent the development of osteoarthritis but also helps to restore scaphoid length. Fixation with a screw to complete the procedure then improves overall stability.

2 Indications (cont)

Choice of implant

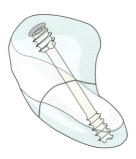

Fig 2.6-6 For scaphoid waist nonunions, a 2.4 mm or 3.0 mm implant using retrograde insertion is advisable. For this patient, a headless compression screw combined with bone grafting was required.

Imaging

Obtaining a full series of scaphoid x-rays of the affected and normal contralateral side is necessary for surgical planning. Also, CT scans in the true longitudinal axis of the scaphoid are helpful in order to identify deformity.

3 Preoperative planning

Equipment

- Headless compression screw set 2.4 or 3.0
- 1.1 mm K-wires
- Pointed reduction forceps
- Autogenous bone graft equipment
- Osteotome
- Image intensifier

Patient preparation and positioning

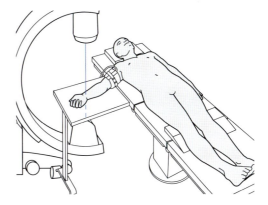

Fig 2.6-7 Position the patient supine and place the forearm on the hand table. Supinate the forearm. A nonsterile pneumatic tourniquet is used. Prophylactic antibiotics are optional.

4 Surgical approach

Approach

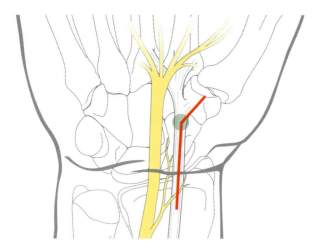

Fig 2.6-8 The surgical approach used was a palmar approach (see chapter 1.1 Palmar approach to the scaphoid).

Hyperextend the wrist

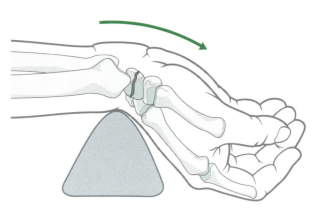

Fig 2.6-9 To assist in the approach, place a rolled towel or bolster under the wrist and hyperextend it. The use of the support helps access the correct entry point for a guide wire. This position also helps to reduce the scaphoid fragments.

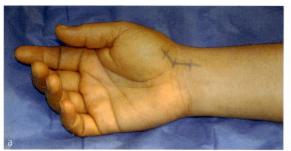
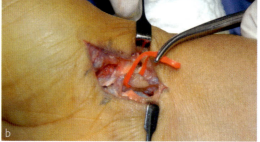

Fig 2.6-10a–b Initially, an incision line was marked crossing the wrist crease at an angle (**a**). After the incision, the superficial palmar branch of the radial artery was protected with a vessel loupe (**b**).

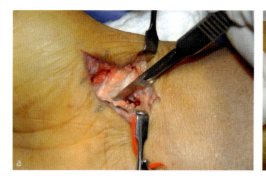
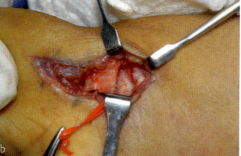

Fig 2.6-11a–b The palmar capsule was then opened in a Z-plasty method (using a Z-shaped incision to relieve tension in scar tissue) (**a**). This was done to preserve the orientation of the radioscaphoid ligament. The nonunion with sclerotic margins was then exposed (**b**).

5 Reduction

Bone graft

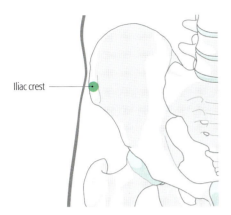

Fig 2.6-12 Harvest the corticocancellous graft material from the iliac crest. For most defects, cancellous or corticocancellous bone graft can be obtained from the distal radius. However, for those nonunions that require substantial debridement of sclerotic bone ends or have fixed rotatory deformities, a larger graft from the iliac crest should be considered.

Harvesting

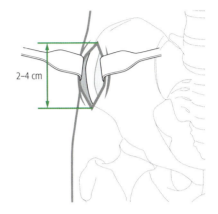

Fig 2.6-13 Make a 2 cm longitudinal incision over the lateral aspect of the palpable iliac crest avoiding the very anterior aspect and the iliofemoral nerve.

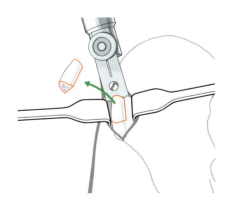

Fig 2.6-14 Expose the crest over a 2–3 cm segment and mark out the preplanned graft size to be harvested. Consider the shape and size of the defect in the scaphoid and how the graft surfaces will contact the two scaphoid pieces. Harvest the selected graft using a sharp osteotome. Control bleeding with a wound pack and use a small suction drain if necessary. Close the skin and apply a pressure dressing.

Insert the bone graft

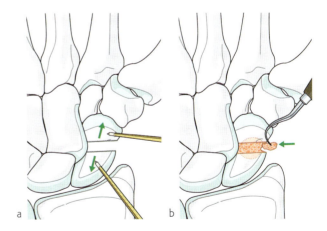

Fig 2.6-15a–b Disimpact the two fragments using a K-wire or dental pick to make room for the graft. Perform the osteotomy and decortication of the nonunion site and ensure the scaphoid is lengthened to its approximate original size (**a**). Use a pusher instrument to impact the bone graft and fill the whole nonunion cavity (**b**). Confirm reduction using image intensification.

5 Reduction (cont)

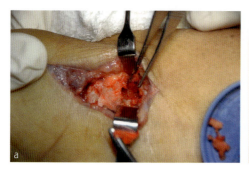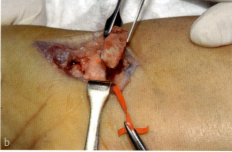

Fig 2.6-16a–b A large nonunion defect was evident. Following decortication of the nonunion site, corticocancellous bone graft was placed into the defect.

Direct reduction

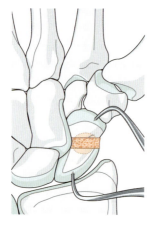

Fig 2.6-17 Use small pointed reduction forceps to reduce the nonunion.

Temporary K-wire

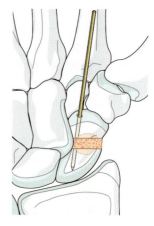

Fig 2.6-18 Alternatively, insert a provisional K-wire to stabilize the fragments and to maintain rotational alignment during drilling. When inserting the K-wire, be careful not to conflict with the planned track of the guide wire for the cannulated screw.

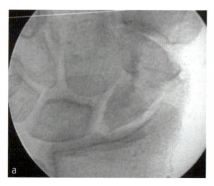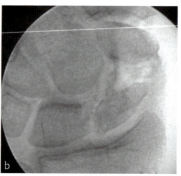

Fig 2.6-19a–b The nonunion was reduced and the scaphoid was given a more normal alignment as seen in the intraoperative images.

5 Reduction (cont)

Determine insertion point for the guide wire

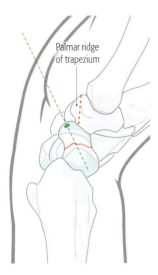

Fig 2.6-20 The correct entry point for the guide wire is the center of the distal pole of the scaphoid. However, to get proper access, it may be necessary to remove the palmar ridge of the trapezium with an osteotome or a bone nibbler/rongeur. This reveals the distal pole of the scaphoid and allows the path of the guide wire to be made more centrally within the bone.

Insert the guide wire

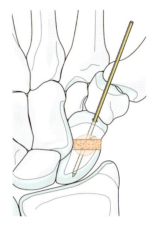

Fig 2.6-21 The guide wire should be inserted through a drill guide. If no drill guide is available, use a protective sleeve. The position of the wire should be as perpendicular as possible to the nonunion plane. Do not penetrate beyond the proximal cortex of the scaphoid.

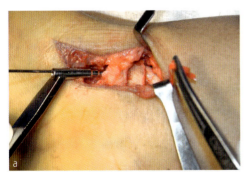
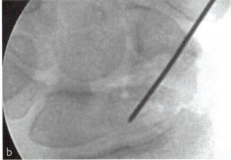

Fig 2.6-22a–b After exposure of the patient's scaphotrapezial joint, a guide wire was placed through a drill guide. The placement of the wire was confirmed with intraoperative imaging.

6 Fixation

Scaphoid fixation

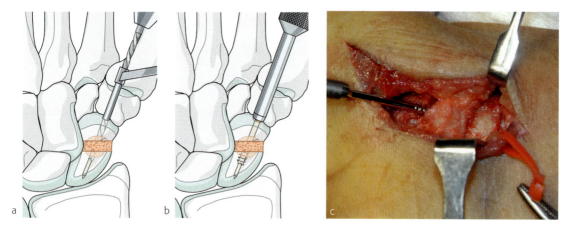

Fig 2.6-23a–c   With the guide wire in place and with care not to damage the graft, the headless screw was inserted across the scaphoid nonunion through the distal pole.

The fixation procedure follows the usual steps of measuring screw length, drilling, selecting the screw, inserting the screw, and advancing and countersinking the screw. For further information on these steps see chapter 2.2 Scaphoid—displaced fracture treated with a headless compression screw.

Ensure correct screw and thread length

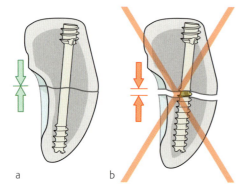

Fig 2.6-24a–b   It is vital that the threaded section of the tip of the screw passes completely beyond the fracture plane if interfragmentary compression is to be achieved. Also ensure that the screw is not too long nor overtightened as it could protrude beyond the cortical surface and lose compression, or endanger the soft tissues, especially tendons and neurovascular structures.

Complete the fixation

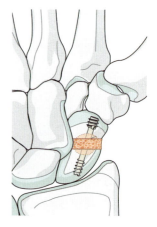

Fig 2.6-25   Before final tightening, remove the guide wire. Make sure that the threads at the near end of the screw are fully buried in the bone at the insertion site. Check the final position of the screw and scaphoid stability using image intensification or x-rays.

6 Fixation (cont)

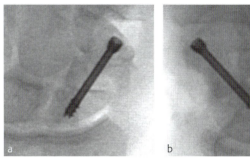
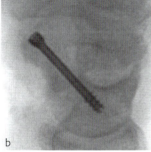
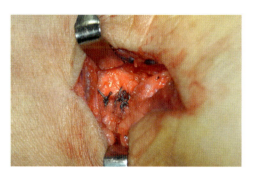

Fig 2.6-26a–b Correct placement of the headless screw was confirmed through intraoperative imaging. Note the large corticocancellous graft.

Fig 2.6-27 During wound closure, the capsular incision was carefully closed to approximate the edges of the capsular ligaments.

7 Rehabilitation

Aftercare, follow-up, and functional exercises

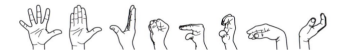

Fig 2.6-28 The patient should receive the standard postoperative rest, injury elevation, follow-up, removal of stitches, and immobilization as required. Following surgery, begin active controlled range of motion exercises. For further information, see the rehabilitation topic in chapter 2.2 Scaphoid—displaced fracture treated with a headless compression screw.

8 Outcome

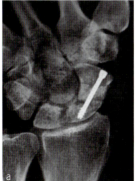
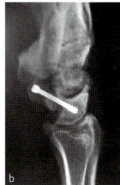
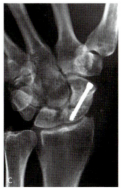
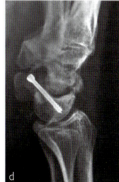

Fig 2.6-29a–d At the 1-month follow-up, the AP and lateral x-rays showed the headless screw and bone graft were in the right position (**a–b**), and at 3-months, the x-rays indicated that partial incorporation of the bone graft had occurred (**c–d**).

8 Outcome (cont)

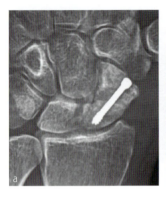
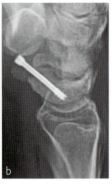

Fig 2.6-30a–b At the 3-year follow-up, the AP and lateral x-rays revealed total incorporation of the bone graft and complete healing of the nonunion.

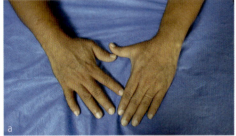
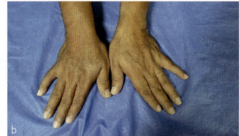
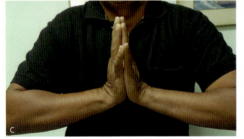
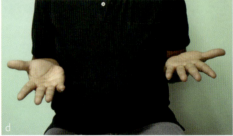

Fig 2.6-31a–d By this stage, the patient had obtained an excellent functional outcome.

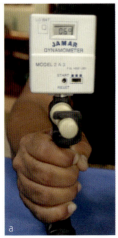
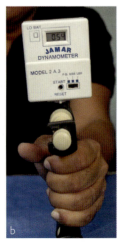

Fig 2.6-32a–b Good grip strength in the injured left hand was also shown.

2.7 Scaphoid, proximal pole—nonunion treated with a vascularized bone graft

1 Case description

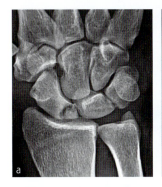
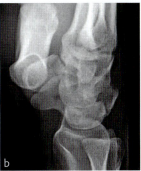

Fig 2.7-1a–b A 30-year-old male shopkeeper presented with wrist pain, functional limitation, and limited range of motion of the right wrist. He recalled an injury to his right hand suffered in a motor vehicle accident 8 months prior. The PA and lateral x-rays revealed a scaphoid proximal pole nonunion with fragmentation at the nonunion site.

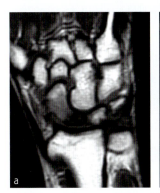
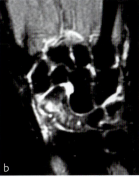
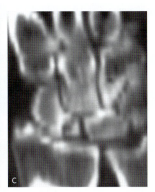

Fig 2.7-2a–c Further investigation with T1 and T2 MRI images demonstrated complete absence of vascularity to the proximal pole fragment, while a 2-D CT image showed the nonunion with a small sclerotic proximal pole fragment.

2 Indications

Proximal pole nonunion with absence of vascularity

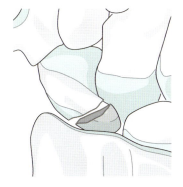

Fig 2.7-3 As has been previously discussed, scaphoid fractures suffer a high rate of nonunion with the poor vascularity of the scaphoid often at fault (refer to the indications topic in chapter 2.1 Scaphoid—nondisplaced fracture treated percutaneously with a headless compression screw). Proximal pole fractures rely largely on a distal to proximal intraosseous blood flow and are therefore especially prone to delayed union and nonunion. Avascular necrosis can also be the cause of scaphoid fracture nonunion, occurring most frequently in the proximal pole. Scaphoid nonunions have a high risk of progressing to osteoarthritis within a few years following the injury, yet effective healing of the nonunion dramatically reduces this risk.

Vascularized bone grafting

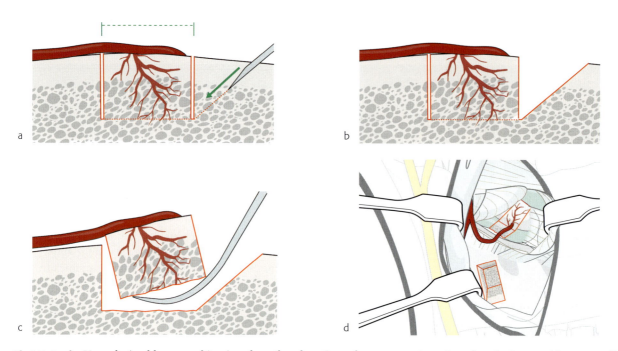

Fig 2.7-4a–d   Vascularized bone grafting involves the elevation of an appropriate size of graft tissue with a centrally located vessel (**a–c**). It is then carefully placed into the prepared fracture or nonunion site (**d**).

Studies have shown that vascularized bone grafting can be used effectively to provide improved blood supply and increase the potential for healing. While evidence continues to be gathered regarding whether vascularized bone grafting is conclusively more effective than standard nonvascularized techniques, it has been considered logical to employ a vascularized graft in situations where vascularity has been compromised. Additionally, vascularized bone graft harvested from the distal radius confers significant theoretical advantages and also reduces the impact of donor site morbidity from a distant site.

Goals of surgical treatment of a scaphoid nonunion

The following are the main goals for the surgical treatment of scaphoid nonunions:

- Restore anatomy (morphology and scaphoid length)
- Obtain healing
- Stop progression of carpal instability
- Reduce progression of osteoarthritis.

2 Indications (cont)

Choice of implant

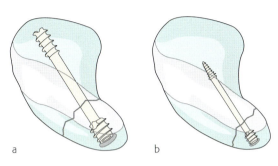

a   b

Fig 2.7-5a–b   For scaphoid nonunions with loss of vascularity, if the proximal fragment is large enough, a 2.4 mm or 3.0 mm implant using antegrade insertion is advised. For smaller proximal fragments, single or multiple mini headless bone screws (1.5 mm) can be used. For this patient, two mini headless bone screws combined with dorsal vascularized bone grafting was required.

Imaging

Obtaining a full series of scaphoid x-rays of the affected and normal contralateral side is necessary for surgical planning. A CT scan in the true longitudinal axis of the scaphoid is also helpful in order to identify deformity. Gadolinium enhanced T1 MRI scans are indicated when assessing the vascularity of the proximal fragment.

3 Preoperative planning

Equipment

- Mini headless screw set 1.5
- 1.1 mm K-wires
- Autogenous bone graft equipment
- Image intensifier
- Knowledge of the technique for dorsal 1,2 intercompartmental supraretinacular artery (1,2 ICSRA) vascularized bone grafting

Patient preparation and positioning

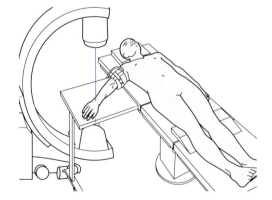

Fig 2.7-6   Position the patient supine and place the forearm on a hand table. Pronate the forearm. A nonsterile pneumatic tourniquet is used. Prophylactic antibiotics are optional.

Approach

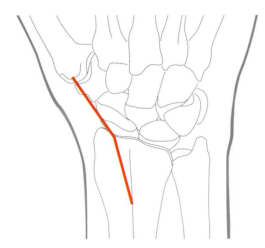

Fig 2.7-7   The surgical approach used was a dorsal approach (see chapter 1.2 Dorsal approach to the scaphoid). However, on this occasion, the incision involved a dorsoradial longitudinal curved skin incision, starting over the base of the thumb and extending proximally for about 6–8 cm. This approach allows for a dorsal pedicled 1,2 ICSRA graft.

5 Reduction

Dorsal vascularized bone grafting

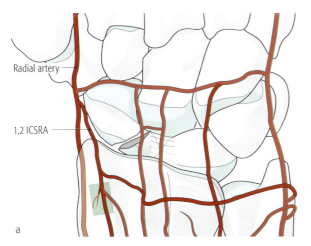

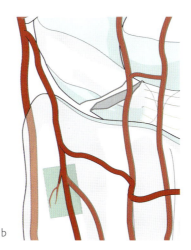

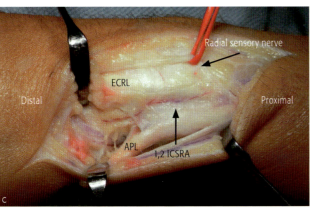

Fig 2.7-8a–c Pedicled vascularized bone grafts used in scaphoid nonunion surgery are based on two different arteries. One vascular pedicle is found on the dorsal surface of the distal radius, the other on the palmar surface. The dorsal pedicle is based on the 1,2 intercompartmental supraretinacular artery (1,2 ICSRA) (**a–b**). A dorsal vascularized graft using these vessels allows excellent mobility to treat nonunions in all regions of the scaphoid, including the proximal pole (**c**).

Excising the nonunion

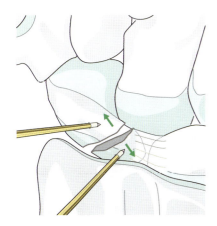

Fig 2.7-9 Prepare the nonunion by excising fibrous tissue to healthy cancellous surfaces. Disimpact the fragments using a K-wire or dental pick to make room for the graft. Ensure scaphoid lengthening to its approximate original size.

5 Reduction (cont)

Elevate the bone graft

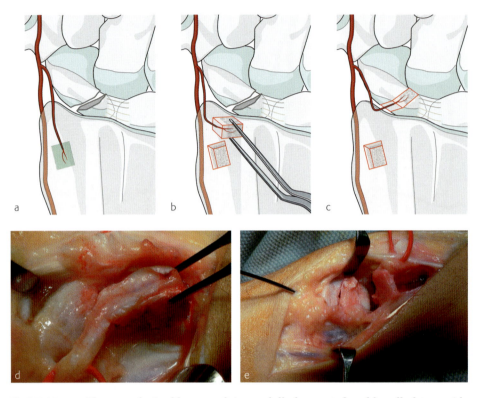

Fig 2.7-10a–e The vascularized bone graft is carefully harvested and handled to avoid twisting of the vascular pedicle (**a–b**). It will later be inserted into the previously prepared defect in the scaphoid (**c–d**). Tension on the vascular pedicle must be avoided. A temporary K-wire is a useful method of stabilizing the reduction and avoids risk of damage to the vascular pedicle (**e**).

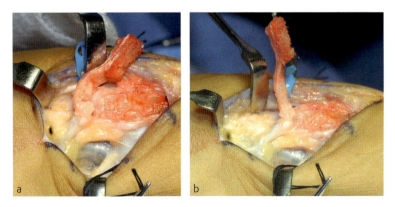

Fig 2.7-11a–b For the patient, the vascularized distal radius bone graft (1,2 ICSRA) was elevated on its pedicle.

5 Reduction (cont)

Prepare a trough if needed

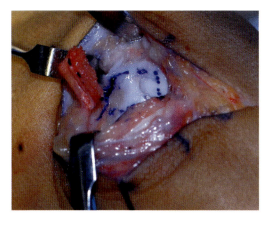

Fig 2.7-12 A trough that crossed the nonunion site for later insertion of the bone graft was planned.

Determine insertion point and insert the guide wire

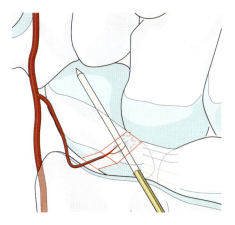

Fig 2.7-13 If cannulated headless bone screws are used, determine the guide wire entry point (in the center of the proximal pole) and insert the guide wire. Do not penetrate the scaphotrapezial joint with the guide wire. Image intensification in at least two planes should be used to confirm accurate advancement of the guide wire in the scaphoid axis and perpendicular to the nonunion.

6 Fixation

Scaphoid fixation

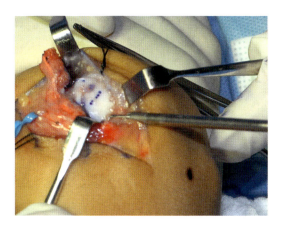

Fig 2.7-14 Following creation of the trough across the nonunion site, two 1.5 mm headless screws were placed across the nonunion through the proximal pole into the body of the scaphoid. However, because the proximal fragment was small it was decided to use an initial screw to guarantee scaphoid shape and stability before creation of the trough.

The fixation procedure follows the usual steps of measuring screw length, drilling, selecting the screw, inserting the screw, and advancing and countersinking the screw. For further information on these steps see chapter 2.4 Scaphoid, proximal pole—fracture treated with a headless compression screw. However, in this particular case, the 1.5 mm mini headless bone screws are noncannulated and therefore require no guide wires.

6   Fixation (cont)

Ensure correct screw and thread length

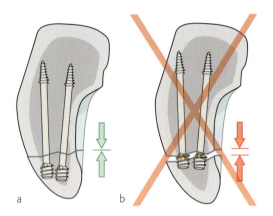

Fig 2.7-15a–b   It is vital that the threaded section of the tip of the screw passes completely beyond the fracture plane if interfragmentary compression is to be achieved. Also ensure that the screw is not too long nor overtightened as it could protrude beyond the cortical surface and lose compression, or endanger the soft tissues, especially tendons and neurovascular structures.

Complete the fixation

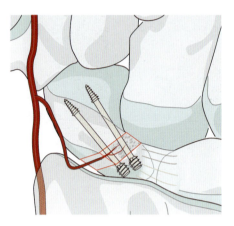

Fig 2.7-16   Before final tightening, remove any guide wires (if cannulated screws were used). Make sure that the threads at the near end of the screws are fully buried in the bone at the insertion site. Check the final position of the screws and scaphoid stability using image intensification or x-rays.

Insert and complete the vascularized graft

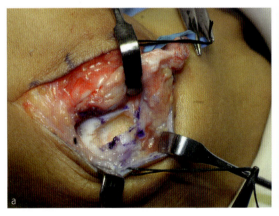
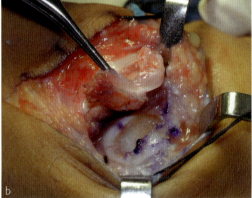

Fig 2.7-17a–b   With the nonunion site now stabilized with one screw previously placed, the vascularized graft was inserted into the trough across the nonunion. This was followed with a second screw used to fix the graft to the scaphoid. The wound was then closed taking care not to damage or compress the vascular pedicle.

Note that in cases where there is bone loss and cyst formation at the nonunion site, the bone graft should be inserted into the defect before stabilization with bone screws. However, when introducing the graft first and then inserting screws, be careful that screw insertion does not force out or damage the graft.

6 Fixation (cont)

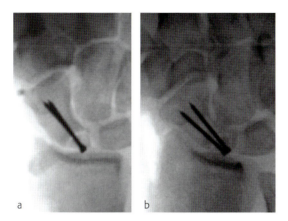

Fig 2.7-18a–b The intraoperative images confirmed the correct placement of the screws.

7 Rehabilitation

Aftercare, follow-up, and functional exercises

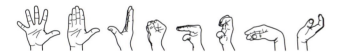

Fig 2.7-19 The patient should receive the standard postoperative rest, injury elevation, follow-up, removal of stitches, and immobilization as required. Following surgery, begin active controlled range of motion exercises. For further information, see the rehabilitation topic in chapter 2.2 Scaphoid—displaced fracture treated with a headless compression screw.

8 Outcome

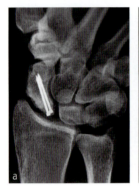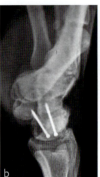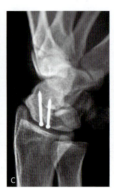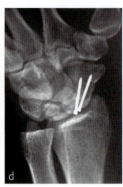

Fig 2.7-20a–d At the 3-year follow-up, the PA and lateral x-rays and the hyperpronation and semipronation oblique x-rays showed complete healing of the nonunion with stable screw fixation and no evidence of avascular necrosis of the proximal pole.

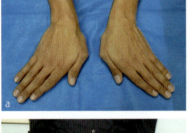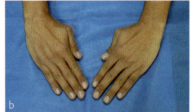
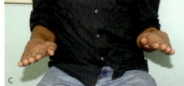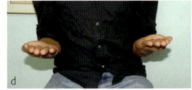
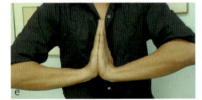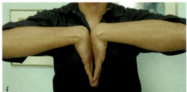

Fig 2.7-21a–f At this stage, the patient had a nearly full range of motion.

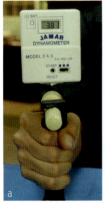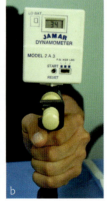

Fig 2.7-22a–b Excellent grip strength had also been restored.

Nonunion treated with a palmar vascularized bone graft

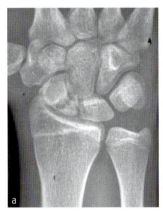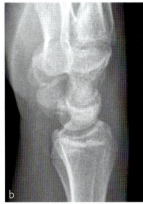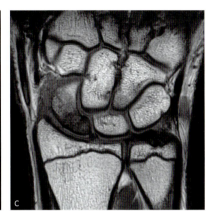

Fig 2.7-23a–c   Just as it is possible to treat a scaphoid nonunion with a dorsal vascularized bone graft, it is also possible to treat such injuries with a palmar vascularized bone graft. A 16-year-old student and recreational skier landed awkwardly while skiing. He had pain and restricted movement in his left wrist but thought it likely to be a soft-tissue injury. After 3 months, he attended his local hospital as he was still experiencing pain with movement, weakness of grip, and a noticeable loss of extension (40 degrees compared with 65 degrees in the opposite wrist). Examination confirmed a "fullness" in the anatomical snuff box and tenderness to firm pressure. Plain PA and lateral x-rays revealed an established nonunion at the proximal waist of the scaphoid with a hump-back deformity (**a–b**). A T1-weighted MRI scan with gadolinium enhancement demonstrated diminished blood flow in the proximal fragment (**c**). On further questioning, he recalled an incident 18 months earlier when he had injured the same wrist falling from his skateboard.

Palmar vascularized bone grafting

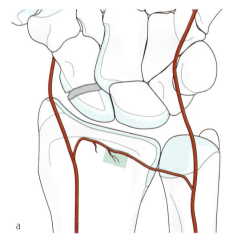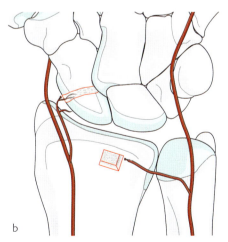

Fig 2.7-24a–b   For palmar vascularized bone graft treatment of scaphoid waist nonunions, the palmar pedicle is used, which is based on the palmar radial carpal artery, an anastomotic (multibranched) vessel between the radial artery and the anterior interosseous artery. The graft provides a strong structural component to the procedure by virtue of the thick cortical bone of the palmar cortex of the distal radius.

9 Alternative technique: case description (cont)

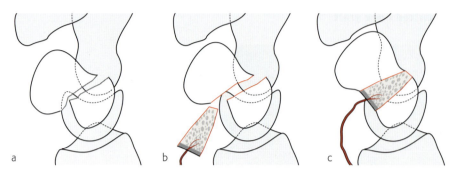

Fig 2.7-25a–c This palmar graft is particularly useful in scaphoid waist nonunions with a hump back deformity, where correction of the deformity is as important as achieving union.

Surgical approach

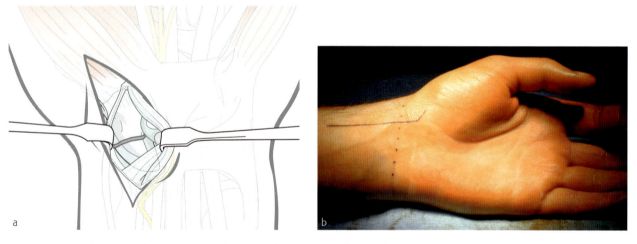

Fig 2.7-26a–b The surgical approach used was a palmar approach (see chapter 1.1 Palmar approach to the scaphoid). Retrograde fixation should be performed with either 1.5 mm mini headless screws or 2.4 mm/3.0 mm cannulated headless compression screws.

10 Alternative technique: reduction and fixation

Excising the nonunion

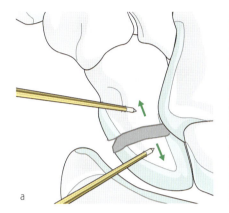
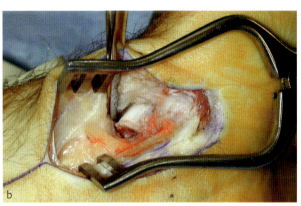

Fig 2.7-27a–b Prepare the nonunion by excising fibrous tissue to healthy cancellous surfaces. For this patient, cyst formation was noted and was removed. Disimpact the fragments using a K-wire or dental pick to make room for the graft (**a**). Ensure scaphoid lengthening to its approximate original size (**b**).

Elevate the bone graft

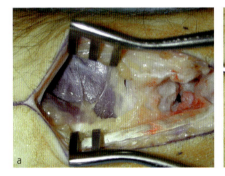
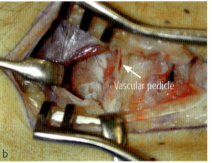
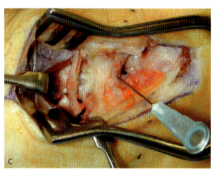

Fig 2.7-28a–c The palmar radial carpal artery pedicle is found distal to the pronator quadratus and is carefully separated from the overlying fascia (**a–b**). The pronator quadratus is retracted (**b**) to reveal the periosteal vessels. The pedicle is cauterized at its ulnar limit and a premeasured rectangular bone graft is harvested from the distal radius, still attached to the pedicle (**c**). A hypodermic needle placed in the radiocarpal joint prevents inadvertent damage to the articular surface during harvest of bone graft.

10 Alternative technique: reduction and fixation (cont)

Insert the vascularized graft

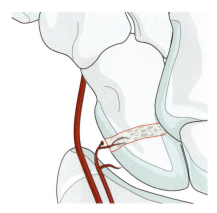

Fig 2.7-29 Insert the bone graft into the prepared defect, correcting the hump back deformity. The vascularized bone graft is carefully handled to avoid twisting of the vascular pedicle attached to the graft, and tension on the vascular pedicle must also be avoided. Confirm reduction using image intensification.

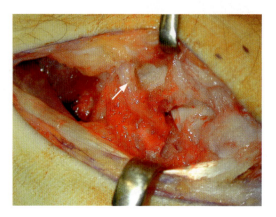

Fig 2.7-30 The patient's vascularized graft can be seen in place.

Determine insertion point and insert the guide wire

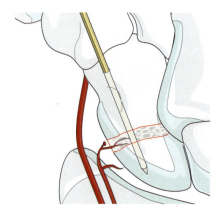

Fig 2.7-31 If cannulated headless bone screws are used, determine the guide wire entry point and insert the guide wire. Image intensification in at least two planes should be used to confirm accurate advancement of the guide wire in the scaphoid axis and perpendicular to the nonunion.

10 Alternative technique: reduction and fixation (cont)

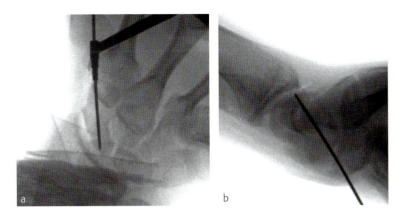

Fig 2.7-32a–b The guide wire should be inserted through a drill guide. If no drill guide is available, use a protective sleeve. Intraoperative images show the guide wire insertion.

Additional temporary K-wire

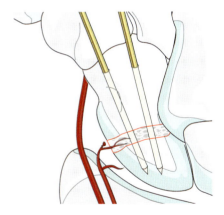

Fig 2.7-33 An additional temporary K-wire can be inserted to stabilize the fragments and to maintain rotational alignment during drilling. When inserting the additional K-wire, be careful not to conflict with the planned track of the guide wire for the cannulated screw.

10 Alternative technique: reduction and fixation (cont)

Scaphoid fixation

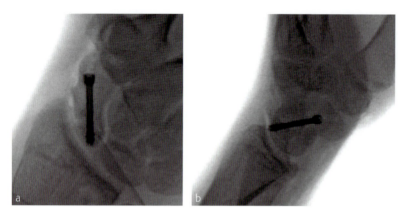

Fig 2.7-34a–b A single headless screw was placed into the body of the scaphoid and through the graft.

The fixation procedure follows the usual steps of measuring screw length, drilling, selecting the screw, inserting the screw, and advancing and countersinking the screw. When an additional temporary K-wire has been used, it must be removed before final tightening of the screw. For further information on these steps see chapter 2.2 Scaphoid—displaced fracture treated with a headless compression screw.

A final check of position and length of the implant was performed from several angles to ensure no overpenetration.

Outcome

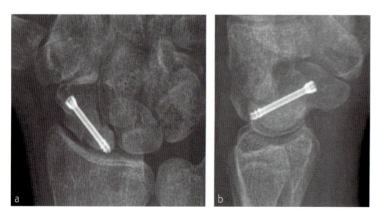

Fig 2.7-35a–b The procedure resulted in healing of the nonunion and return to normal movement and activity levels.

2.8 Perilunate dislocation treated with K-wires

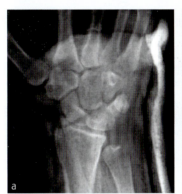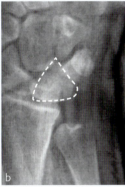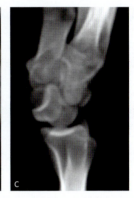

Fig 2.8-1a–c A 28-year-old salesman and amateur surfer was swept off his surfboard while riding a large wave. He presented to the emergency department experiencing pain, deformity, and edema of his right wrist, accompanied by numbness of the fingers. On the PA x-rays, a triangular profile of the lunate was shown rather than a normal quadrilateral shape (**a–b**). This was due to an anterior dislocation and widening between the scaphoid and lunate. The lateral x-ray also showed the palmar dislocation of the lunate. The capitate was displaced proximally toward the distal radial articular surface. The "spilled teacup" configuration of the lunate was a classic sign of a lunate dislocation (**c**).

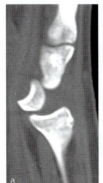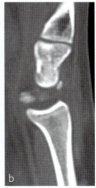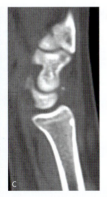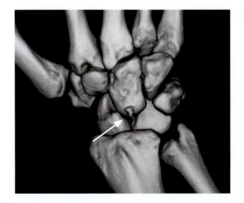

Fig 2.8-2a–c The sagittal 2-D CT scans showed the palmar dislocation of the lunate (**a**) and the empty lunate facet of the radius with some small chip fractures of the lunate (**b**). However, there was a normal anatomical relationship between the hamate and the triquetrum (**c**).

Fig 2.8-3 The dorsal view 3-D CT scan confirmed the palmar dislocation of the lunate, although the scaphoid kept its normal anatomical relationship with the radius and the distal carpal row. A small chip fracture of the dorsal aspect of the lunate (arrow) presented the possibility (later confirmed) that there was an avulsion of the dorsal scapholunate ligament.

2 Indications

Perilunate dislocations

Perilunate dislocations are ligamentous injuries that result from high-energy trauma and involve damage to the capsuloligamentous connections of the lunate to its adjacent carpal bones and the radius. They can lead to severe disruption of carpal anatomy, resulting in profound changes in wrist biomechanics. Of all wrist dislocations, perilunate dislocations are the most common.

Carpal ligament anatomy and rupture

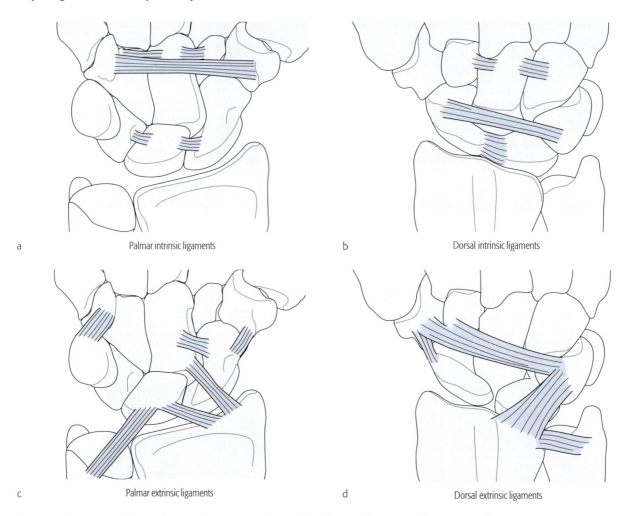

a Palmar intrinsic ligaments	b Dorsal intrinsic ligaments
c Palmar extrinsic ligaments	d Dorsal extrinsic ligaments

Fig 2.8-4a–d   Bones of the wrist are given supporting stability by a wide range of ligaments. The carpal rows are supported by stout intrinsic ligaments (**a–b**), which begin and end within the same carpal row. These ligaments are reinforced by a complex system of palmar and dorsal extrinsic ligaments (**c–d**), which begin and end in different rows. Rupture of the intrinsic ligaments is called "dissociation". Rupture of the extrinsic ligaments alone causes a "nondissociative" injury.

2   Indications (cont)

The Perilunate Instability Classification

The progression of ligamentous damage and the sequence of injuries that can occur in a perilunate dislocation were investigated by Mayfield and colleagues in anatomical specimen experimentation. Their findings confirmed that most carpal dislocations around the lunate are the consequence of a similar pathomechanical event, the so-called progressive perilunate instability. The four types (or stages) of carpal destabilization were identified as follows:

- Stage I: Scapholunate dissociation
- Stage II: Lunocapitate dislocation
- Stage III: Midcarpal dislocation
- Stage IV: Lunate dislocation.

Stage I: Scapholunate dissociation

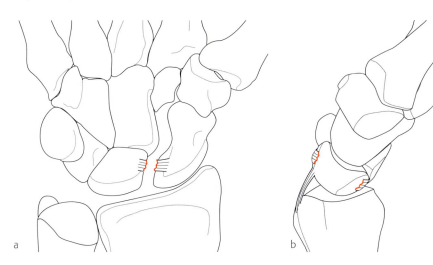

Fig 2.8-5a–b   Stage I: Scapholunate dissociation involves tearing of the scapholunate ligament. Any increased separation between the scaphoid and lunate is known as the Terry Thomas or David Letterman sign, named after famous entertainers with pronounced gaps in their front teeth.

Stage II: Lunocapitate dislocation

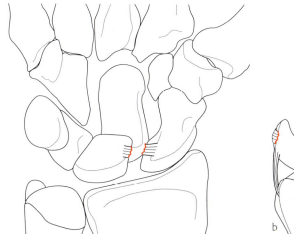
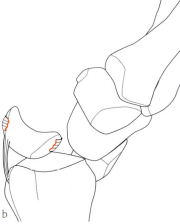

Fig 2.8-6a–b   Stage II: Lunocapitate dislocation is where the lunate remains aligned normally with the distal radius but the surrounding carpal bones are dislocated. The lunocapitate joint becomes disrupted.

159

2 Indications (cont)

Stage III: Midcarpal dislocation

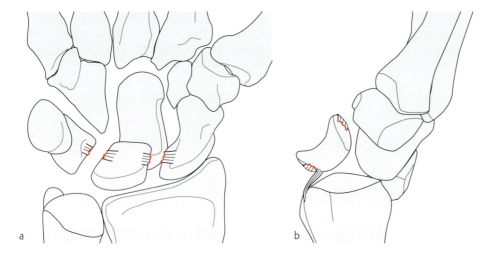

a b

Fig 2.8-7a–b Stage III: Midcarpal dislocation is where both the lunate and capitate have lost alignment with the distal radius. The lunotriquetral ligament and or triquetral bone are affected.

Stage IV: Lunate dislocation

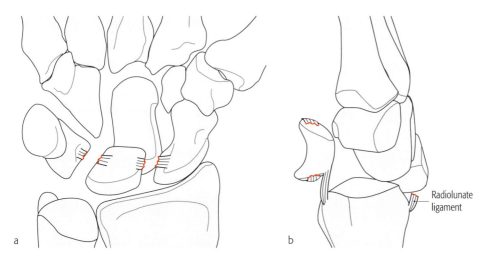

a b

Radiolunate ligament

Fig 2.8-8a–b Stage IV: A lunate dislocation is where there is dislocation of the lunate and injury to the dorsal radiolunate ligament. The unique teacup appearance of the lunate and the extreme angle that can result in this injury creates what is known as the spilled teacup sign.

2   Indications (cont)

Complete dislocations of the lunate

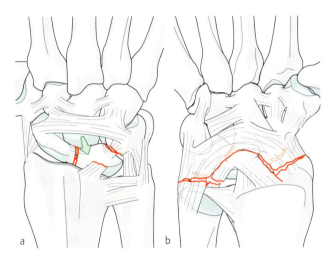

a   b

Fig 2.8-9a–b   In stage IV complete dislocations of the lunate, the luxation is usually in a palmar direction. The greater force required to produce this injury is responsible for massive disruption of both the dorsal and palmar ligaments.

Disruption of the dorsal radiolunotriquetral ligament complex

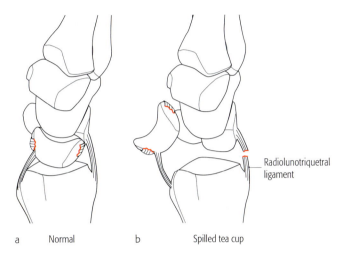

a   Normal   b   Spilled tea cup

Radiolunotriquetral ligament

Fig 2.8-10a–b   There can also be a disruption of the dorsal radiolunotriquetral ligament complex.

Imaging

Diagnosis of simple ligament dissociation can be difficult as there might be no immediate carpal bone movement or dislocation, and x-rays may appear normal. Taking stress x-rays with the hand holding a pencil, for example, may cause gaps between the carpals to open and be more clearly identified.

Perilunate dislocations should be suspected when a patient presents with a painful and swollen wrist after a high-energy hyperextension injury and signs of median nerve compression. The final diagnosis needs to be based on a careful radiographic examination. Although in the coronal view abnormal overlapping of the carpal bones and alteration of "Gilula´s arcs" can be observed, a true lateral view is the best way to make the diagnosis (for further information on using arcs to determine carpal injury see the indications topic in chapter 2.10 Transtriquetral transscaphoid perilunate fracture dislocation treated with screws). Lateral x-rays can also show the spilled teacup configuration of a dislocated lunate. Additionally, as the capitate displaces proximally toward the distal radial articular surface, on x-rays thc displaced lunate has a triangular profile (**Fig 2.8-1a–b**), rather than its normal quadrilateral shape. These can be difficult injuries to manage, with many going on to have ligament repair failure and developing some osteoarthritis of the wrist.

A CT scan is also of great help offering more precise detail of the injury in order to plan the surgery in a more logical and accurate way.

3 Preoperative planning

Equipment

- 1.4 mm to 1.6 mm K-wires
- Pointed reduction forceps
- Bone anchors
- Image intensifier

Patient preparation and positioning

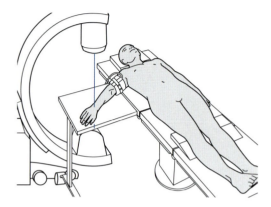

Fig 2.8-11 Position the patient supine and place the forearm on a hand table. Pronate the forearm. A nonsterile pneumatic tourniquet is used. Prophylactic antibiotics are optional.

4 Surgical approach

Approach

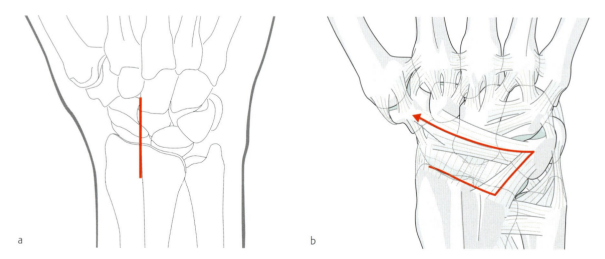

a   b

Fig 2.8-12a–b The surgical approach used was a dorsal approach (see chapter 1.3 Combined approach to the lunate and perilunate injuries, however, only the dorsal approach was required with this patient). This approach involves a radially based capsular ligamentous flap to be elevated and a capsulotomy incision.

5 Reduction

Preliminary reduction of the lunate

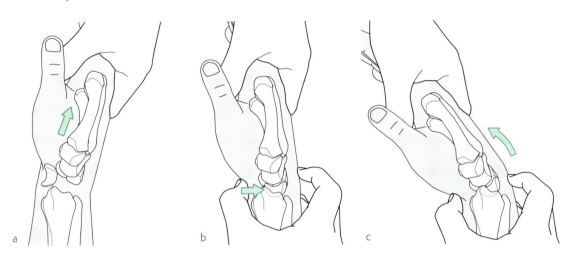

a   b   c

Fig 2.8-13a–c   Closed reduction is a preliminary to operative treatment and has three benefits:
- It restores carpal alignment
- It improves the patient's comfort
- It reduces pressure on the median nerve.

Reduction of the dislocated lunate is achieved by distracting the wrist (**a**) and applying direct thumb pressure over the lunate from palmar to dorsal (**b**). The hand is then gently flexed, and once reduction has occurred, the distraction is gently relaxed (**c**).

Open reduction of the lunate

If closed reduction is not successful, open reduction is necessary as soon as possible due to the risk of median nerve compromise, of pain, and to preserve blood supply to the lunate.

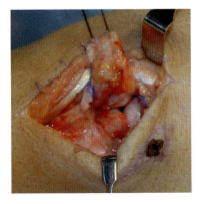

Fig 2.8-14   For this patient, a radially based capsulotomy was performed and the flap was elevated and held with two sutures exposing the dorsal aspect of the carpus. The lunate was reduced by longitudinal traction and by the use of a periosteal elevator with care taken not to damage the articular cartilage.

5 Reduction (cont)

Assessment of dorsal and proximal ligament remnants

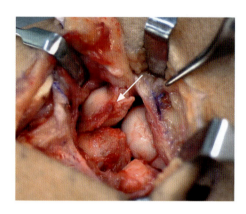

Fig 2.8-15 The scapholunate ligament can be avulsed from either the scaphoid or from the lunate. In this case, the ligament was avulsed from the lunate, remaining attached to the scaphoid as is shown by the arrow. The avulsion site was appropriately debrided to improve contact and healing.

Open reduction of the scapholunate joint

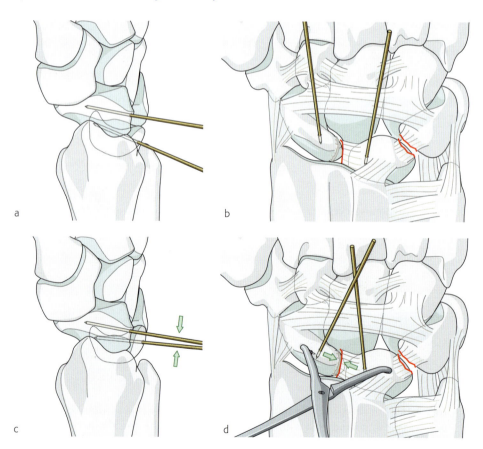

Fig 2.8-16a–d Use two joystick K-wires, inserting them deep into the bone, to extend the scaphoid and flex the lunate, and then close the gap. A pointed reduction forceps helps to secure the reduction temporarily. Confirm reduction using image intensification in two planes.

5 Reduction (cont)

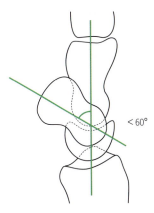

Fig 2.8-17 On the lateral view, with the wrist neutral, check that the radius, lunate, and capitate are in line, that the scapholunate angle is < 60 degrees, and that there is no dorsal tilt of the lunate.

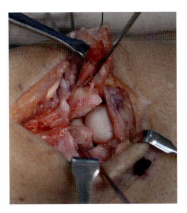

Fig 2.8-18 The clinical image shows the joystick K-wires being inserted into each of the scaphoid and the lunate. They were used to complete the closure of the scapholunate diastasis.

6 Fixation

Scapholunate ligament repair

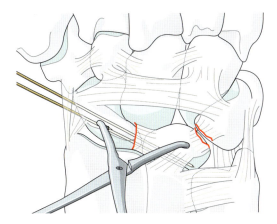

Fig 2.8-19 The scaphoid and lunate bones should be secured by transfixation with two K-wires inserted percutaneously, from scaphoid to lunate. Confirm the position of the wires using image intensification.

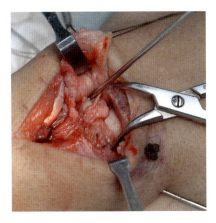

Fig 2.8-20 After the gap between the scaphoid and the lunate was reduced using the two joysticks and maintained by the pointed reduction forceps, percutaneous K-wires were introduced between the scaphoid and lunate, between the triquetrum and lunate, and between the scaphoid and the capitate.

6 Fixation (cont)

Pearl: alternative K-wire insertion

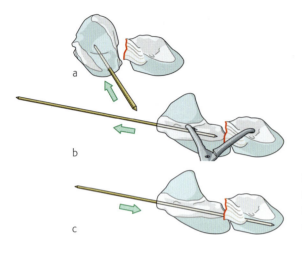

Fig 2.8-21a–c The transfixation K-wires can be inserted into the scaphoid from inside outward prior to the reduction and then advanced into the lunate across the scapholunate articulation once reduction has been achieved.

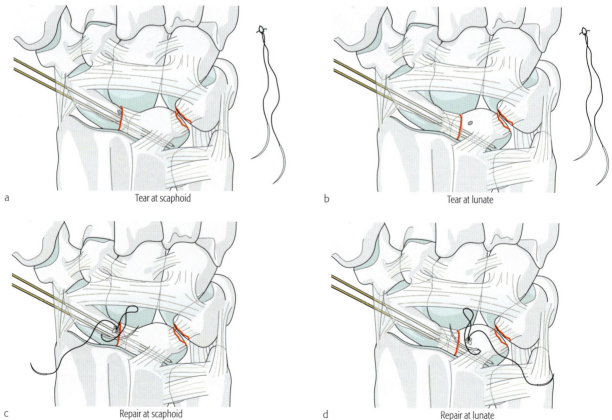

a   Tear at scaphoid   b   Tear at lunate

c   Repair at scaphoid   d   Repair at lunate

Fig 2.8-22a–d The anchor is inserted dorsally into the debrided area of the scaphoid (**a**) or into the lunate if the ligament is avulsed from that bone (**b**). The entry point for the anchor must be placed in such a position that the line of pull of the suture is slightly oblique, to resist rotational forces between both bones. Often one anchor will be sufficient but occasionally two anchors are needed. The anchor suture is inserted into the torn end of the ligament (**c–d**).

6 Fixation (cont)

Option: transosseous ligament refixation

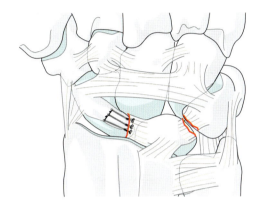

Fig 2.8-23   If bone anchors are not available, the avulsed ligament is attached using sutures that are passed through small tunnels drilled into the proximal pole of the scaphoid.

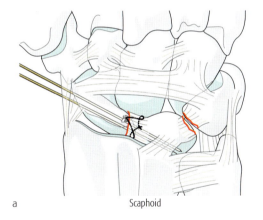

a   Scaphoid

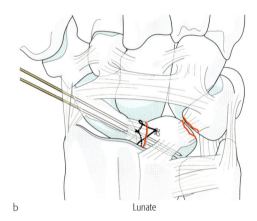

b   Lunate

Fig 2.8-24a–b   The anchor sutures in the ligament are then tied.

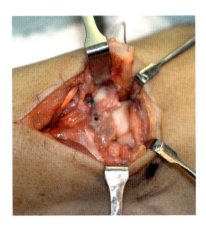

Fig 2.8-25   For this patient, two anchors were inserted into the debrided area of the dorsal aspect of the lunate, and the anchor sutures were passed through the ligament and tied.

6 Fixation (cont)

Lunotriquetral ligament repair

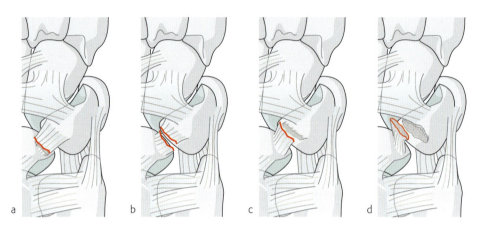

Fig 2.8-26a–d   In perilunate injuries, the lunotriquetral ligament can also be torn. This can occur from the lunate (most common) (**a**), in its midsubstance (**b**), or from the triquetrum (**c**), and there can be a bony avulsion from either bone (**d**).

There must be sufficient ligament remnant for repair with bone anchors, otherwise it is repaired by direct suture or transfixation of both bones with either K-wires or a small screw depending on the nature of the injury. Regardless of the repair technique used, it is recommended to support the soft-tissue repair using transfixation with two K-wires (for approximately 6–10 weeks).

Reduction and fixation of the lunotriquetral alignment is usually possible using a dorsal approach.

6   Fixation (cont)

Repair with bone anchors

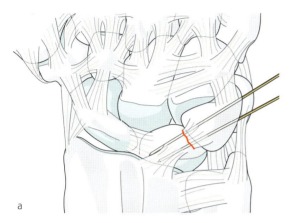

a

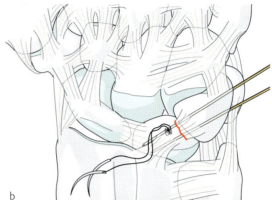

b

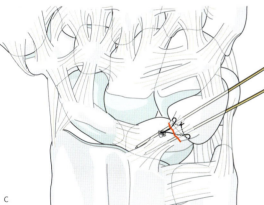

c

Fig 2.8-27a–c   When there is sufficient ligament remnant, the lunotriquetral joint is reduced and two K-wires are inserted percutaneously from the ulnar side of the triquetrum across the lunotriquetral joint into the lunate (**a**). Confirm the position of the wires using image intensification. If the detachment occurs from the lunate, the anchor is placed on the lunate (**b**) so the ligament can be reattached using the sutures of the anchor (**c**). If the detachment occurs from the triquetrum, the anchor is placed on that bone instead.

6   Fixation (cont)

Repair with a screw

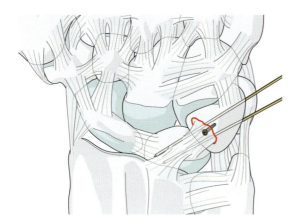

Fig 2.8-28   When there is bony avulsion of the lunotriquetral ligament from either bone, the fragment can be fixed with fine K-wires or a small screw.

Repair with direct suture

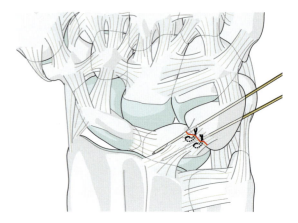

Fig 2.8-29   Direct suture of the ligament may also be possible.

Complete the fixation

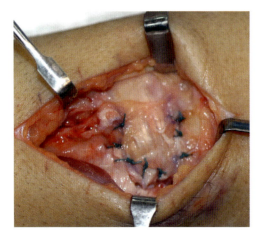

Fig 2.8-30   The capsulotomy flap was then fixed using multiple sutures.

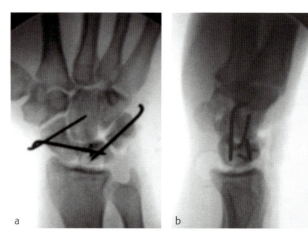

Fig 2.8-31a–b   Intraoperative images showed normal relationships in the lunotriquetral and scapholunate joints, and in the lateral view, there was a normal colinear relationship between the capitate the lunate and the radius.

7 Rehabilitation

Aftercare

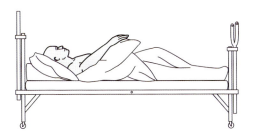

Fig 2.8-32 While the patient is in bed, use pillows to keep the hand elevated above the level of the heart to reduce swelling.

Immobilization

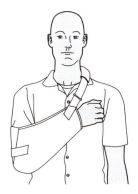

Fig 2.8-33 In perilunate injuries involving K-wire fixation, the K-wires can be removed at 6–8 weeks. It may also be necessary to rest the wrist for 8–12 weeks in a short arm splint or cast. Until removal of the cast, attention must be paid to ensure active mobilization of the associated joints of the fingers, elbow, and shoulder.

Follow-up

See the patient after 2–5 days to change the dressing. After 10 days, remove the sutures and confirm with x-rays that no secondary displacement has occurred.

Functional exercises

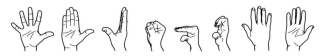

Fig 2.8-34 When both cast and K-wires have been removed, active controlled range of motion exercises can begin at the wrist. Load-bearing activities are usually delayed until radiological evidence of bone healing. The importance of mobilization must be emphasized to the patient and rehabilitation should be supervised by a physical therapist.

8 Outcome

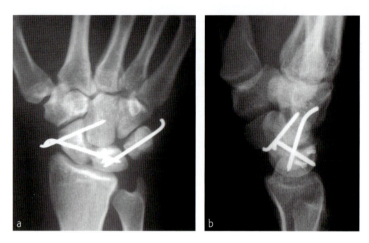

Fig 2.8-35a–b At the 8-week follow-up, the x-rays showed normal anatomical relationships within the carpus. As a result, the K-wires were removed and the patient was sent for physical therapy.

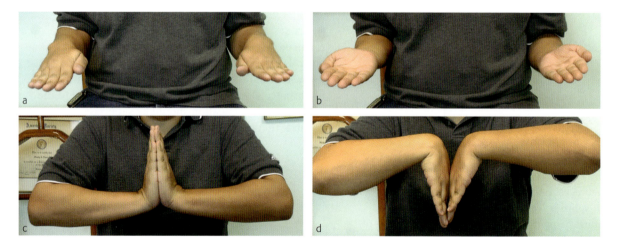

Fig 2.8-36a–d The patient later regained near normal range of motion.

2.9 Transscaphoid perilunate fracture dislocation treated with K-wires and a headless screw

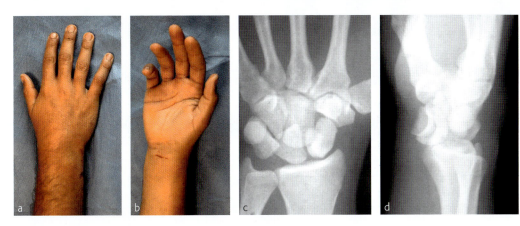

1 Case description

Fig 2.9-1a–d A 19-year-old man sustained an injury to his right hand during an amateur motocross race accident, presenting with noticeable swelling at the wrist. The AP and lateral x-rays demonstrated anterior dislocation of the lunate with the classic spilled teacup positioning. The images also showed a markedly displaced fracture of the waist of the scaphoid.

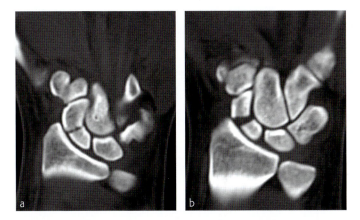

Fig 2.9-2a–b Following closed reduction of the lunate dislocation, the 2-D CT scans in the frontal plane showed the displaced scaphoid fracture.

1 Case description (cont)

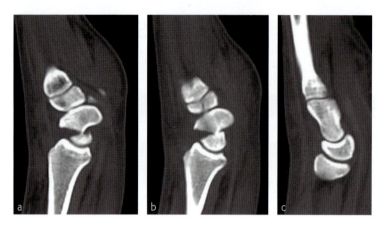

Fig 2.9-3a–c Sagittal view 2-D scans also showed displacement in the frontal plane.

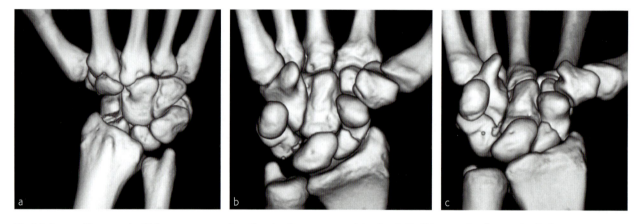

Fig 2.9-4a–c The scaphoid fracture was also clearly demonstrated in the 3-D CT scans in the sagittal plane.

2   Indications

Perilunate fracture dislocations

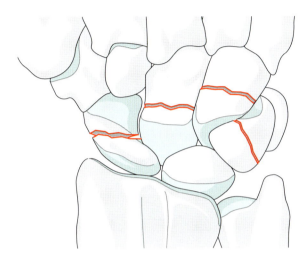

Fig 2.9-5   Of all wrist dislocations, perilunate dislocations are the most common. They are characterized by a progressive disruption of capsuloligamentous connections of the lunate to the adjacent carpal bones and radius. There are many clinical forms of perilunate dislocation and they can be conveniently classified into two major groups: the pure perilunate dislocation and the perilunate fracture dislocation, where the ligament disruption is associated with a variety of carpal fractures around the lunate.

Perilunate fracture dislocations present an extensive array of injuries. Fractures of carpal bones adjacent to the lunate can occur instead of only ligamentous ruptures when the disrupting force propagates around the midcarpal joint. However, it is recognized that more than 90% of all perilunate fractures involve the scaphoid. Recognition and repair of all bony and soft-tissue components are essential in order to restore carpal stability and to prevent posttraumatic degenerative joint disease. Concurrent bony and soft-tissue lesions of the carpus are not mutually exclusive (eg, concomitant scaphoid fracture and scapholunate rupture). But unlike the pure ligamentous injury of the perilunate dislocation, perilunate fracture dislocation injuries can be well treated by careful attention to the bony elements.

2   Indications (cont)

Lunate dislocations with transscaphoid fracture

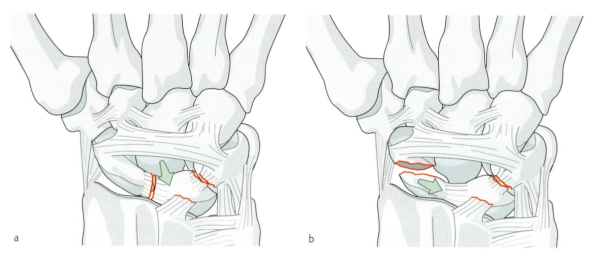

a   b

Fig 2.9-6a–b   In stage IV complete dislocations of the lunate, the luxation is usually in a palmar direction (**a**). When there is an additional transscaphoid fracture, the proximal scaphoid fragment can follow the dislocated lunate (**b**).

Disruption of the dorsal radiolunotriquetral ligament complex

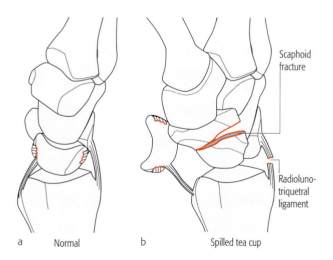

a   Normal   b   Spilled tea cup

Fig 2.9-7a–b   There can also be a disruption of the dorsal radiolunotriquetral ligament complex.

Choice of implant

For perilunate injuries with a scaphoid fracture, if the proximal fragment is large enough, 2.4 mm or 3.0 mm implants using antegrade insertion can be considered.

Imaging

Diagnosis of perilunate fracture dislocations is based on the history of trauma, clinical examination, and radiographic examination. In the coronal view, abnormal overlapping of carpal bones and alteration of "Gilula's arcs" can be observed, but a true lateral view is also recommended (for further information on using arcs to determine carpal injury see the indications topic in chapter 2.10 Transtriquetral transscaphoid perilunate fracture dislocation treated with screws). Lateral x-rays can show the spilled teacup configuration of a dislocated lunate (as shown in **Fig 2.9-1d**). Also look for the triangular profile of a displaced lunate when the capitate displaces proximally toward the distal radial articular surface. Obtaining CT scans can offer more precise detail of the injury, in this case demonstrating this patient's scaphoid fracture in the frontal plane (**Fig 2.9-2a–b**) and in the sagittal view (**Fig 2.9-3a–c**).

3 Preoperative planning

Equipment

- Headless compression screw set 2.4 or 3.0
- 1.4 mm to 1.6 mm K-wires
- Pointed reduction forceps
- Bone anchors
- Image intensifier

Patient preparation and positioning

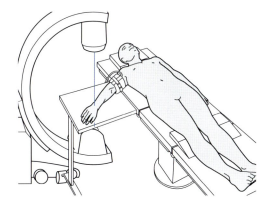

Fig 2.9-8 Position the patient supine and place the forearm on a hand table. Pronate the forearm. A nonsterile pneumatic tourniquet is used. Prophylactic antibiotics are optional.

4 Surgical approach

Approach

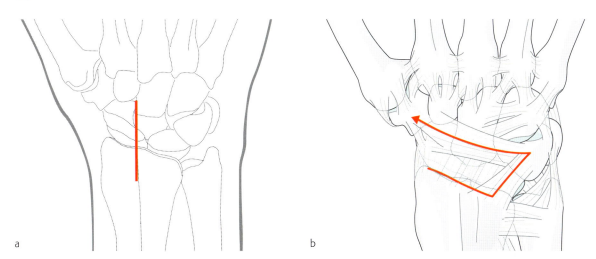

a   b

Fig 2.9-9a–b The surgical approach used was a dorsal approach (see chapter 1.3 Combined approach to the lunate and perilunate injuries, however, only the dorsal approach was required with this patient). This approach involves a radially based capsular ligamentous flap to be elevated and a capsulotomy incision. The dorsal approach can also be utilized to repair other carpal injuries.

4 Surgical approach (cont)

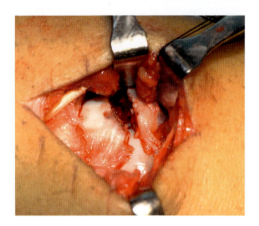

Fig 2.9-10 The scaphoid fracture was exposed through the dorsal approach.

5 Reduction

Preliminary reduction of the lunate

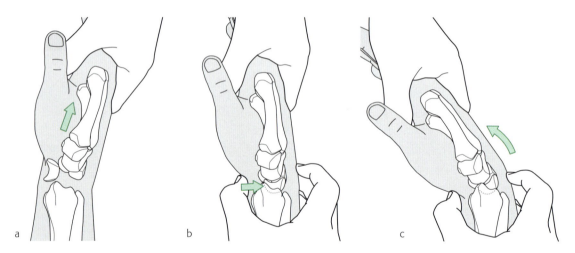

a   b   c

Fig 2.9-11a–c Closed reduction is preliminary to operative treatment and has three benefits:
• It restores carpal alignment
• It improves the patient's comfort
• It reduces pressure on the median nerve.

Reduction of the dislocated lunate is achieved by distracting the wrist and applying direct thumb pressure over the lunate from palmar to dorsal. The hand is then gently flexed, and once reduction has occurred, the distraction is gently relaxed.

Open reduction of the lunate

If closed reduction is not successful, open reduction is necessary as soon as possible due to the risk of median nerve compromise, of pain, and to preserve blood supply to the lunate.

5   Reduction (cont)

Direct reduction of the scaphoid

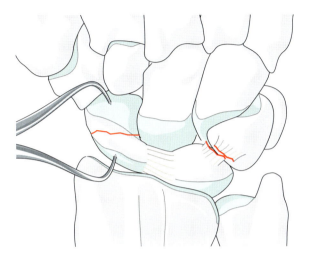

Fig 2.9-12   Use small pointed reduction forceps to reduce the scaphoid fracture.

Determine insertion point for the guide wire

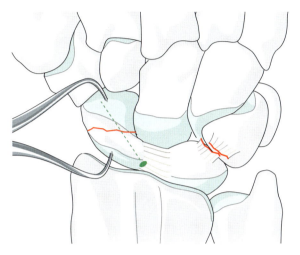

Fig 2.9-13   The correct entry point for the guide wire is at the center of the proximal pole, directly adjacent to the scapholunate ligament insertion.

Insert the guide wire

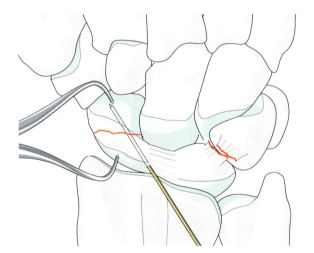

Fig 2.9-14   The guide wire is inserted in the axis of the shaft of the first metacarpal, in radial abduction. During the introduction of the guide wire, the wrist should be in flexion otherwise the entry point cannot be reached. Do not penetrate the scaphotrapezial joint with the guide wire.

Image intensification in at least two planes should be used to confirm accurate advancement of the guide wire in the scaphoid axis and perpendicular to the fracture.

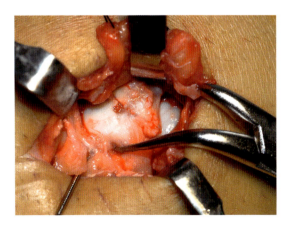

Fig 2.9-15   The fracture was reduced and held with a pointed reduction forceps and the K-wire was inserted under image guidance.

179

6 Fixation

Scaphoid fixation

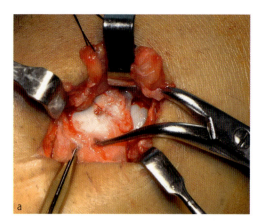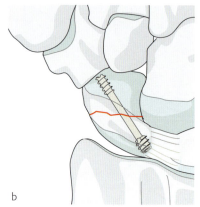

Fig 2.9-16a–b Using a dorsal approach for this scaphoid waist fracture, stable fixation was achieved with insertion of a 3.0 mm headless screw.

The fixation procedure follows the usual steps of measuring screw length, drilling, selecting the screw, inserting the screw, and advancing and countersinking the screw. For further information on these steps see chapter 2.3 Scaphoid—multifragmentary fracture treated with a headless compression screw and lag screw.

Lunotriquetral ligament repair

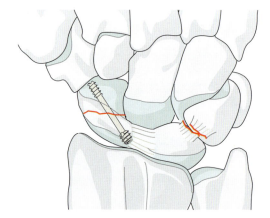

Fig 2.9-17 In transscaphoid perilunate fracture dislocations, the lunotriquetral ligament can also be torn. This can occur from the lunate (most common), in its midsubstance, or from the triquetrum, and there can be a bony avulsion from either bone.

There must be sufficient ligament remnant for repair with bone anchors otherwise it is repaired by direct suture or transfixation of both bones with either K-wires or a small screw depending on the nature of the injury. Regardless of the repair technique used, it is recommended to support the soft-tissue repair using transfixation with two K-wires (for approximately 6–10 weeks).

Reduction and fixation of the lunotriquetral alignment is usually possible using a dorsal approach.

6 Fixation (cont)

Repair with bone anchors

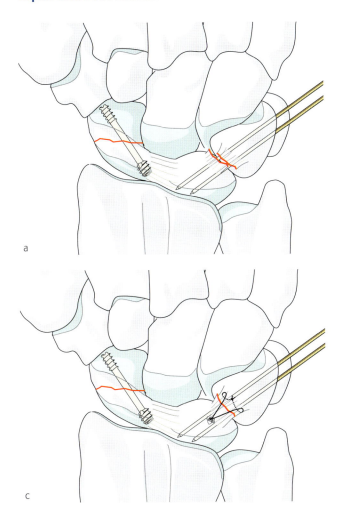

a

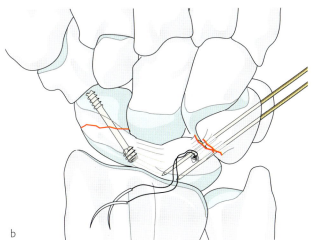

b

c

Fig 2.9-18a–c When there is sufficient ligament remnant, the lunotriquetral joint is reduced and two K-wires are inserted percutaneously from the ulnar side of the triquetrum across the lunotriquetral joint into the lunate (**a**). Confirm the position of the wires using image intensification. If the detachment occurs from the lunate, the anchor is placed on the lunate (**b**) so the ligament can be reattached using the sutures of the anchor (**c**). If the detachment occurs from the triquetrum, the anchor is placed on that bone instead.

6 Fixation (cont)

Repair with a screw

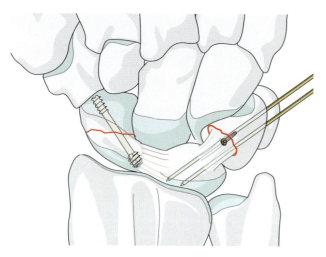

Fig 2.9-19 When there is bony avulsion of the lunotriquetral ligament from either bone, the fragment can be fixed with fine K-wires or a small screw.

Repair with direct suture

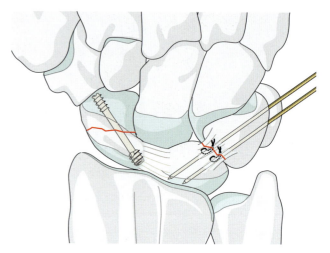

Fig 2.9-20 Direct suture of the ligament may also be possible.

Complete the fixation

The capsulotomy flap is then closed.

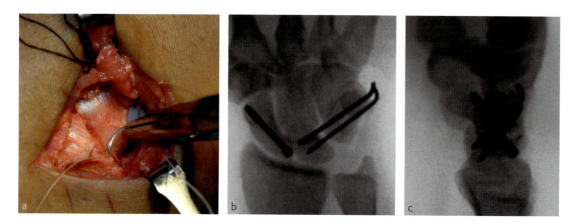

Fig 2.9-21a–c Intraoperative images show the direct repair of the dorsal lunotriquetral ligament and placement of two K-wires across the joint.

6 Fixation (cont)

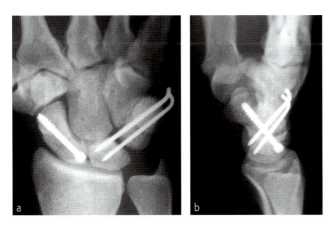

Fig 2.9-22a–b Immediate postoperative x-rays demonstrate the anatomical reduction and K-wire fixation.

7 Rehabilitation

Aftercare, follow-up, and functional exercises

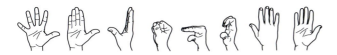

Fig 2.9-23 The patient should receive the standard postoperative rest, injury elevation, follow-up, removal of stitches, and immobilization as required. Following surgery, begin active controlled range of motion exercises. For further information, see the rehabilitation topic in chapter 2.8 Perilunate dislocation treated with K-wires.

8 Outcome

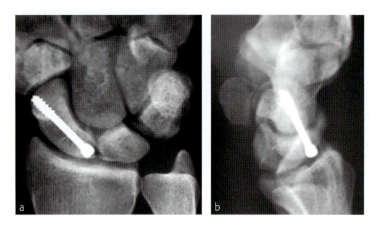

Fig 2.9-24a–b   At the 12-month follow-up, the x-rays showed a healed scaphoid fracture and normal lunate alignment.

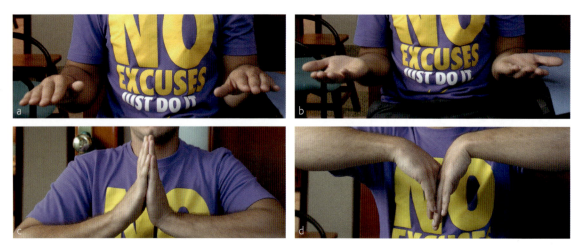

Fig 2.9-25a–d   The patient had achieved near full functional recovery.

9 Alternative technique: case description

Transscaphoid perilunate fracture dislocation treated using multiple screws and via both dorsal and palmar surgical approaches

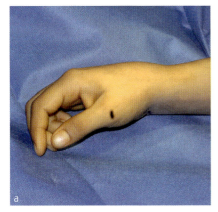 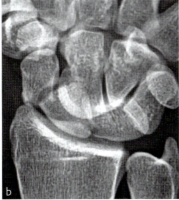 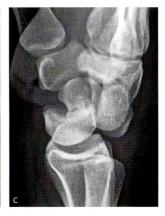

Fig 2.9-26a–c   A 21-year-old man sustained a transscaphoid perilunate fracture dislocation as a result of a motorcycle injury. The clinical appearance of the hand and wrist showed severe dorsal deformity and swelling. The AP and lateral x-rays demonstrated that the capitate was dorsally dislocated over the lunate, and there was a displaced proximal pole fracture of the scaphoid.

Indications

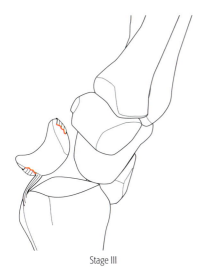

Stage III

Fig 2.9-27   In this perilunate injury, the capitate has become dislocated from its normal positioning, and the lunate has lost its normal alignment with the distal radius. The lunotriquetral ligament was also affected. This makes it a stage III midcarpal fracture dislocation.

In cases of extensive displacement, multifragmentation, or scaphoid bone defect, fixation with a single screw alone is unlikely to give enough stability. In these cases, a combination of two screws or a screw and a K-wire may be necessary to achieve the required stability. In addition, both dorsal and palmar surgical approaches may be necessary. Before the final fixation, reduce all displaced fragments. In cases of multifragmentation, bone grafting may be indicated.

9 Alternative technique: case description (cont)

Combined dorsal and palmar surgical approaches

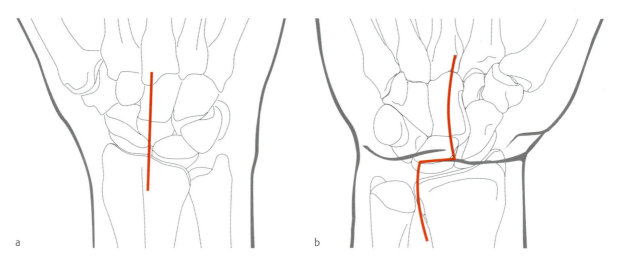

a   b

Fig 2.9-28a–b   Along with the usual dorsal approach, an additional palmar approach will reveal the characteristic disruptions of the extrinsic palmar ligaments. A palmar approach should be considered when there is median nerve disfunction or when it is not possible to do effective reduction by a dorsal only approach. By doing this, it also allows better access to the palmar band of the lunotriquetral ligament (see chapter 1.3 Combined approach to the lunate and perilunate injuries).

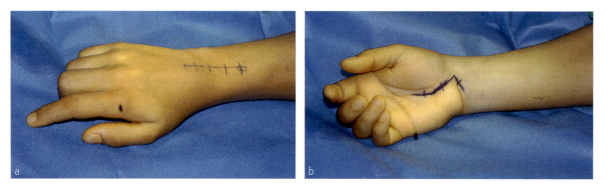

Fig 2.9-29a–b   The dorsal (**a**) and palmar (**b**) approaches to the wrist were outlined on the skin.

9   Alternative technique: case description (cont)

Palmar side

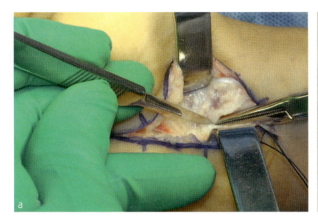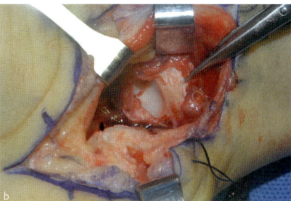

Fig 2.9-30a–b   Because of the specific nature of this injury, the initial surgical approach was on the palmar side with release of the transverse carpal ligament and median nerve (**a**). The contents of the carpal tunnel are carefully retracted in order to see the tear in the palmar capsular ligaments and the positioning of the lunate and capitate bones (**b**).

Dorsal side

A standard dorsal approach is then also performed (as described earlier in this chapter).

10 Alternative technique: reduction and fixation

Reduction of carpals

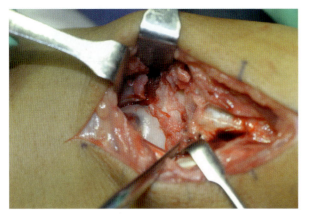

Fig 2.9-31 Once the dorsal approach was performed, the carpal bones were reduced in relation to the lunate (as seen through the dorsal exposure).

Reduction of the scaphoid

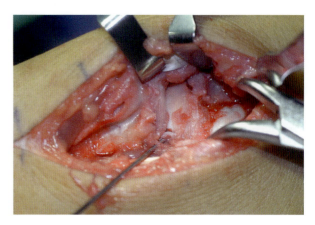

Fig 2.9-32 The scaphoid fracture was then reduced and held with a pointed reduction forceps. A guide wire was placed through a drill guide and confirmed with intraoperative imaging.

Fixation of the scaphoid

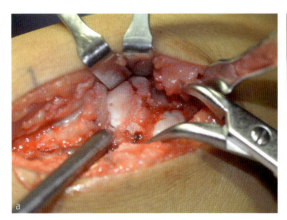
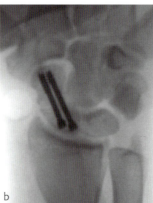

Fig 2.9-33a–b Stable fixation of the scaphoid fracture was achieved with insertion of two 2.4 mm headless compression screws.

The fixation procedure follows the usual steps of measuring screw length, drilling, selecting the screw, inserting the screw, and advancing and countersinking the screw. For further information on these steps see chapter 2.4 Scaphoid, proximal pole—fracture treated with a headless compression screw.

10 Alternative technique: reduction and fixation (cont)

Fixation of the palmar ligaments

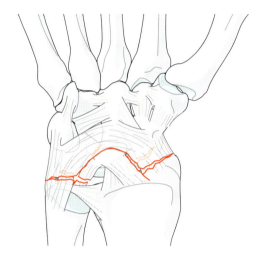

Fig 2.9-34 The palmar approach reveals the disruptions of the extrinsic palmar ligaments, which occur through the space of Poirier (an anatomical weak spot in the floor of the carpal tunnel that can allow movement of the distal carpal row away from the lunate). A rent or tear in the palmar capsule, between proximal and distal ligament arches, exposes the midcarpal joint and the lunotriquetral ligament.

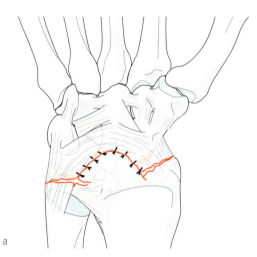

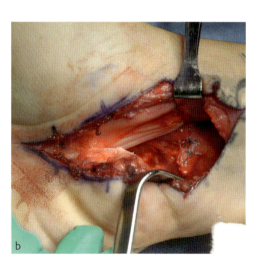

a

b

Fig 2.9-35a–b The midcarpal joint is irrigated, loose bodies or subchondral flakes are removed, and the rent is repaired anatomically using interrupted resorbable sutures.

10 Alternative technique: reduction and fixation (cont)

Lunotriquetral ligament repair

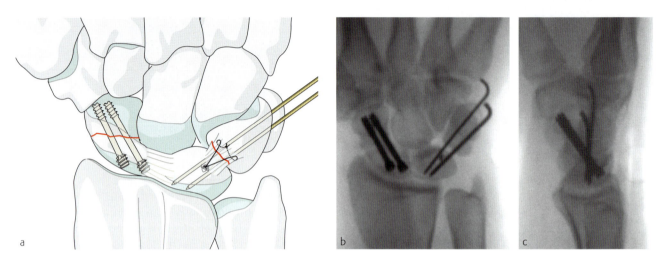

Fig 2.9-36a–c The lunotriquetral joint was stabilized with two smooth K-wires and the lunotriquetral ligament was then repaired using a bone anchor in the lunate.

The fixation procedure follows the usual steps of assessing ligament remnant, percutaneous insertion of K-wires, placing of bone anchor, and reattaching the ligament using the anchor sutures. This procedure is explained more fully earlier in this chapter.

Outcome

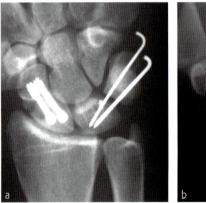
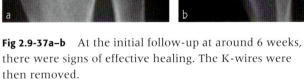
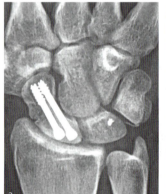
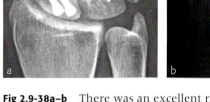
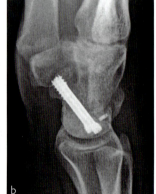

Fig 2.9-37a–b At the initial follow-up at around 6 weeks, there were signs of effective healing. The K-wires were then removed.

Fig 2.9-38a–b There was an excellent radiological result by the 1-year follow-up.

10 Alternative technique: reduction and fixation (cont)

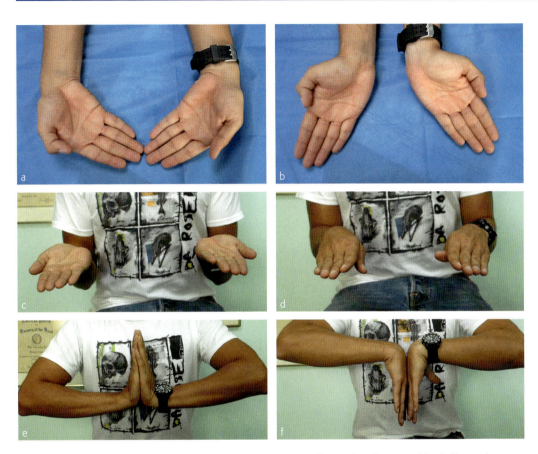

Fig 2.9-39a–f At this stage, near full wrist motion was achieved with no residual discomfort.

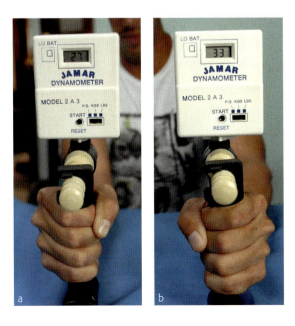

Fig 2.9-40a–b Good grip strength had also returned.

2.10 Transtriquetral transscaphoid perilunate fracture dislocation treated with screws

1 Case description

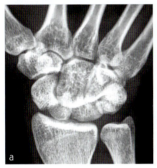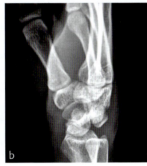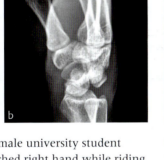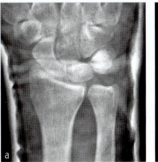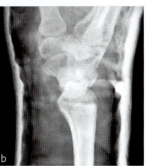

Fig 2.10-1a–b A 23-year-old male university student suffered a fall on his outstretched right hand while riding a bicycle. He presented to the emergency department with numbness in the fingers, severe pain, and deformity of the wrist. The x-rays revealed overlapping of the carpal bones, loss of continuity of Gilula's arcs, and a displaced fracture of the scaphoid. In the lateral view, the capitate was dislocated dorsally while the lunate maintained its normal anatomical relationship with the radius.

Fig 2.10-2a–b Reduction was achieved under sedation in the emergency department providing immediate improvement to patient pain and numbness of the fingers. The subsequent x-rays revealed perfect reduction to the carpal bones and the scaphoid fracture.

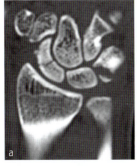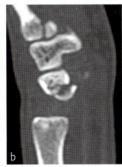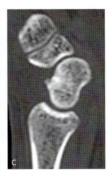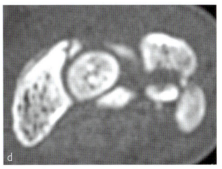

Fig 2.10-3a–d In addition, CT scans revealed a perfect anatomical relationship between the carpal bones. However, while there was perfect reduction of the scaphoid proximal pole fracture, the CT scan revealed a previously undetected fracture of the triquetrum. The triquetral fracture appeared displaced, raising the suspicion (and later proved) that there was also an avulsion of the lunotriquetral ligament. The axial view CT scan showed the fracture of the triquetrum was on the palmar aspect, which is where the stronger part of the lunotriquetral ligament is attached.

1 Case description (cont)

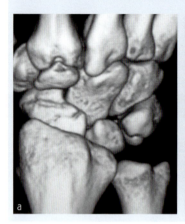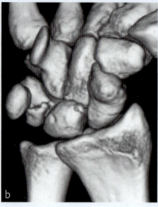

Fig 2.10-4a–b The dorsal and palmar view 3-D CT scans offered a more precise perspective of both the scaphoid and triquetral fractures.

2 Indications

Perilunate fracture dislocations involving the triquetrum

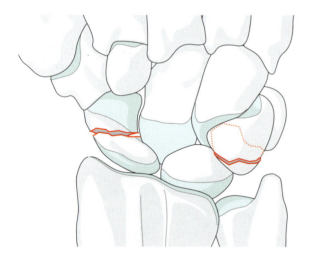

Fig 2.10-5 Perilunate fracture dislocations present an extensive array of injuries. Fractures of the carpal bones adjacent to the lunate can occur instead of isolated ligament ruptures, when the disrupting force propagates around the midcarpal joint. While most perilunate fractures involve the scaphoid, other carpal bones including the triquetrum can be involved. Recognition and repair of all bony and soft-tissue components are essential in order to restore carpal stability and to prevent posttraumatic degenerative joint disease.

Arcs

Arcs are lines that can be drawn or imagined on x-ray/CT images of the hand and wrist to help assess the alignment of the carpus. Countless variations of injury patterns can be identified depending on which carpal bones are affected and the direction of any dislocation or fracture displacement.

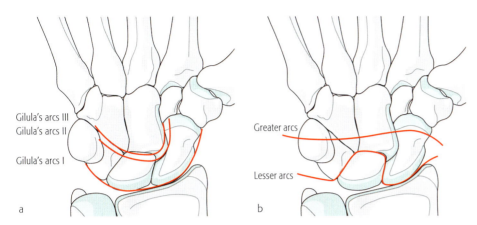

Fig 2.10-6a–b   As an example, Gilula's arcs outline the borders of the proximal and distal carpal rows (**a**). A deviation in the normal smooth line contour along the rows indicates disruption or dislocation among the carpals. This is common in cases of perilunate fracture dislocation. Greater arc injuries indicate fracture dislocations of the scaphoid, capitate, hamate, and/or triquetrum, while lesser arc injuries are pure ligamentous injuries around the lunate (**b**). These various arcs help greatly in identifying the location of any carpal injury.

3   Preoperative planning

Equipment

- Headless compression screw set 2.4 or 3.0
- Modular screw set 1.5 or 2.0
- 1.4 mm to 1.6 mm K-wires
- Pointed reduction forceps
- Bone anchors
- Image intensifier

Patient preparation and positioning

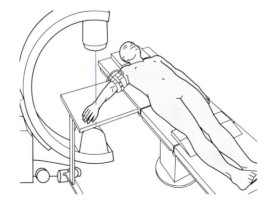

Fig 2.10-7   Position the patient supine and place the forearm on a hand table. Pronate the forearm. A nonsterile pneumatic tourniquet is used. Prophylactic antibiotics are optional.

4 Surgical approach

Approach

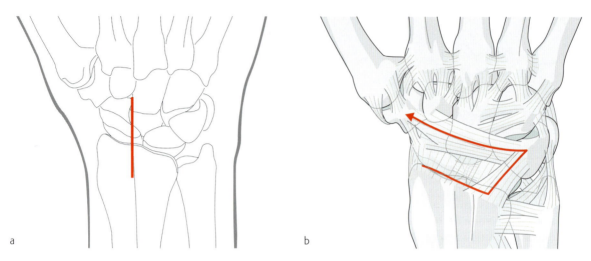

a   b

Fig 2.10-8a–b The surgical approach used was a dorsal approach (see chapter 1.3 Combined approach to the lunate and perilunate injuries, however, only the dorsal approach was required with this patient). This approach involves a radially based capsular ligamentous flap to be elevated and a capsulotomy incision.

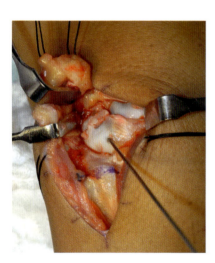

Fig 2.10-9 The intraoperative image shows the dorsal approach to the carpus, which allows reduction and stabilization of the scaphoid fracture to be clearly seen while ensuring integrity of the scapholunate ligament.

5 Reduction

Scaphoid reduction

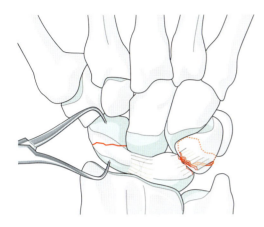

Fig 2.10-10 Use small pointed reduction forceps to reduce the scaphoid fracture.

Determine scaphoid insertion point and insert the guide wire

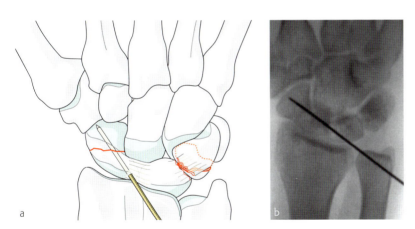

Fig 2.10-11a–b The correct entry point for the guide wire is in the center of the proximal pole, directly adjacent to the scapholunate ligament insertion. The guide wire is inserted in the axis of the shaft of the first metacarpal, in radial abduction. During the introduction of the guide wire, the wrist should be in flexion otherwise the entry point cannot be reached (**a**). Do not penetrate the scaphotrapezial joint with the guide wire. Image intensification should be used to confirm accurate advancement of the guide wire in the scaphoid axis and perpendicular to the fracture (**b**).

6 Fixation

Scaphoid fixation

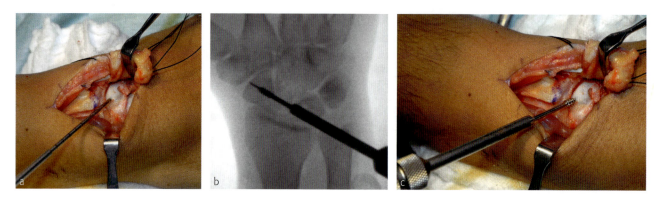

Fig 2.10-12a–c Following measuring and drilling, and using image intensification, a cannulated headless compression screw was introduced into the scaphoid bone until the fracture gap was closed and compressed.

The fixation procedure follows the usual steps of measuring screw length, drilling, selecting the screw, inserting the screw, and advancing and countersinking the screw. For further information on these steps see chapter 2.4 Scaphoid, proximal pole—fracture treated with a headless compression screw.

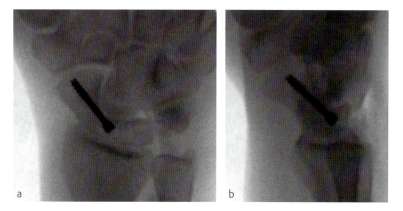

Fig 2.10-13a–b Intraoperative images showed there was correct positioning of the screw.

6 Fixation (cont)

Triquetrum fixation

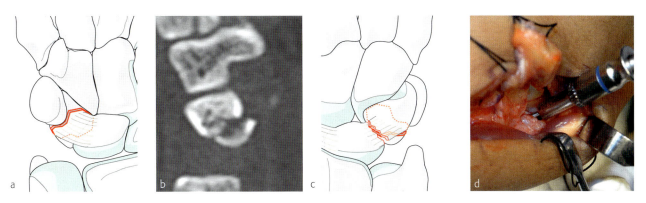

Fig 2.10-14a–d The triquetrum had been split into palmar and dorsal components. Although the palmar fracture fragment was the bigger fragment (**a–b**), it was reduced and stabilized by introducing a 1.5 mm lag screw via the dorsal aspect of the bone (**c–d**).

Use of lag screws

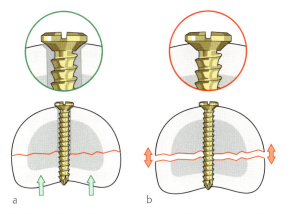

Fig 2.10-15a–b Be sure to insert the screw as a lag screw, with a gliding hole in the near cortex, and a threaded hole in the far cortex (**a**). Inserting a screw across a fracture plane that is threaded in both cortices (position screw) will hold the fragments apart and apply no interfragmentary compression (**b**).

Countersinking

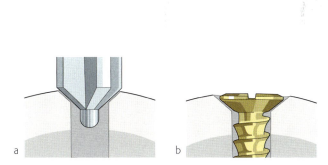

Fig 2.10-16a–b Also ensure to countersink the screw to reduce the risk of soft-tissue irritation, so that the screw head has maximal contact area with the bone.

6 Fixation (cont)

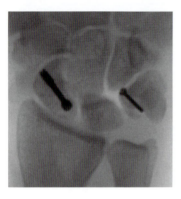

Fig 2.10-17 The reduction and fixation of the triquetral fracture was then also checked intraoperatively.

Lunotriquetral ligament repair

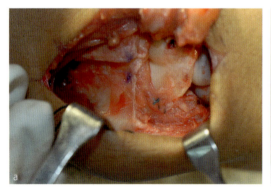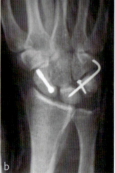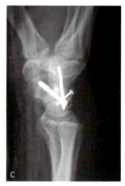

Fig 2.10-18a–c The palmar component of the lunotriquetral ligament was reduced through a dorsal approach. The palmar component is the thicker and stronger aspect, and it is important to ensure its repair. However, as the fracture fixations in this case were made by a dorsal approach, an additional palmar approach was not necessary. The dorsal portion of the lunotriquetral ligament was then repaired with sutures. The lunotriquetral joint was stabilized with a K-wire.

Complete the fixation

The capsulotomy flap is then closed. The patient was immediately immobilized using a plaster splint.

7 Rehabilitation

Aftercare, follow-up, and functional exercises

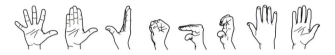

Fig 2.10-19 The patient should receive the standard postoperative rest, injury elevation, follow-up, removal of stitches, and immobilization as required. Following surgery, begin active controlled range of motion exercises. For further information, see the rehabilitation topic in chapter 2.8 Perilunate dislocation treated with K-wires.

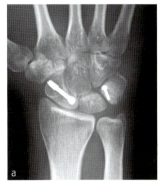
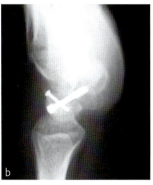

Fig 2.10-20a–b For this patient, both the K-wire and the cast were removed at the 8-week follow-up. The patient was then referred for physical therapy.

8 Outcome

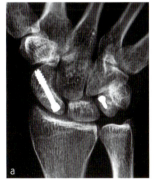
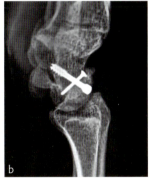

Fig 2.10-21a–b At the 1-year follow-up, the x-ray images showed perfect alignment of the carpus and complete healing of both the scaphoid and triquetral fractures.

8 Outcome (cont)

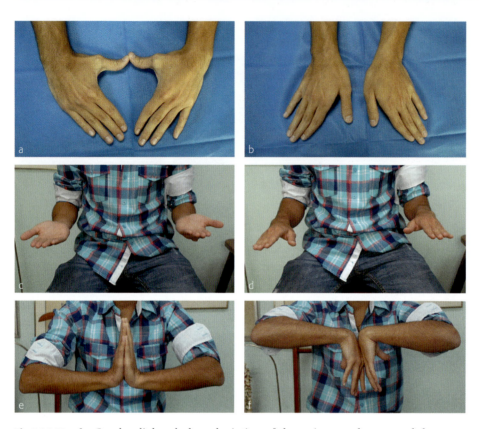

Fig 2.10-22a–f   Good radial and ulnar deviation of the wrist was shown, and there was an excellent functional outcome.

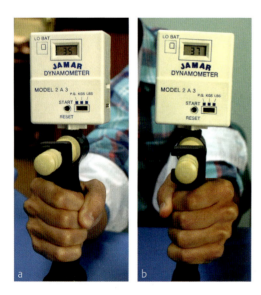

Fig 2.10-23a–b   The patient had achieved good grip strength compared with the uninjured hand, allowing him to return to his previous activities without limitation.

2.11 Multiple carpal perilunate fracture dislocation and scaphocapitate syndrome treated with screws

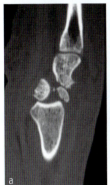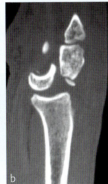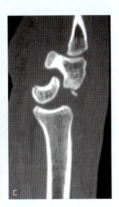

Fig 2.11-1a–c A 21-year-old semiprofessional BMX bicycle rider sustained a high-energy injury to his dominant right wrist after a fall during a racing competition. He presented to the emergency department complaining of severe pain, wrist deformity, and median nerve distribution numbness.

Following examination, a wide range of images were taken. The following injuries were indicated:
- Dorsal perilunate dislocation of the carpus
- Fracture of the scaphoid proximal third
- Fracture of the proximal pole of the hamate
- Fracture of the head of the capitate
- Displacement of the capitate fracture in the dorsal aspect of the carpus and rotated 90 degrees
- The lunate remained articulated with the proximal pole of the scaphoid and with the distal radius but it was subluxed palmarly on the lunate facet
- Fracture of the ulnar styloid base.

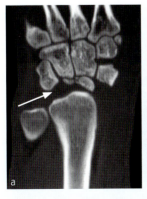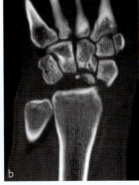

Fig 2.11-2a–b The coronal view 2-D CT scans showed greater detail of this complex injury, including the fracture of the scaphoid, the fracture of the head of the capitate, the fracture of the hamate, and evidence of dissociation between the triquetrum and the lunate (arrow).

1 Case description (cont)

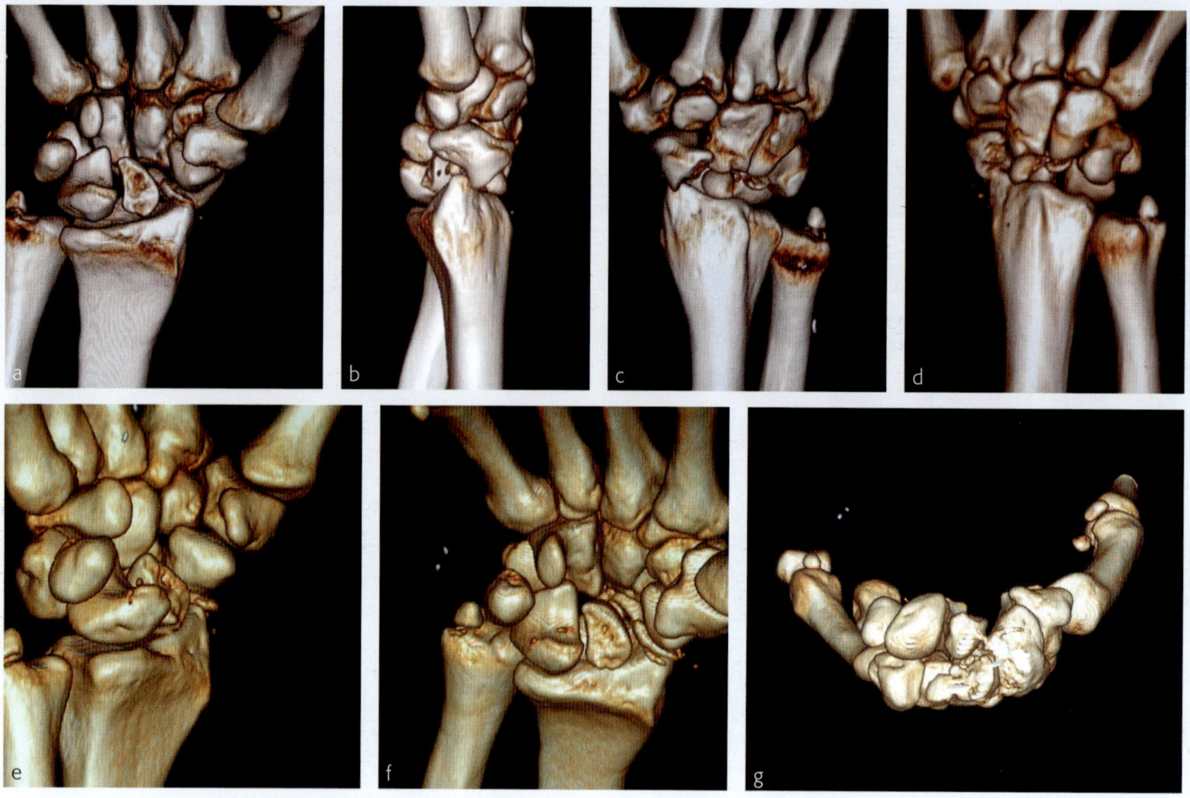

Fig 2.11-3a–g The AP view 3-D CT scan (**a**) showed the dorsal dislocation of the carpus, while the lunate remained articulated with the radius and to the proximal pole of the scaphoid. The radial view CT scan (**b**) showed the scaphoid fracture. The 3-D images also showed that the proximal third of the scaphoid was deeply displaced, the head of the capitate had rotated 90 degrees, and that there were fractures of the hamate and the ulnar styloid (**c–d**). The lunotriquetral ligament disruption was evidenced (**e–f**). The axial view 3-D CT scans showed the dorsal dislocation of the carpus with more detail (**g**).

After evaluating all the images, it was concluded that the patient had received a dorsal perilunate fracture dislocation that involved scaphoid, capitate, hamate, and ulnar styloid fractures.

2 Indications

Perilunate fracture dislocation with scaphocapitate syndrome

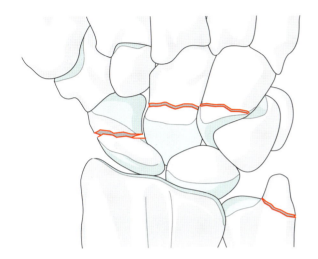

Fig 2.11-4 As previously discussed, perilunate fracture dislocations present an extensive array of injuries and include fractures of carpal bones and ligamentous injury adjacent to the lunate. While most perilunate fractures involve the scaphoid, other carpal bones including the capitate and the hamate can be involved. Additional fractures can also occur at the radial styloid and, as with this patient, the ulnar styloid.

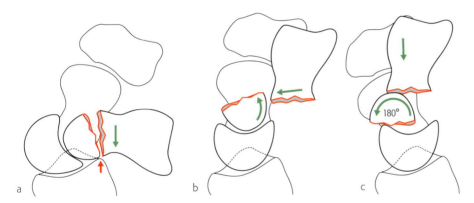

a   b   c

Fig 2.11-5a–c The injury to this patient also represents a specific variation of multiple carpal perilunate fracture dislocation known as scaphocapitate (or naviculocapitate) syndrome, and is rare. In this injury, the high-energy force passes through the neck of the capitate, fracturing both the scaphoid and the capitate. The result is that the proximal portion of the capitate can rotate 90 to 180 degrees, with the articular surface of the head of the capitate directed distally. Open reduction and internal fixation is almost always required in order to restore carpal stability.

3   Preoperative planning

Equipment

- Headless compression screw set 2.4 or 3.0
- Modular screw set 1.3 or 1.5
- 1.4 mm to 1.6 mm K-wires
- A toothed forceps
- Bone anchors
- Image intensifier

Patient preparation and positioning

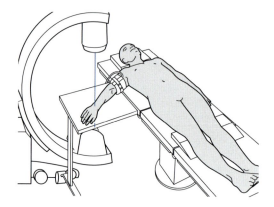

Fig 2.11-6   Position the patient supine and place the forearm on a hand table. Pronate the forearm. A nonsterile pneumatic tourniquet is used. Prophylactic antibiotics are optional.

4   Surgical approach

Approach

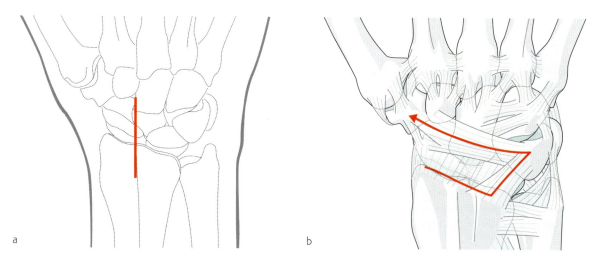

a   b

Fig 2.11-7a–b   The surgical approach used was a dorsal approach (see chapter 1.3 Combined approach to the lunate and perilunate injuries, however, only the dorsal approach was required with this patient). This approach involves a radially based capsular ligamentous flap to be elevated and a capsulotomy incision.

4 Surgical approach (cont)

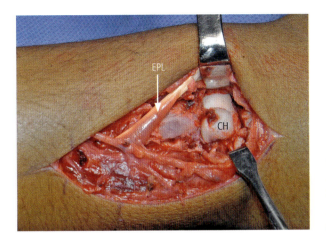

Fig 2.11-8 The wrist was exposed through a dorsal approach and capsular incision. The fracture of the head of the capitate became evident (CH), as was its displacement in the dorsal aspect of the carpus with 90 degree rotation. The extensor pollicis longus (EPL) was retracted.

5 Reduction

Capitate reduction

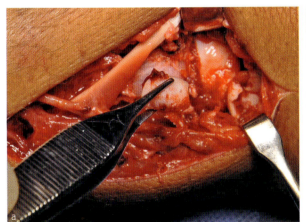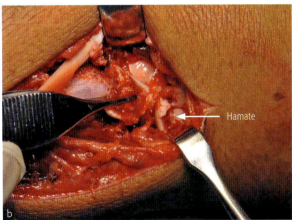

Fig 2.11-9a–b Using a toothed forceps, the displaced proximal head of the capitate is reapproximated to its correct anatomical location. The intraoperative images show the head of the capitate being held by the forceps (**a**), which were used to reduce the fracture. An arrow identifies the hamate fracture (**b**).

5 Reduction (cont)

Hamate reduction

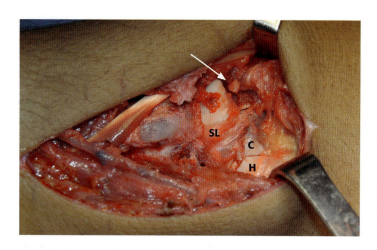

Fig 2.11-10 Once the capitate is reduced, the hamate is then stabilized and reduced. The intraoperative image shows the reduction of the midcarpal joint, including the capitate (C) and hamate (H) reduction. The scapholunate ligament (SL) remained unaffected. The scaphoid waist fracture remained displaced at this stage (arrow).

Scaphoid reduction

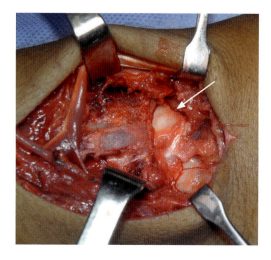

Fig 2.11-11 Further traction on the area permitted the scaphoid fracture to be reduced. Note that no compression is yet applied (arrow).

Determine scaphoid insertion point and insert the guide wire

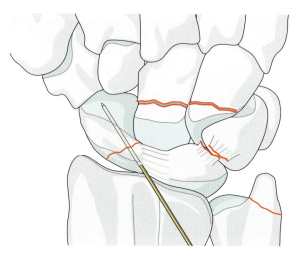

Fig 2.11-12 The correct entry point for the guide wire is in the center of the proximal pole, directly adjacent to the scapholunate ligament insertion. The guide wire is inserted in the axis of the shaft of the first metacarpal, in radial abduction. During the introduction of the guide wire, the wrist should be in flexion otherwise the entry point cannot be reached. Do not penetrate the scaphotrapezial joint with the guide wire. Image intensification should be used to confirm accurate advancement of the guide wire in the scaphoid axis and perpendicular to the fracture.

6 Fixation

Capitate fixation

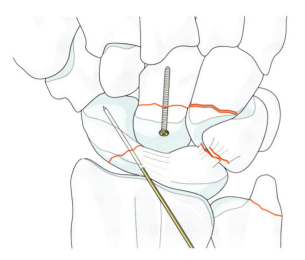

Fig 2.11-13 The head of the capitate was devoid of any attachment, so it was anatomically reduced. The capitate fragment can then be stabilized with either a 1.5 mm headless compression screw or a 1.5 mm fully threaded cortex screw applied as a lag screw. In this case, a 1.5 mm lag screw was inserted in antegrade direction.

Hamate fixation

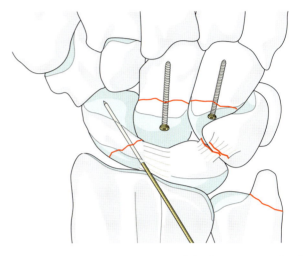

Fig 2.11-14 The proximal pole of the hamate was fixed with a 1.3 mm lag screw in antegrade direction. Care was taken to bury both the capitate and hamate screw heads under the articular cartilage.

Use of lag screws

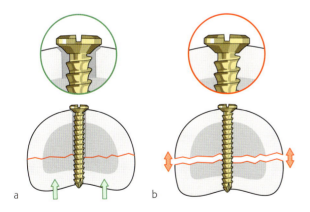

Fig 2.11-15a–b Be sure to insert the screw as a lag screw, with a gliding hole in the near cortex, and a threaded hole in the far cortex (**a**). Inserting a screw across a fracture plane that is threaded in both cortices (position screw) will hold the fragments apart and apply no interfragmentary compression (**b**).

Countersinking

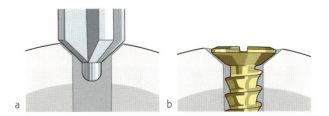

Fig 2.11-16a–b Also ensure to countersink the screw to reduce the risk of soft-tissue irritation, so that the screw head has maximal contact area with the bone.

6 Fixation (cont)

Scaphoid fixation

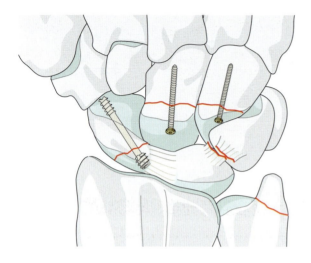

Fig 2.11-17 Attention was then brought to the scaphoid proximal third fracture. After anatomical reduction was performed, fixation was achieved with a 3.0 mm headless compression screw. The dorsal scapholunate ligament was uninjured.

The fixation procedure follows the usual steps of measuring screw length, drilling, selecting the screw, inserting the screw, and advancing and countersinking the screw. For further information on these steps see chapter 2.4 Scaphoid, proximal pole—fracture treated with a headless compression screw.

Lunotriquetral ligament repair

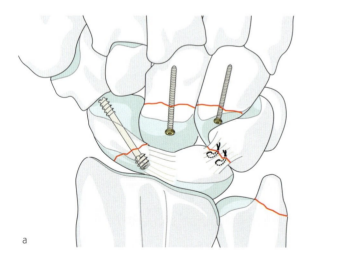

a

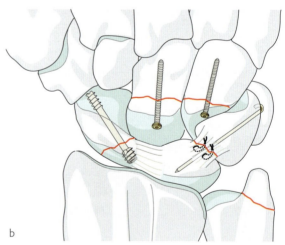

b

Fig 2.11-18a–b A midsubstance tear of the lunotriquetral ligament was noted and repaired directly with nonabsorbable sutures (**a**). The lunotriquetral joint was stabilized with a percutaneous K-wire (**b**).

The ligament repair procedure follows the usual steps of determining if the tear is midsubstance or bony avulsion, determining size of ligament remnant for bone anchors or direct suture, and insertion of K-wires. For further information on these steps see chapter 2.8 Perilunate dislocation treated with K-wires.

6 Fixation (cont)

Ulnar styloid repair

The DRUJ was stable during intraoperative examination so on this occasion the ulnar styloid fracture was not fixed.

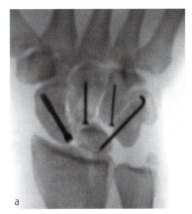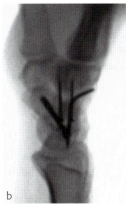

Fig 2.11-19a–b The intraoperative images show the various fracture reductions and fixations.

7 Rehabilitation

Aftercare, follow-up, and functional exercises

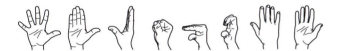

Fig 2.11-20 The patient should receive the standard postoperative rest, injury elevation, follow-up, removal of stitches, and immobilization as required. Following surgery, begin active controlled range of motion exercises. For further information, see the rehabilitation topic in chapter 2.8 Perilunate dislocation treated with K-wires.

The patient in this chapter was immediately placed into a short arm plaster splint. There were no intraoperative or postoperative complications, and median nerve distribution numbness resolved completely in the immediate postoperative period. Sutures were removed 2 weeks after surgery and the splint was replaced with a removable orthosis. Nine weeks after surgery there was radiographic evidence of healing of all fractures thus the K-wire was removed. The patient was cleared for active and passive range of motion exercises at 12 weeks and returned to impact bike riding sports at 4 months.

8 Outcome

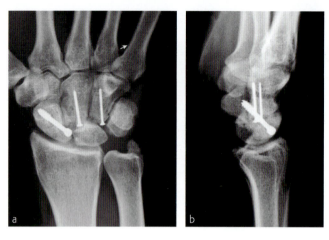

Fig 2.11-21a–b At the 8-month follow-up, the x-rays demonstrated healing of all fractures without evidence of avascular necrosis or collapse.

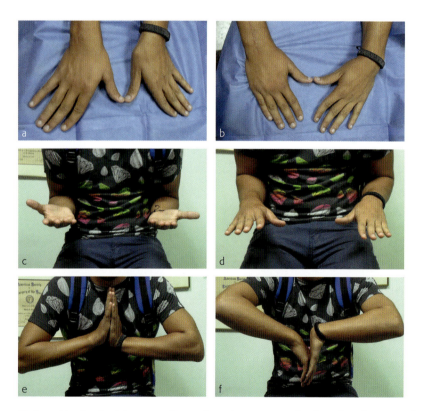

Fig 2.11-22a–f At this stage, the patient demonstrated a functional range of motion. Note the flexion limitation of the wrist, which can be expected in this severe type of injury. The patient went on to achieve excellent recovery by the 1-year follow-up, eventually returning to prior levels of activity without limitations.

2.12 Trapezium—displaced fracture treated with lag screws

| 1 | Case description |

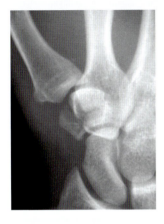

Fig 2.12-1 A 44-year-old male retail worker injured his left dominant thumb when he tried to catch a large heavy object as it fell toward him at work. His thumb was forcibly hyperextended. The initial x-rays revealed a displaced fracture in the body of the trapezium.

| 2 | Indications |

Trapezium fractures

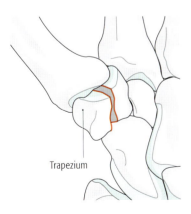

Trapezium

Fig 2.12-2 Fractures of the trapezium are rare and account for only 3–5% of all carpal fractures. The trapezium is an important bone and contributes to the stability and pain-free function of the thumb in pinching and gripping. Fractures of the trapezium are either avulsion fractures of the peripheral aspects of the bone sustained during a carpometacarpal (CMC) joint dislocation (the most common type of trapezial fracture), or a compression fracture affecting the body of the bone. The latter mechanism, illustrated in this case, is almost always the consequence of a high-energy injury. Displaced body fractures of the trapezium involve the CMC joint of the thumb and will heal in articular malunion, if not adequately reduced and stabilized.

Choice of implant

The bone quality in the trapezium is almost always good. As a consequence, fractures are suitable for stabilization with lag screws (usually 1.5 mm) unless there are central areas of fragmentation and effective bone loss. In these circumstances, K-wires are a useful option if compression of the fragments is contraindicated due to multifragmentation.

213

3 Preoperative planning

Equipment

- Modular hand set 1.3 or 1.5
- Pointed reduction forceps
- Image intensifier

Patient preparation and positioning

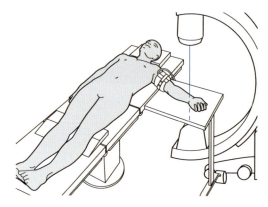

Fig 2.12-3   Position the patient supine and place the forearm on the hand table. Supinate the forearm. A nonsterile pneumatic tourniquet is used. Prophylactic antibiotics are optional.

4 Surgical approach

Approach

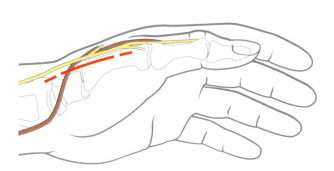

Fig 2.12-4   The surgical approach used was a radiopalmar approach to the thumb (see chapter 1.4 Radiopalmar approach to the thumb base). This approach allowed access to the trapezium immediately proximal to the metacarpal.

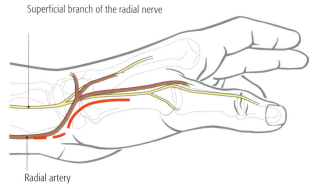

Superficial branch of the radial nerve

Radial artery

Fig 2.12-5   Of the two incision options available for this approach, on this occasion a Wagner incision was used, which follows the thenar eminence in a gentle curve toward its palmar aspect.

5   Reduction

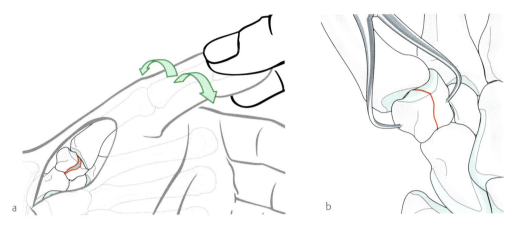

a   b

Fig 2.12-6a–b   As part of the surgical approach, the joint capsule has been opened (**a**). This now allows for direct inspection of the articular reduction. Pointed reduction forceps are used to stabilize the reduction temporarily (**b**).

6   Fixation

Drilling

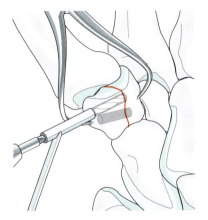

Fig 2.12-7   Leaving the reduction forceps in place, drill a gliding hole as perpendicular to the fracture plane as possible, using a 1.5 mm drill bit for a 1.5 mm screw. Insert a 1.5 mm drill guide into the gliding hole. Use a 1.1 mm drill bit to drill a threaded hole in the opposite fragment, just through the far cortex. Repeat the above for a second screw.

Screw insertion

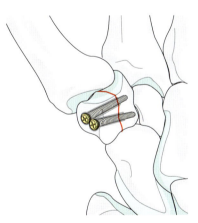

Fig 2.12-8   A minimum of two screws used as lag screws are necessary to provide sufficient stability in compression and rotation. While 1.5 mm screws are recommended, 1.3 mm screws may also be used if fragment size does not permit.

6   Fixation (cont)

Use of lag screws

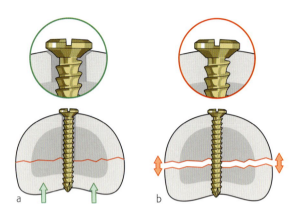

Fig 2.12-9a–b   Be sure to insert the screw as a lag screw, with a gliding hole in the near cortex, and a threaded hole in the far cortex (**a**). Inserting a screw across a fracture plane that is threaded in both cortices (position screw) will hold the fragments apart and apply no interfragmentary compression (**b**).

Countersinking

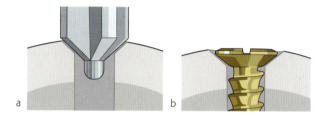

Fig 2.12-10a–b   Also ensure to countersink the screw to reduce the risk of soft-tissue irritation, so that the screw head has maximal contact area with the bone.

Complete the fixation

Confirmation of reduction and fixation should be obtained using image intensification or x-rays. It will be necessary to take several images at various angles in order to ensure there is no articular penetration with a lag screw tip. Confirmation of this can be obtained by direct inspection through the previously created capsulotomy.

7　Rehabilitation

Aftercare

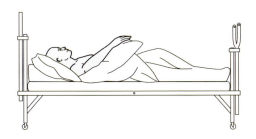

Fig 2.12-11　While the patient is in bed, use pillows to keep the hand elevated above the level of the heart to reduce swelling.

Follow-up

See the patient after 2–5 days to change the dressing. After 10 days, remove the sutures and confirm with x-rays that no secondary displacement has occurred.

Immobilization

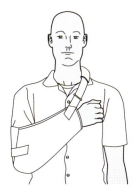

Fig 2.12-12　The wrist and thumb are immobilized for 4 to 6 weeks in a short arm splint. A removable wrist splint including the thumb to the interphalangeal joint can be used from 2 weeks, during which time the patient is encouraged to remove the splint for short periods during the day to allow gentle thumb motion.

Functional exercises

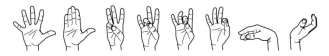

Fig 2.12-13　As pain and swelling recede, controlled flexion and extension exercises for the thumb and hand gently progress. The importance of mobilization must be emphasized to the patient and rehabilitation should be supervised by a physical therapist. A return to normal activities can be encouraged after 6 weeks.

8   Outcome

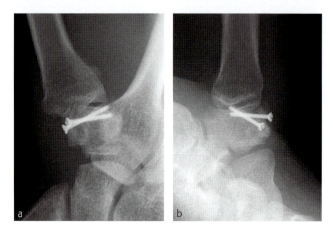

Fig 2.12-14a–b   Congruent reduction was confirmed on review of the 6-week postoperative follow-up images. The patient was then able to return to normal retailing work activities.

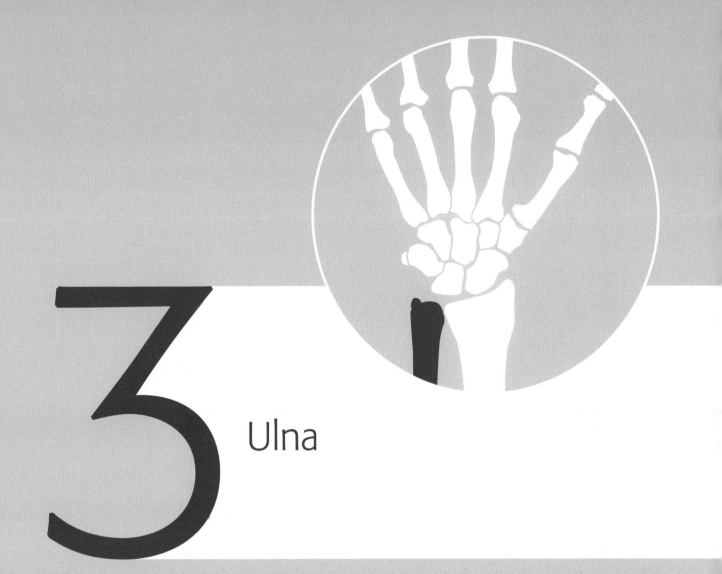

3

Ulna

3.1 Ulnar styloid–fracture treated with tension band wiring

1 Case description

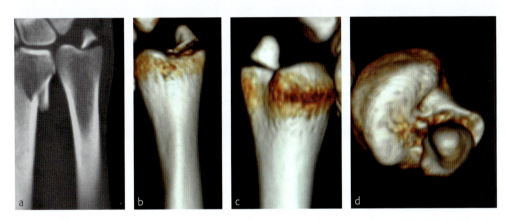

Fig 3.1-1a–d A 38-year-old engineer was injured while participating in a dirt bike competition. When he arrived in the emergency department he complained of pain in his nondominant left wrist, and there was evidence of edema and deformity. The x-rays and 3-D CT scans indicated a fracture at the base of the ulnar styloid.

There was also extensive multifragmentation in both the intermediate and radial columns of the distal radius, however, treatment for this patient's distal radial fractures are discussed in detail in chapter 4.6 Distal radius—multifragmentary intraarticular fracture treated with a palmar plate. For the purposes of this chapter, only the ulnar styloid fracture is discussed.

2 Indications

Fractures of the ulnar styloid

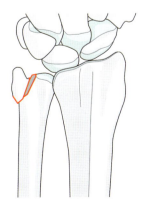

Fig 3.1-2 The ulnar styloid can be avulsed at its tip, through the body, or at its base. The level at which the avulsion occurred has implications on the integrity of the attachment of the triangular fibrocartilage complex (TFCC) and the stability of the distal radioulnar joint (DRUJ). If the injury involves these structures they may also require repair.

2 Indications (cont)

Distal radioulnar joint assessment

Fractures of the ulnar styloid that require fixation are those that produce evident DRUJ instability. The DRUJ should be assessed for both forearm rotation and stability. The following two methods are recommended to determine if instability exists.

Method 1: DRUJ ballottement

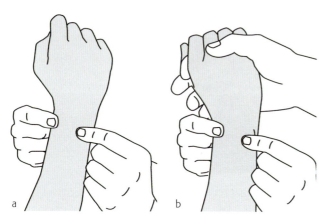

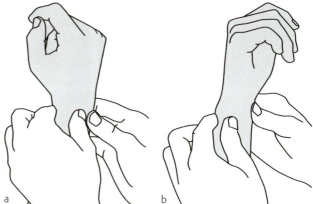

Fig 3.1-3a–b The elbow is flexed 90 degrees on the arm table with the forearm in neutral rotation and displacement in a dorsal/palmar direction is assessed. This is repeated with the wrist in radial deviation, which stabilizes the DRUJ, if the ulnar collateral complex is not disrupted.

Fig 3.1-4a–b This is again repeated with the wrist in full supination and full pronation.

Method 2: ulnar compression test

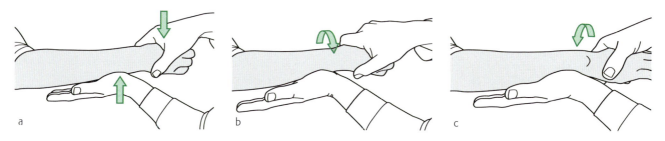

Fig 3.1-5a–c In this test, the ulna is compressed against the radius (**a**). The forearm is rotated passively through full supination (**b**) and pronation (**c**).

If there is a palpable "clunk", instability of the DRUJ is present. This is an indication to consider internal fixation of the ulnar styloid fracture by tension band wire, lag screw, or plate. A DRUJ instability can also result from soft-tissue injury to the TFCC.

3   Preoperative planning

Equipment

- 0.4 mm cerclage wire
- 1.0 mm K-wires
- Pointed reduction forceps
- Hypodermic needle

Patient preparation and positioning

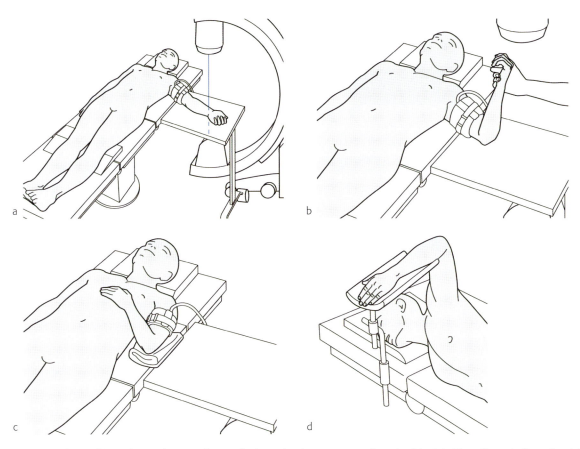

Fig 3.1-6a–d   Position the patient supine and place the forearm on a hand table (**a**). The elbow is flexed, which holds the forearm in neutral rotation and allows for a direct approach to the distal ulna (**b**). In some fractures, it may also be possible to simply rest the patients forearm on their chest (**c**). Alternatively, positioning patients on their side and resting the affected forearm in a padded trough with the elbow flexed will allow the ulnar styloid to be perfectly visible when the forearm is rotated into full supination (**d**). A nonsterile pneumatic tourniquet is used. Prophylactic antibiotics are optional.

Approach

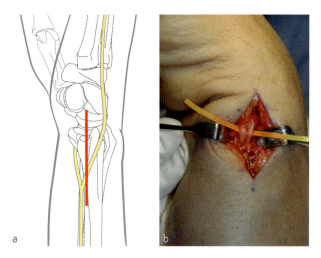

Fig 3.1-7a–b   The surgical approach used was an ulnar approach (see chapter 1.10 Ulnar approach to the distal ulna) (**a**). Care was taken to avoid damaging the dorsal cutaneous branch of the ulnar nerve during the approach (**b**).

5   Reduction

Reduction with stay suture

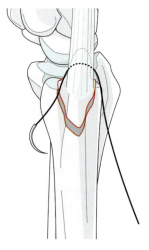

Fig 3.1-8   A strong stay suture can be inserted around the tip of the styloid to help with reduction in preparation for the later application of a tension band wire.

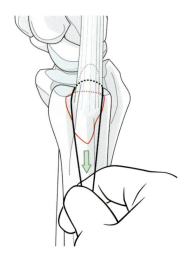

Fig 3.1-9   By pulling proximally on this suture, the ulnar styloid is reduced.

5 Reduction (cont)

Direct reduction

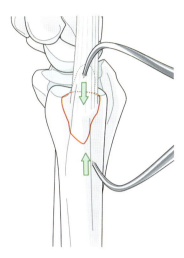

Fig 3.1-10 Reduction can also be achieved using a dental pick or a pointed reduction forceps.

6 Fixation

Drill hole

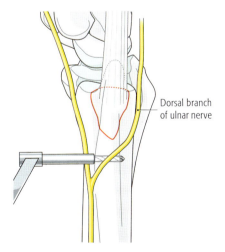

Dorsal branch
of ulnar nerve

Fig 3.1-11 Drill a hole through the ulna approximately 2 cm proximal from the tip of the styloid. Care needs to be taken to avoid injury to the dorsal cutaneous branch of the ulnar nerve.

6 Fixation (cont)

Insert the cerclage wire

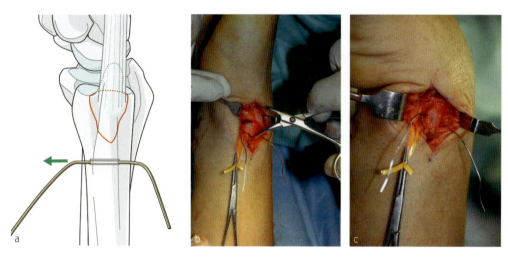

Fig 3.1-12a–c Pass a wire through the hole made proximal to the ulnar styloid fracture (**a**). The clinical images show the wire placed through the hole made into the ulna (**b–c**).

Insert the K-wires

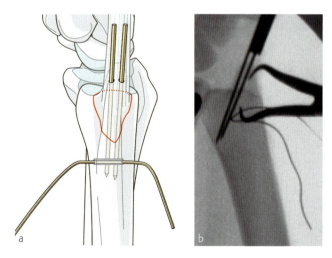

Fig 3.1-13a–b If there is enough room, insert two K-wires from the tip of the styloid in such a direction as to engage their tips in the opposite cortex of the ulna, proximal to the DRUJ (**a**). Image intensification should be used to ensure correct placement of the K-wires (**b**).

Create a figure-of-eight

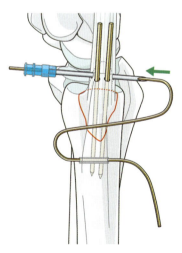

Fig 3.1-14 Continue the wire through the drill hole and, using a hypodermic needle as a guide, pass the wire around the K-wires distally to create a figure-of-eight loop.

6 Fixation (cont)

Apply tension to the wire

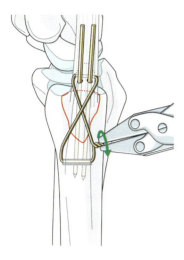

Fig 3.1-15 After creating the figure-of-eight, the wire twist is begun, ensuring that each end of the wire spirals equally. The wire is tensioned by pulling on the twist until the desired tension is achieved and then twisted to take up the slack created. Cut the twist and bend it toward the bone so as to not irritate the soft tissues.

Bury the K-wires

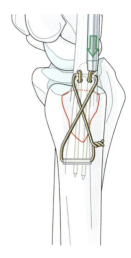

Fig 3.1-16 Using the bending iron for K-wires, the wires are bent at the level of the tip of the styloid through 180 degrees and cut short. They are then impacted into the bone using a small punch or other appropriate tool. Confirm using image intensification to ensure that the proximal tips of the K-wires are not in the interosseous space.

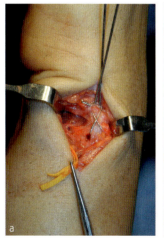
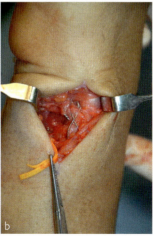

Fig 3.1-17a–b The intraoperative images show the location of the K-wires (**a**) and the cut K-wires embedded into the bone (**b**).

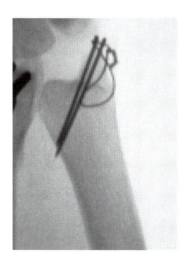

Fig 3.1-18 Intraoperative image intensification also ensures that the proximal tips of the wires are not in the interosseous space and that there is perfect reduction of the fracture.

6 Fixation (cont)

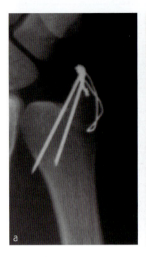 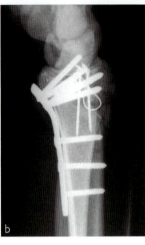

Fig 3.1-19a–b The AP and lateral x-rays (also showing the distal radial fracture) 1 week after surgery shows perfect reduction of the fractures and correct location of the implants.

7 Rehabilitation

Aftercare

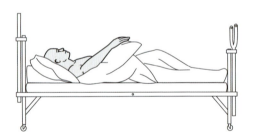

Fig 3.1-20 While the patient is in bed, use pillows to keep the hand elevated above the level of the heart to reduce swelling.

Follow-up

See the patient after 2–5 days to change the dressing. After 10 days, remove the sutures and confirm with x-rays that no secondary displacement has occurred.

7 Rehabilitation (cont)

Immobilization

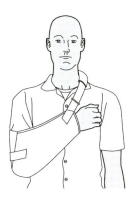

Fig 3.1-21   The type and duration of postoperative immobilization for distal ulnar fractures depends on a number of factors including the quality of the internal fixation as well as patient activity and reliability. It may be necessary to rest the wrist for several weeks in a cast or removable splint. During that time, the patient is encouraged to remove the immobilization for short periods to allow gentle wrist motion.

Functional exercises

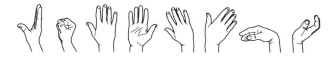

Fig 3.1-22   Following surgery, begin active controlled range of motion exercises. Active motion exercises and later resistance exercises should be initiated based upon the surgeon's decision as to time after surgery and patient compliance. Load-bearing activities are usually delayed until radiological evidence of bone healing. The importance of mobilization must be emphasized to the patient and rehabilitation should be supervised by a physical therapist.

8 Outcome

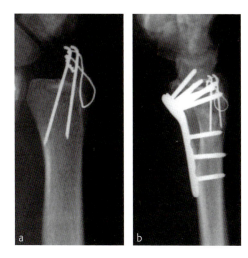

Fig 3.1-23a–b   The x-rays at the 1-year follow-up confirmed anatomical healing.

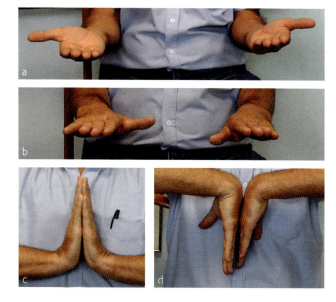

Fig 3.1-24a–d   The patient had no pain and could achieve full range of motion. He had returned to normal work and sporting activities.

9 Alternative technique

Alternative fixation with a screw

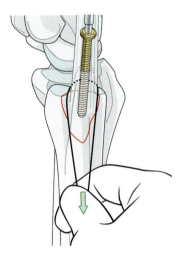

Fig 3.1-25 While reduction is maintained by pulling on the suture, or by pressure with a dental pick, the styloid can also be fixed with an appropriate sized screw introduced from the tip of the styloid into the lateral cortex of the ulnar shaft.

The ulnar styloid needs to be overdrilled for the screw to have a lag screw effect.

Assessment of DRUJ

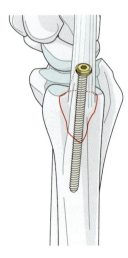

Fig 3.1-26 Stable reattachment of the ulnar styloid with correct tension of the TFCC should be achieved with this single screw. The stability of the radioulnar joint is tested after insertion of the screw. The suture can now be withdrawn.

3.2 Ulna, head and neck—multifragmentary fracture treated with a hook plate

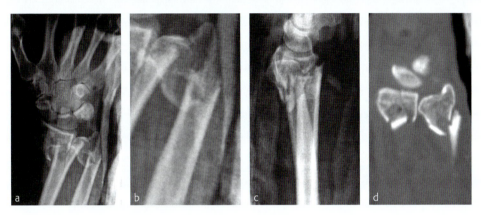

Fig 3.2-1a–d   A 62-year-old salesman injured his left wrist in a motor vehicle accident. He suffered a type II Gustillo fracture that involved both the ulna and distal radius. The AP and lateral x-rays and coronal CT scan demonstrated complex ulnar head and neck fractures with marked displacement and a multifragmentary fracture of the distal radius.

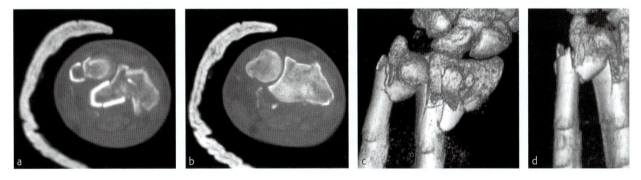

Fig 3.2-2a–d   Further 2-D axial CT scans demonstrated substantial metaphyseal fragmentation within both the ulna and distal radius, while 3-D CT reconstructions identified the extent of displacement of each fracture. However, for the purposes of this chapter, only the ulnar fractures are discussed.

2   Indications

Fractures of the distal ulna

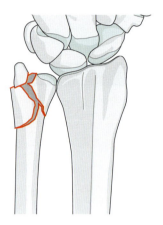

Choice of implant

Multifragmentary fractures of the distal ulna can be treated with bridge or hook plating or with a minicondylar plate. Hook plating with a locking compression plate (LCP) distal ulna plate allows better control of smaller distal fragments and was selected for this patient.

Fig 3.2-3   In multifragmentary ulnar fractures there is instability and shortening. Anatomical restoration of the ulnar head and neck is essential to restore normal distal radioulnar joint (DRUJ) function. Restoration of the DRUJ creates intrinsic stability.

3   Preoperative planning

Equipment

- LCP distal ulna plate 2.0
- 1.1 mm K-wire
- Image intensifier

Patient preparation and positioning

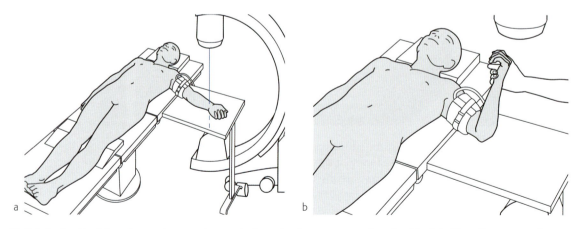

Fig 3.2-4a–b   Position the patient supine and place the forearm on a hand table (**a**). The elbow can also be flexed, which holds the forearm in neutral rotation and allows for a direct approach to the distal ulna (**b**). A nonsterile pneumatic tourniquet is used. Prophylactic antibiotics are optional.

4 Surgical approach

Approach

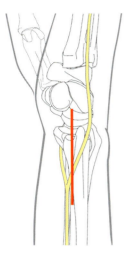

Fig 3.2-5 The surgical approach used was an ulnar approach (see chapter 1.10 Ulnar approach to the distal ulna).

5 Reduction

Reduce the ulnar head

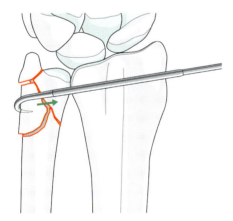

Fig 3.2-6 Under direct vision, the ulnar head is reduced to the ulnar shaft using a small periosteal elevator or a dental pick. In multifragmentary subcapital fractures, correct alignment and correct rotational alignment of the head is verified. A reduction forceps is usually not applicable due to the small fragments and the soft bone quality at this level.

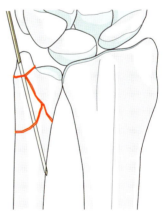

Fig 3.2-7 Temporary stabilization with a small K-wire may be necessary, especially if there is a separate ulnar styloid fragment.

6 Fixation

Select the plate

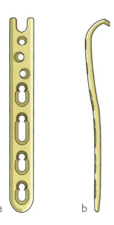

Fig 3.2-8a–b The distal ulna plate is a precontoured plate that fits to the surface of the distal ulna and allows grasping of the ulnar styloid with the pointed hooks.

Apply the plate

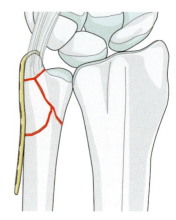

Fig 3.2-9 The pointed hooks are placed around the tip of the ulnar styloid and the plate is aligned on the ulnar shaft. If a K-wire has been inserted, it would ideally sit between the distal hooks of the plate.

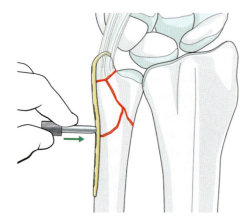

Fig 3.2-10 Handling of the plate may be facilitated using the LCP drill guide inserted in one of the LCP plate holes. Image intensification can be used to verify correct plate position.

Insert the first screw

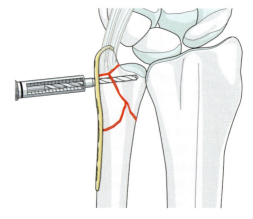

Fig 3.2-11 An LCP drill guide is used to drill a hole for a locking screw in the ulnar head. Avoid drilling through the opposite cortex, as the screw tip would penetrate into the distal radioulnar joint. Screw length is measured pushing the hook of the depth gauge against the opposite cortex. A slightly shorter screw is then chosen.

6 Fixation (cont)

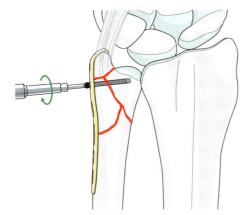

Fig 3.2-12 The first locking head screw is inserted into the ulnar head.

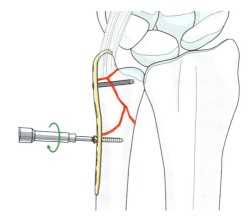

Fig 3.2-13 A standard screw is inserted through the oblong plate hole to reduce the shaft fragment to the plate. At this point reduction is verified under image intensification and unrestricted pronation and supination is checked.

Insert additional screws

Additional locking head screws are inserted into the ulnar head and fixation at the shaft fragment is completed using standard or locking head screws. The multiple options for screw insertion in the plate allow a wide range of fracture patterns to be securely stabilized.

Option 1: fractures requiring length adjustment

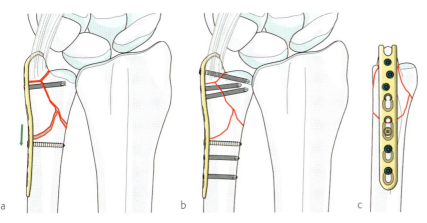

a   b   c

Fig 3.2-14a–c In fractures that require length adjustment, place one or two 2.0 mm locking screws in the ulnar head to securely fix the implant distally, then place a 2.0 mm cortex screw in the oblong hole of the shaft and obtain the correct length of reduction (**a**). Use a combination of cortex and locking screws in the surrounding holes to stabilize the fracture securely, as dictated by bone quality (**b–c**).

Option 2: fractures requiring stability of the ulnar styloid

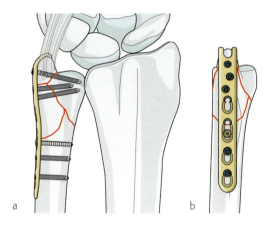

Fig 3.2-15a–b In the case of unstable fractures of the base of the ulnar styloid, a 2.0 mm locking screw can be applied through the most distal hole in the plate. A locking screw does not need to reach the far cortex for stable fixation.

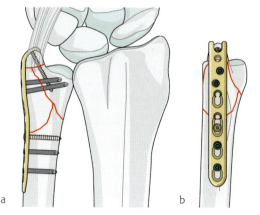

Fig 3.2-16a–b In unstable fractures of the tip of the ulnar styloid, the distal plate hole is left empty. Remove the K-wire if used for preliminary fixation. Overdrill the near fragment with a 1.5 mm drill bit. Insert a 1.5 mm cortex screw in lag mode between the arms of the distal hooks.

Pitfall: locking head screw too long

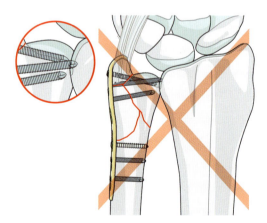

Fig 3.2-17 If a screw penetrates the opposite cortex of the ulnar head, the screw tip will damage the cartilage of the radioulnar joint.

Pearl: retaining the K-wire

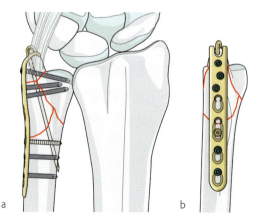

Fig 3.2-18a–b If a K-wire has been used for fixation of the ulnar styloid, and has not been removed for distal screw placement, it may be left in place if it enters the ulnar styloid between the pointed hooks. The K-wire is then bent and cut short.

6 Fixation (cont)

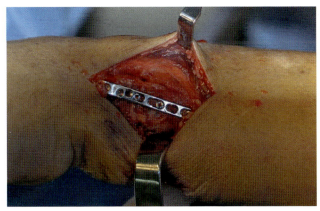

Fig 3.2-19 The intraoperative image shows the ulnar fractures stabilized using the LCP distal ulna plate.

7 Rehabilitation

Aftercare, follow-up, and functional exercises

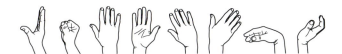

Fig 3.2-20 The patient should receive the standard postoperative rest, injury elevation, follow-up, removal of stitches, and immobilization as required. Following surgery, begin active controlled range of motion exercises. For further information, see the rehabilitation topic in chapter 3.1 Ulnar styloid–fracture treated with tension band wiring.

8 Outcome

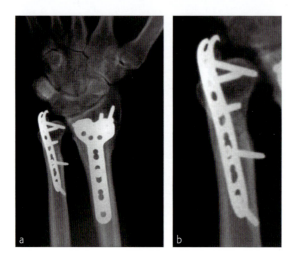

Fig 3.2-21a–b   At the 6-month follow-up, there was healing of the ulnar fractures in good position.

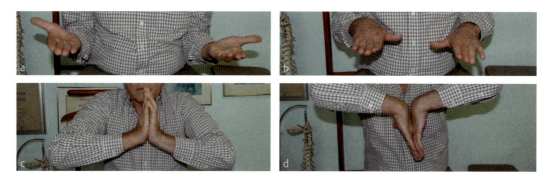

Fig 3.2-22a–d   There was a successful functional result showing good range of motion.

Video

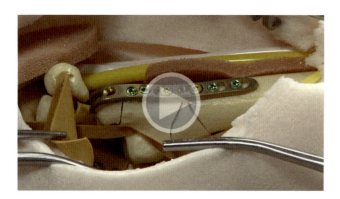

Video 3.2-1   This video demonstrates a distal ulna subcapital fracture with diaphyseal comminution and styloid fracture treated with an LCP distal ulna plate.

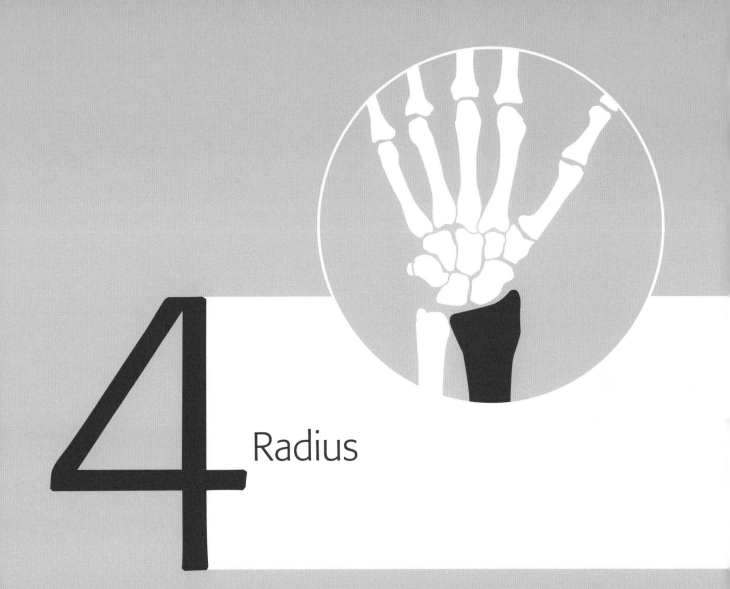

4 Radius

4.1 Radial styloid–fracture treated with a radial column plate

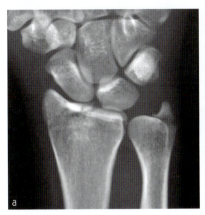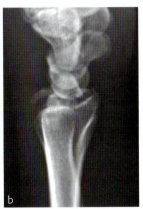

Fig 4.1-1a–b A 23-year-old female university student suffered an injury to her right wrist in a traffic accident and was initially treated for a wrist sprain by cast immobilization. She returned to the hand clinic for cast removal 3 weeks later, however, the follow-up PA and lateral x-rays showed an apparently benign nondisplaced fracture of the radial styloid. As there was suspicion of intraarticular displacement in the lateral view, a CT scan was requested.

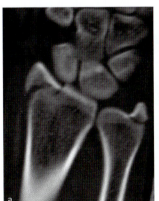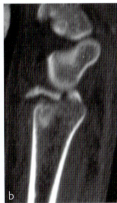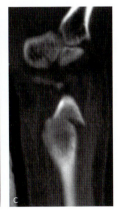

Fig 4.1-2a–c The CT scans revealed a displaced intraarticular fracture with a step-off of the dorsal aspect of the radial styloid.

A displaced fracture of the ulnar styloid was also evident; however, for the purposes of this chapter, only the radial styloid is discussed. For further information on treating ulnar styloid fractures see chapter 3.1 Ulnar styloid–fracture treated with tension band wiring.

2 Indications

Radial styloid fractures

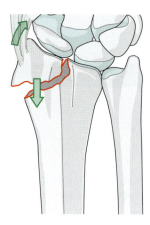

Fig 4.1-3 Simple radial styloid fractures are fractures without multifragmentation. They can occur as a result of shearing or compression forces. As they involve an articular split of the radial styloid, they are partial articular fractures. These fractures demand accurate reduction since they involve the articular surface. Often the fracture exists in the sagittal plane.

Associated median nerve compression

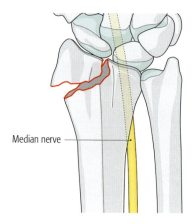

Median nerve

Fig 4.1-4 If there is dense sensory loss or other signs of median nerve compression, the median nerve should be decompressed.

Associated carpal injuries

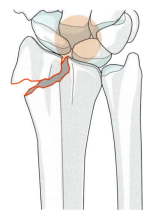

Fig 4.1-5 These injuries may be associated with shearing injuries of the articular cartilage, scaphoid fractures, and ruptures of the scapholunate ligament. Every patient should be assessed for these injuries.

2 Indications (cont)

Associated ulnar injuries

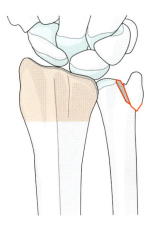

Fig 4.1-6 These injuries can also be accompanied by avulsion of the ulnar styloid and/or disruption of the distal radioulnar joint (DRUJ). If there is gross instability after the fixation of the radial fracture, it is recommended that the ulnar styloid and/or the triangular fibrocartilage disc (TFC) is reattached. This is not common in simple fractures but can occur in some high-energy injuries. The uninjured side should be tested as a reference for the injured side. However, it may not be possible to assess DRUJ stability until the fracture has been stabilized.

Contraindications

Throughout the chapters in the remaining two sections of the book, patient treatment mostly involves open reduction and internal fixation with a variety of plate and screw technology. The reader is reminded that in some instances surgical treatment for a distal radial fracture is not recommended, and these can include but are not limited to the type of displacement of the fracture, nerve compromise, severe swelling, poor state of soft tissues, and the patient not being fit for surgery.

Choice of implant

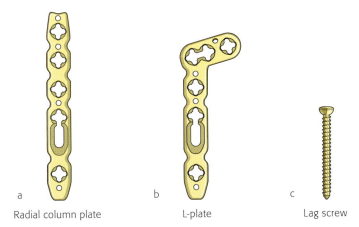

a
Radial column plate

b
L-plate

c
Lag screw

Fig 4.1-7a–c A variety of plate and screw options are available for radial styloid fractures depending on fracture pattern, the state of the affected soft tissues, and stability. Plates with variable angle (VA) locking screw options can be useful. For this patient, a straight radial column plate was selected and further supported with an additional lag screw.

3 Preoperative planning

Equipment

- VA LCP distal radius set
- VA LCP radial column plate 2.4
- 1.1 mm or 1.2 mm K-wires
- 2.4 mm cortex screw
- Osteotome
- Pointed reduction forceps
- Image intensifier

Patient preparation and positioning

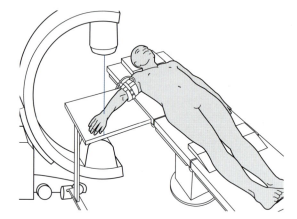

Fig 4.1-8   Position the patient supine and place the forearm on the hand table. Pronate the forearm. The position of the limb should allow complete imaging in the frontal and sagittal plane of the distal radius. A nonsterile pneumatic tourniquet is used. Prophylactic antibiotics are optional.

4 Surgical approach

Approach

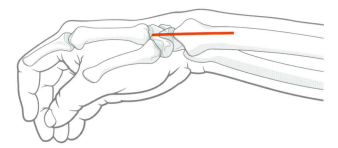

Fig 4.1-9   The surgical approach used was a dorsoradial approach between the first and second extensor compartments (see chapter 1.5 Dorsoradial approach to the distal radius).

4 Surgical approach (cont)

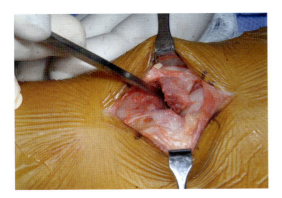

Fig 4.1-10 To improve visibility of the joint surface, an arthrotomy of the dorsal capsule was performed. This revealed a bigger fragment than suspected from the x-rays. Additionally, because the surgery was performed 3 weeks after the initial trauma, opening of the early callus with an osteotome was required.

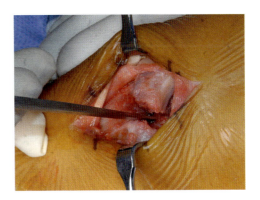

Fig 4.1-11 Further examination of the surface revealed that the articular fracture was oriented in the sagittal and in the coronal plane.

5 Reduction

Provisional reduction

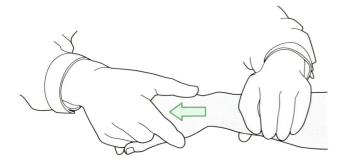

Fig 4.1-12 Reduction is achieved by applying longitudinal traction either manually or using finger traps. The reduction is maintained by a temporary splint. If definitive surgery is planned but cannot be performed within a reasonable time scale, a temporary external fixator may be helpful.

Provisional fixation

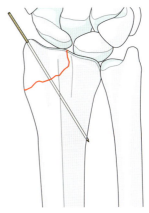

Fig 4.1-13 Insert a K-wire through the tip of the radial styloid to provisionally hold the fragments. Confirm using image intensification.

6 Fixation

Contour the plate

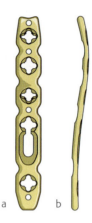

Fig 4.1-14a–b Plates used in treating radial and intermediate column injuries are available precontoured. However, some additional contouring may be necessary to accommodate the individual anatomy of the patient.

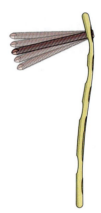

Fig 4.1-15 Variable angle locking plates enable precise positioning of the distal screws in desired directions because there is 30 degrees of freedom for each screw inside the plate hole in order to address the individual fracture patterns.

Pitfall: screw hole distortion

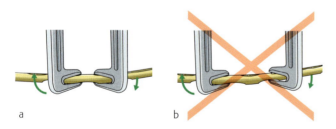

Fig 4.1-16a–b Avoid contouring the plate through the locking holes, otherwise the locking head screw might no longer fit.

Fixation of radial column
Select and apply the plate

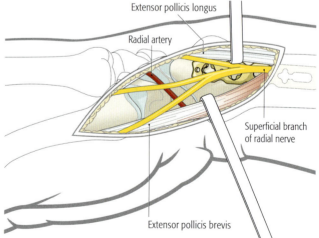

Extensor pollicis longus

Radial artery

Superficial branch of radial nerve

Extensor pollicis brevis

Fig 4.1-17 The appropriate plate is selected according to the fracture configuration and contoured if necessary. Slide the plate underneath the first compartment and apply it onto the radial column.

6 Fixation (cont)

Stabilize the radial column

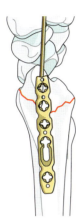

Fig 4.1-18 Ideally while applying the plate, the notch in the distal tip of the implant is placed against the temporary K-wire.

Pitfall: incorrect placement

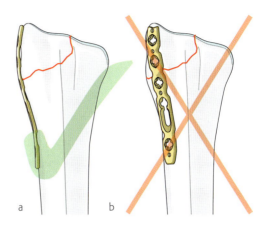

Fig 4.1-19a–b Placement of the plate on the dorsal aspect of the radial column is to be avoided, as it will not buttress the reduction adequately against axial shear forces.

Insert the first screw

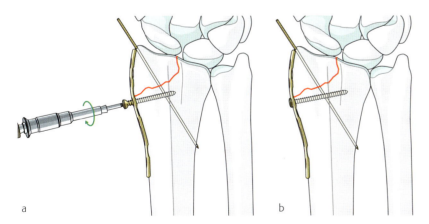

Fig 4.1-20a–b Insert a standard cortex screw into the oblong plate hole proximal to the fracture (**a**). It is preferable that the screw should engage the far cortex, but in this case this would result in penetration of the DRUJ. The dense subchondral bone in this region allows secure fixation if bone quality is good. The position of the plate may be adjusted before the screw is tightened. Tightening this screw will reduce the radial styloid (**b**).

6 Fixation (cont)

Insert the first locking head screw

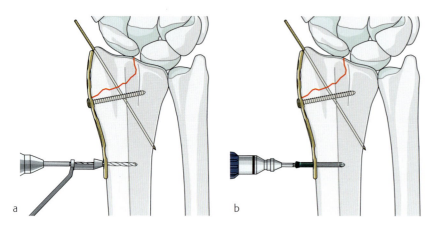

Fig 4.1-21a–b To prevent rotation of the plate during distal subchondral locking screw fixation, the plate should be secured to the bone by inserting the most proximal screw. To avoid overtightening the locking screw a torque limiting device should be used.

Insert the distal locking head screw

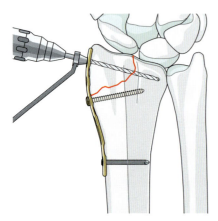

Fig 4.1-22 If a K-wire was used, it is now removed. Insert a locking head screw into the distal locking hole of the plate. The screw should be placed in a subchondral position.

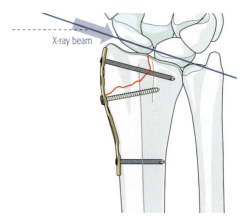

Fig 4.1-23 Confirm that the screw does not protrude into the joint using the image intensifier, with the beam angled 20 degrees from the true lateral. This projection will profile the radial articular surface and show any encroachment of the screw into the joint.

6 Fixation (cont)

Complete the fixation

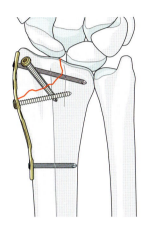

Fig 4.1-24 To complete the fixation, it may be necessary to insert a lag screw. In order to obtain the lag effect, use either partially threaded screws or prepare a gliding hole in the radial styloid. Use a drill guide to ensure that the soft tissues are protected during drilling.

Distal radioulnar joint assessment

After fixation, the DRUJ should be assessed for both forearm rotation and stability. The following two methods are recommended to determine if instability exists.

Method 1: DRUJ ballottement

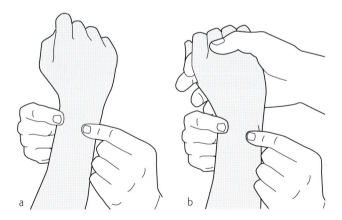

Fig 4.1-25a–b The elbow is flexed 90 degrees on the arm table with the forearm in neutral rotation and displacement in a dorsal/palmar direction is assessed. This is repeated with the wrist in radial deviation, which stabilizes the DRUJ, if the ulnar collateral complex is not disrupted.

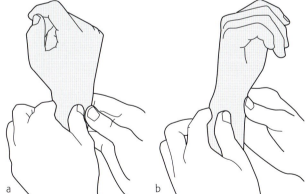

Fig 4.1-26a–b This is again repeated with the wrist in full supination and full pronation.

6 Fixation (cont)

Method 2: ulna compression test

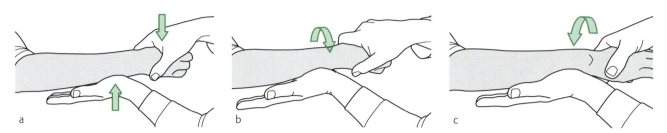

a b c

Fig 4.1-27a–c   In this test, the ulna is compressed against the radius (**a**). The forearm is rotated passively through full supination (**b**) and pronation (**c**). If there is a palpable "clunk", instability of the DRUJ is present. This is an indication to consider internal fixation of an ulnar styloid fracture by tension band wire, lag screw, or plate. A DRUJ instability can also result from soft-tissue injury to the triangular fibrocartilage complex (TFCC).

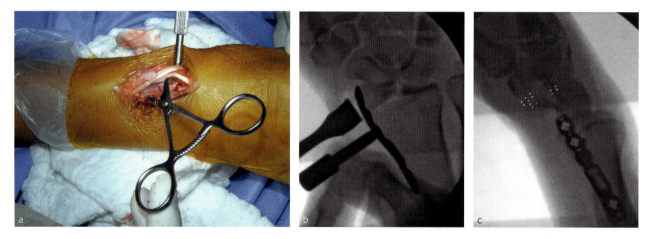

Fig 4.1-28a–c   With the pointed reduction forceps used to reduce the fracture, the plate was placed on the radial column and the screws inserted (**a**). Intraoperative image intensification showed the displacement of the fracture and helped to determine the right location for the plate (**b–c**).

6 Fixation (cont)

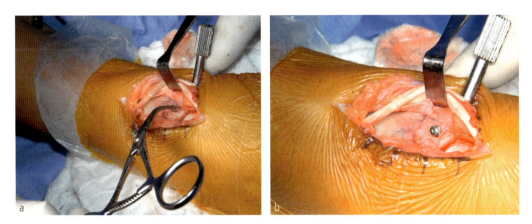

Fig 4.1-29a–b Following plate fixation, a 2.4 mm lag screw was inserted perpendicular to the fracture in the coronal plane to further stabilize the fracture (**a**). The pointed reduction forceps was then removed (**b**).

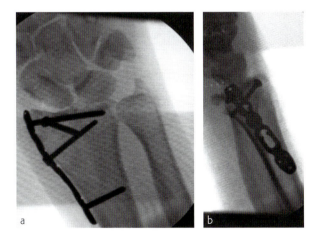

Fig 4.1-30a–b Intraoperative imaging showed the fracture reduction with the VA LCP straight plate acting as a buttress to the joint surface and the lag screw placed through the plate into the subchondral bone.

7 Rehabilitation

Aftercare

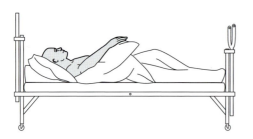

Fig 4.1-31 While the patient is in bed, use pillows to keep the hand elevated above the level of the heart to reduce swelling.

Follow-up

See the patient after 2–5 days to change the dressing. After 10 days, remove the sutures and confirm with x-rays that no secondary displacement has occurred.

Immobilization

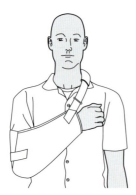

Fig 4.1-32 The type and duration of postoperative immobilization depends on a number of factors including the quality of the internal fixation as well as patient activity and reliability. It may be necessary to rest the wrist for several weeks in a plaster or removable splint. During that time, the patient is encouraged to remove the splint for short periods to allow gentle wrist motion.

Functional exercises

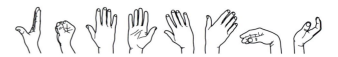

Fig 4.1-33 Following surgery, begin active controlled range of motion exercises. Active motion exercises and later resistance exercises should be initiated based upon the surgeon's decision as to time after surgery and patient compliance. Load-bearing activities are usually delayed until radiological evidence of bone healing. The importance of mobilization must be emphasized to the patient and rehabilitation should be supervised by a physical therapist.

8 Outcome

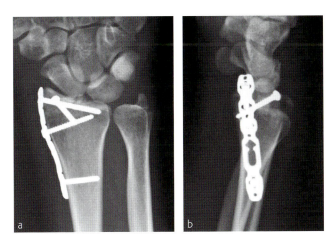

Fig 4.1-34a–b At the 3-month follow-up, the PA and lateral x-rays showed healing of the fracture.

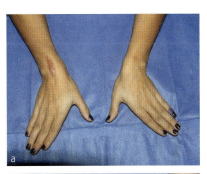

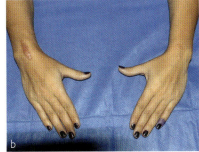

Fig 4.1-35a–b There was also normal ulnar and radial deviation of the wrist.

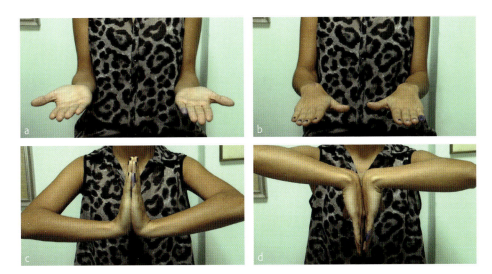

Fig 4.1-36a–d There was an excellent functional result.

9 Alternative technique

Radial styloid fracture treated with percutaneous fixation

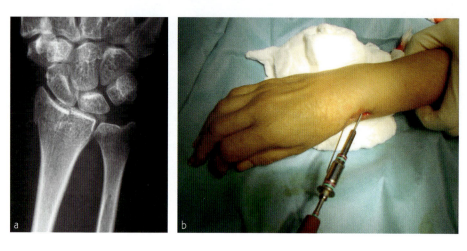

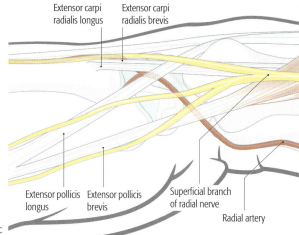

Extensor carpi radialis longus

Extensor carpi radialis brevis

Extensor pollicis longus

Extensor pollicis brevis

Superficial branch of radial nerve

Radial artery

Fig 4.1-37a–c In some cases of simple radial styloid fracture (**a**), it can be possible to reduce and fix the fracture through a small percutaneous approach over the tip of the styloid (**b**). The advantages of percutaneous treatment include preserving soft tissue and reducing immobilization time. However, care must still be taken to avoid damaging important structures in this region (**c**).

9 Alternative technique (cont)

Closed reduction

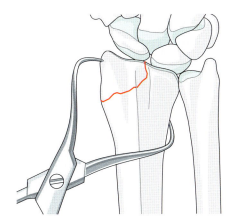

Fig 4.1-38 Reduce the fracture using percutaneous pointed reduction forceps, inserted through small stab incisions, or the main small incision over the styloid process. Confirm the reduction using image intensification.

Fixation

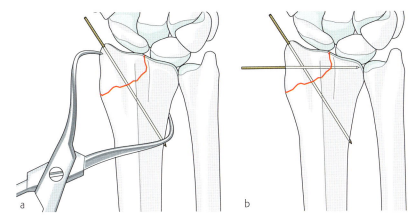

Fig 4.1-39a–b Insert a guide wire into the styloid fragment as perpendicular as possible to the fracture site (**a**). Pass the wire across the fracture site, gaining purchase in the ulnar cortex of the radius. If the fragment is large enough, place a second guide wire as parallel to the joint surface as possible (**b**).

9 Alternative technique (cont)

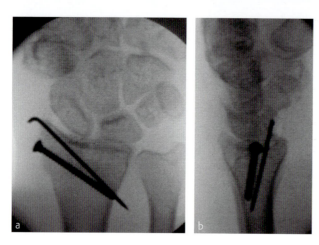

Fig 4.1-40a–b Drill over the guide wires and insert the appropriate screws. Fracture treatment can involve screw and/or K-wire fixation.

4.2 Distal radius—dorsally displaced extraarticular fracture treated with a palmar plate

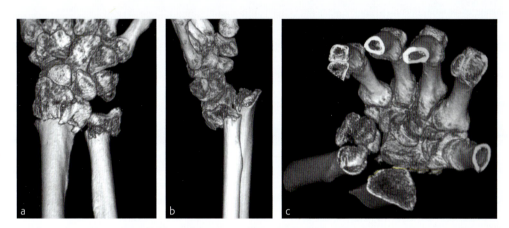

Fig 4.2-1a–c   A 76-year-old woman suffered a fall onto her outstretched right hand. She went to the emergency department having severe pain, numbness of the fingers, and gross deformity of the wrist. The PA and lateral 3-D CT scan showed dorsal displacement of a nonarticular distal radial fracture with some dorsal metaphyseal multifragmentation (**a–b**). There was also a displaced fracture of the ulna neck. An axial view 3-D CT scan more clearly demonstrated the marked fracture displacement (**c**).

For this patient, both the distal ulna and radius were involved, with the ulna being treated using a distal ulna (hook) plate. However, for the purposes of this chapter, only the distal radius is discussed. For further information on treating distal ulnar fractures see chapter 3.2 Ulna, head and neck—multifragmentary fracture treated with a hook plate.

2 Indications

Extraarticular fractures

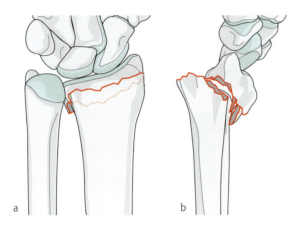

Fig 4.2-2a–b Fractures of the distal radius can involve a dorsally displaced extraarticular fracture of the distal metaphysis (proximal to but not including the articular surface). This is the most common type of wrist fracture.

Extraarticular distal radial fractures are common among elderly patients with lesser quality bone whereas stronger younger patients tend to suffer these only after high-energy impact, often involving intraarticular fractures as well. Fractures angulated dorsally at > 25 degrees and associated with osteoporosis or residual void after reduction can prove unstable. Therefore, primary palmar plating is often the best treatment option.

Before palmar plating became a commonly used treatment, most of these fractures were treated with closed reduction, which was then maintained with either K-wires or a plaster cast. Many surgeons now treat most these fractures with a palmar plate and often use the plate as an aid to reduction.

Associated median nerve compression

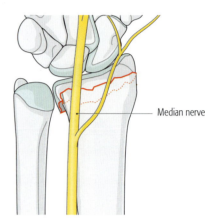

Median nerve

Fig 4.2-3 If there is dense sensory loss or other signs of median nerve compression, the median nerve should be decompressed.

2 Indications (cont)

Associated ulnar injuries

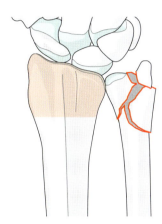

Fig 4.2-4 Head, neck, and multifragmentary fractures of the distal ulna often occur in combination with distal radial fractures. With these ulnar fractures there is instability and shortening, so the distal ulnar hook plate can be used to hold the fracture. Attention should be paid to restoring correct rotation and length in relation to the radius. Complete dislocation of the radiocarpal joint is often associated with disruption of the distal radioulnar joint (DRUJ).

Choice of implant

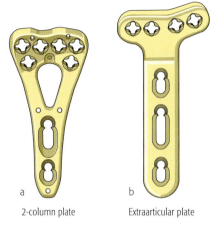

a 2-column plate   b Extraarticular plate

Fig 4.2-5a–b A variety of plate options are available for extraarticular distal radial fractures. Advances in plate design have provided angular stable fixation, which allows enhanced stability and ease of application even in the presence of osteoporotic bone. Plates with variable angle (VA) locking screw options can be useful. For this patient, a VA locking compresion plate (LCP) 2-column palmar plate was selected.

3 Preoperative planning

Equipment

- VA LCP distal radius set
- VA LCP 2-column plate 2.4
- 1.1 mm or 1.2 mm K-wires
- Image intensifier

Patient preparation and positioning

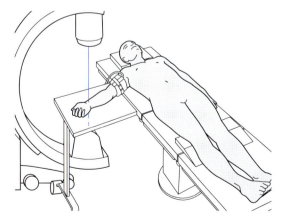

Fig 4.2-6 Position the patient supine and place the forearm on a hand table. Supinate the forearm. The position of the limb should allow complete imaging in the frontal and sagittal plane of the distal radius. A nonsterile pneumatic tourniquet is used. Prophylactic antibiotics are optional.

4 Surgical approach

Approach

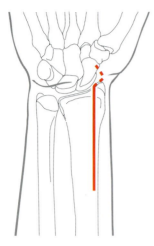

Fig 4.2-7 The surgical approach used was a palmar approach (see chapter 1.6 Modified Henry palmar approach to the distal radius).

5 Reduction and fixation

Provisional reduction

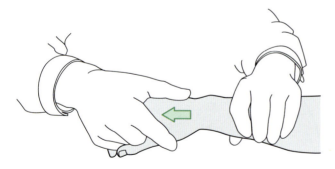

Fig 4.2-8 Reduction is achieved by applying longitudinal traction either manually or using finger traps. The reduction is maintained by a temporary splint. If definitive surgery is planned but cannot be performed within a reasonable time scale a temporary external fixator may be helpful.

5   Reduction and fixation (cont)

Reduction using the plate

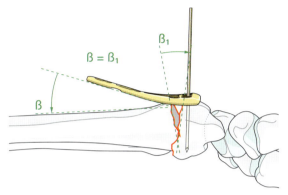

Fig 4.2-9   Select and apply the plate to the distal fragment. The distal end of the plate should end at the anatomical watershed line of the distal radius. Insert a K-wire through a screw hole as close to the subchondral bone as possible and parallel to the articular surface. The resultant angle of the plate to the shaft should equal the angle of the displacement. Confirm using image intensification.

Alternative reduction

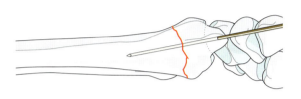

Fig 4.2-10   Some surgeons believe that using the plate for reduction in patients with osteoporosis may cause the screws to loosen in the bone. In such cases, manual reduction and preliminary fixation with K-wires may be preferable.

Insert the first distal screw

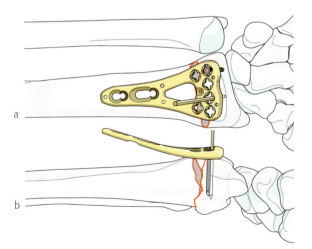

Fig 4.2-11a–b   The initial screw is inserted in the most ulnar screw hole. The reason is that if the initial screw is placed on the radial side it will block accurate imaging of the ulnar screw placement. Choose a locking head screw 2–4 mm shorter than measured. Provided the screw is parallel to the K-wire it should not enter the radiocarpal joint.

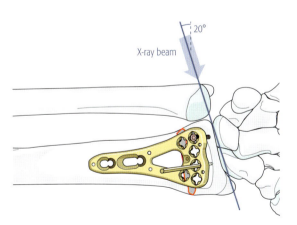

Fig 4.2-12   Confirm screw position with a lateral view under image intensification, with the beam aimed at an angle of 20 degrees to the true lateral, clearly showing the joint surface.

5 Reduction and fixation (cont)

Insert additional locking head screws

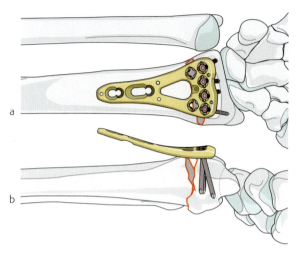

Fig 4.2-13a–b Insert at least two other distal locking head screws.

Pitfall: screw tip protrusion

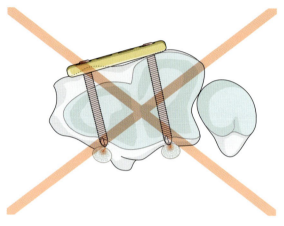

Fig 4.2-14 Due to the prominence of Lister tubercle, as seen on the lateral image projection, a screw placed on either side of the tubercle may appear not to protrude through the far cortex. Protrusion of such a screw may result in extensor tendon irritation and rupture.

Apply the plate to the shaft

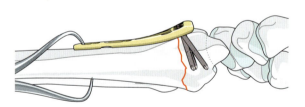

Fig 4.2-15 The implant is then used to reduce the fragments by pushing it onto the surface of the radius. Bring the plate onto the shaft and hold it with a forceps. Check correct placement with imaging and adjust the position of the distal fragment if necessary by moving the plate.

Insert the first proximal screw

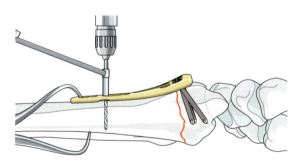

Fig 4.2-16 Once satisfactory reduction is confirmed, insert an appropriate cortex screw through the oblong plate hole.

5 Reduction and fixation (cont)

Complete the fixation

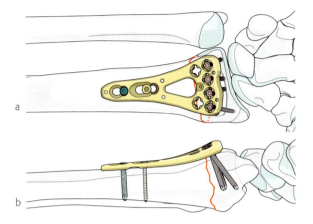

Fig 4.2-17a–b Insert further proximal screws to complete the fixation.

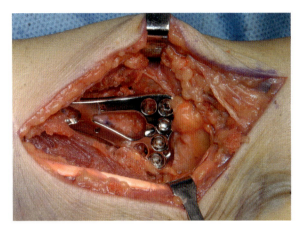

Fig 4.2-18 Intraoperative picture of the reduced fracture fixed with the VA LCP 2-column palmar plate 2.4.

Distal radioulnar joint assessment

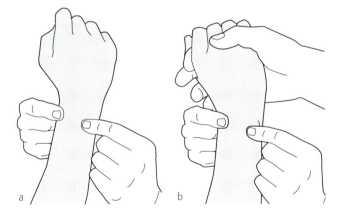

Fig 4.2-19a–b After fixation, the DRUJ should be assessed for both forearm rotation and stability. The methods for determining if DRUJ instability exists are shown in the fixation topic in chapter 4.1 Radial styloid—fracture treated with a radial column plate.

6 Rehabilitation

Aftercare, follow-up, and functional exercises

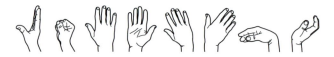

Fig 4.2-20 The patient should receive the standard postoperative rest, injury elevation, follow-up, removal of stitches, and immobilization as required. Following surgery, begin active controlled range of motion exercises. For further information see the rehabilitation topic in chapter 4.1 Radial styloid—fracture treated with a radial column plate.

7 Outcome

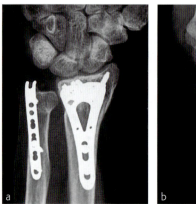
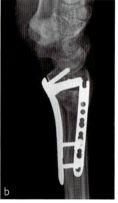

Fig 4.2-21a–b At the 1-year follow-up, the x-rays revealed full healing with anatomical reduction of both the distal radial and ulnar neck fractures.

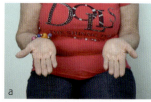
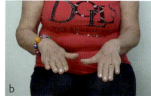
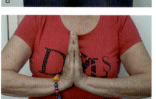
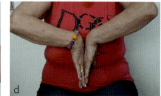

Fig 4.2-22a–d There was an excellent functional result with full forearm and wrist motion possible.

4.3 Distal radius—lunate facet fracture treated with a buttress plate

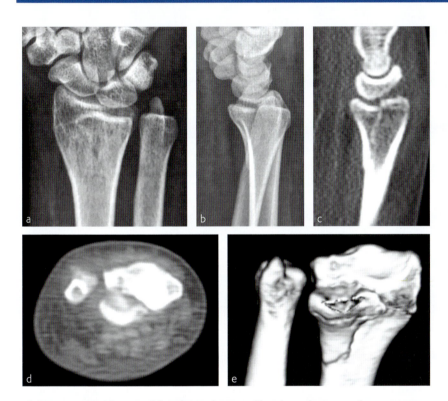

Fig 4.3-1a–e A 48-year-old male engineer suffered a polytrauma in a motor vehicle injury sustaining femoral fractures, fractures of the distal humerus, and a fracture of the shaft of the left ulna. All fractures were treated surgically. However, the patient was seen in the hand clinic 2 months after the injury having pain, signs of median nerve compression, and functional limitation of the right wrist. New PA and lateral x-rays then indicated a previously undetected lunate facet fracture of the radius (**a–b**). Sagittal and coronal 2-D scans along with a 3-D CT scan clearly showed the displaced lunate facet fracture as an isolated distal radial injury (**c–e**).

2 Indications

Lunate facet fractures

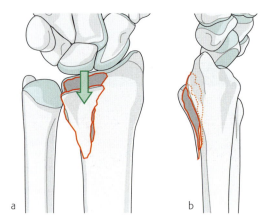

Fig 4.3-2a–b Following high-energy impact a lunate facet fracture can occur, which is a partial articular fracture where the rim of the distal radius at the radiocarpal joint is sheared off. This often occurs at the palmar rim, as the palmar lunate facet projects anteriorly to the flat palmar surface of the distal radius and is therefore relatively vulnerable to injury. The result of the injury is joint incongruity and palmar sublux-ation of the carpus. Displaced lunate facet fractures affect both radiocarpal and radioulnar alignment and function. Buttress plating is the recommended treatment option.

Imaging

As shown with this case, the fracture pattern may not always be clear on standard x-rays, so additional CT scanning is strongly recommended.

Associated median nerve compression

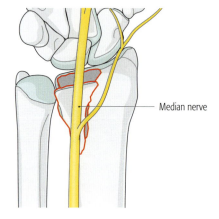

Median nerve

Fig 4.3-3 If there is dense sensory loss or other signs of median nerve compression, the median nerve should be decompressed.

Choice of implant

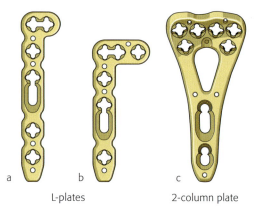

L-plates   2-column plate

Fig 4.3-4a–c A variety of plate options are available for palmar buttress plating, and the size of the palmar rim fragment/s will influence the choice of plate. Plates with variable angle (VA) locking screw options can be useful. For this patient, a VA locking compression plate (LCP) L-shaped plate with two holes in the distal limb was selected to reduce and buttress the fracture.

---

3 Preoperative planning

Equipment

- VA LCP distal radius set
- VA LCP L-plate 2.4
- Pointed reduction forceps
- Image intensifier

Patient preparation and positioning

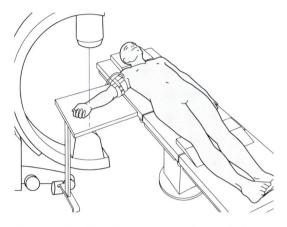

Fig 4.3-5 Position the patient supine and place the forearm on a hand table. Supinate the forearm. The position of the limb should allow complete imaging in the frontal and sagittal plane of the distal radius. A nonsterile pneumatic tourniquet is used. Prophylactic antibiotics are optional.

---

4 Surgical approach

Approach

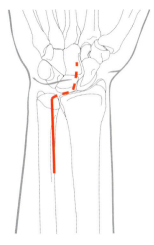

Fig 4.3-6 The surgical approach used was an ulnar palmar approach (see chapter 1.7 Ulnar palmar approach to the distal radius).

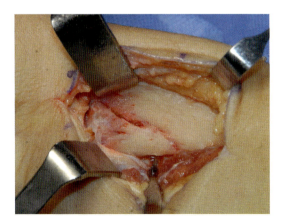

Fig 4.3-7 Once the fracture was exposed it was noted that the fracture line extended to the middle of the distal radial surface.

---

5 Reduction

Hyperextend the wrist

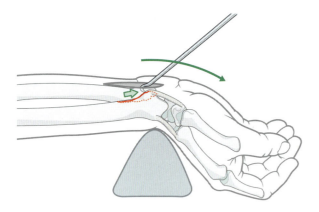

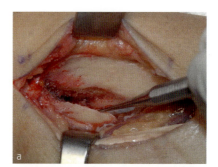

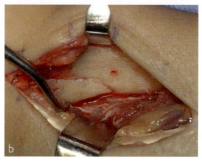

Fig 4.3-8   To assist in the approach and to help reduce the fracture, place a rolled towel or bolster under the wrist and hyperextend it. Perfect anatomical reduction can be achieved by direct manipulation of the distal fragment using a dental pick or a fine hook. Reduction can be maintained using a pointed reduction forceps.

Fig 4.3-9a–b   The fracture was disimpacted to define the articular injury. The reduced fracture was held with a pointed reduction forceps. Note that a carpal tunnel release was also performed through a separate incision.

---

6 Fixation

Contour the plate

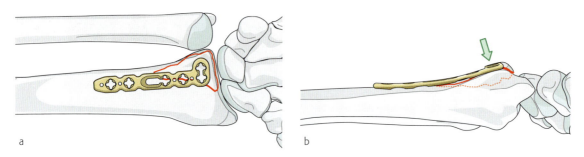

Fig 4.3-10a–b   The distal end of the plate should end at the anatomical watershed zone of the distal radius (**a**). Once positioned, ensure that the plate is contoured so that its distal limb exerts even pressure over the fragment or fragments of the palmar rim of the radius (**b**).

6   Fixation (cont)

Apply the plate in buttress mode

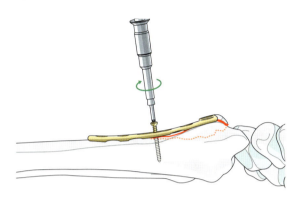

Fig 4.3-11   Attach the plate to the distal radial shaft using an appropriate cortex screw through the oblong plate hole. Before fully tightening it, check the plate position using intraoperative imaging, adjusting the position of the plate as necessary so as to provide an optimal buttress effect.

Insert second screw

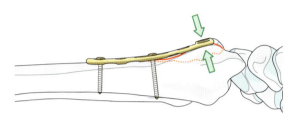

Fig 4.3-12   Now tighten the first screw and insert a second cortex screw. Check for adequate buttress pressure on the palmar rim fragment(s).

Insert distal screws and complete the fixation

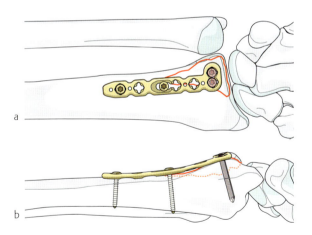

Fig 4.3-13a–b   Secure the distal fragment(s) with at least two screws through the appropriate distal holes, as dictated by the fracture pattern. The screws must not penetrate the dorsal radial cortex. If a plate is selected with threaded holes in the distal limb, then locking head screws are used. Confirm reduction using image intensification.

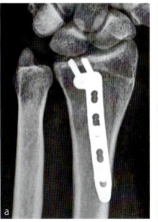
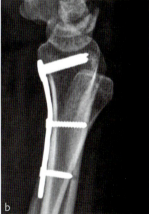

Fig 4.3-14a–b   Definitive fixation was achieved with a VA LCP L-plate 2.4.

7 Rehabilitation

Aftercare, follow-up, and functional exercises

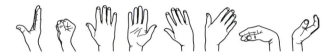

Fig 4.3-15 The patient should receive the standard postoperative rest, injury elevation, follow-up, removal of stitches, and immobilization as required. Following surgery, begin active controlled range of motion exercises. For further information see the rehabilitation topic in chapter 4.1 Radial styloid—fracture treated with a radial column plate.

8 Outcome

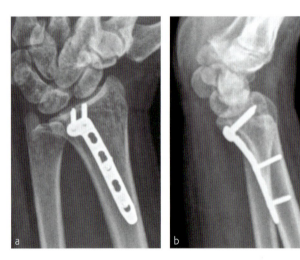

Fig 4.3-16a–b At the 12-month follow-up, the x-rays showed effective healing had been achieved.

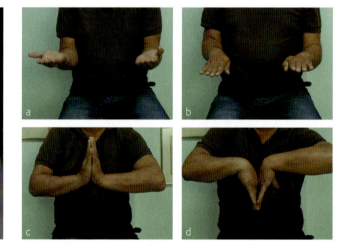

Fig 4.3-17a–d The patient had nearly full hand, wrist, and forearm range of motion.

8 Outcome (cont)

Video

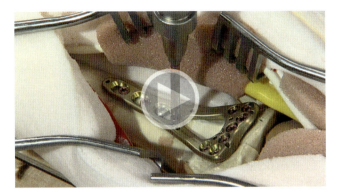

Video 4.3-1 This video demonstrates a reverse Barton (ie, palmar) distal radial fracture treated using an LCP 2-column plate.

9 Alternative technique: case description

Lunate facet fracture treated with screws

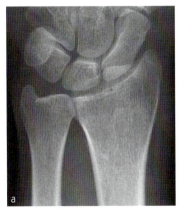 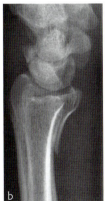

Fig 4.3-18a–b A classical concert guitarist had a fall onto his left hand while riding his bicycle when it became stuck in tramway lines. He presented to the emergency department the following day with concerns about his playing future and asked for a perfect functional result. The PA and lateral x-rays indicated a shearing type of lunate facet fracture.

9 Alternative technique: case description (cont)

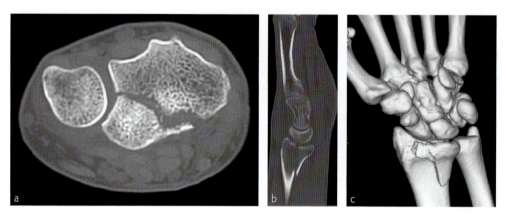

Fig 4.3-19a–c Axial and sagittal 2-D CT scans (**a–b**) showed the displacement of the isolated lunate facet fracture. A 3-D CT scan more clearly showed the morphology of the facet fracture (**c**).

10 Alternative technique: reduction and fixation

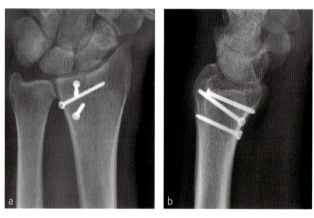

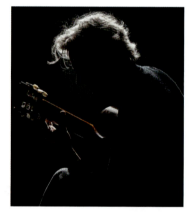

Fig 4.3-20a–b   As the patient was a professional guitarist, and following discussion of potential perioperative and postoperative problems, he was considered reliable for receiving treatment with less stable fixation. Therefore, just a few days after presentation, he was treated with three cannulated 2.7 mm screws. Screws rarely interfere with soft tissues, especially flexor tendons, which allowed the patient to resume guitar playing quickly and with consideration that implant removal was unlikely to be necessary in the future.

Fig 4.3-21   The highly motivated patient undertook immediate functional after-treatment in the hand therapy department and quickly regained full mobility to his wrist joint. He was soon able to play the guitar again without pain and performed his next concert 8 weeks postoperatively.

4.4 Distal radius—shearing fracture treated with a buttress plate

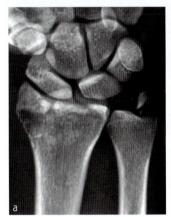
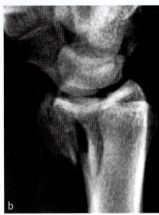

Fig 4.4-1a–b A 35-year-old sales consultant suffered a fall from his motorcycle while riding to work. He was seen in the emergency department having pain and swelling of the right wrist. The PA and lateral x-rays demonstrated a shearing fracture of the distal radius with palmar displacement, with the carpus also subluxated from its normal position.

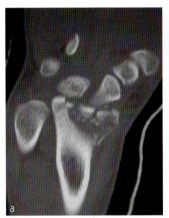
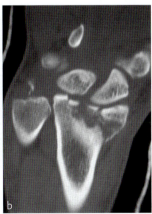
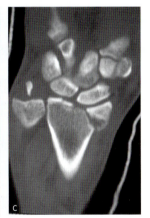

Fig 4.4-2a–c Three 2-D CT frontal plane images demonstrated multifragmentation of the palmar articular surface. There was a fracture of the radial styloid, multifragmentation of the scaphoid facet, and partial involvement of the lunate facet. On the ulna there was a displaced avulsion fracture of the ulnar styloid.

1   Case description (cont)

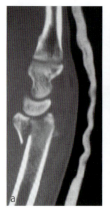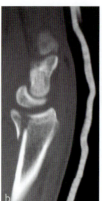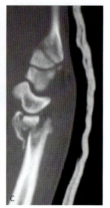

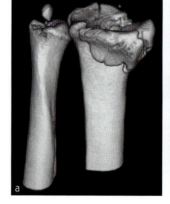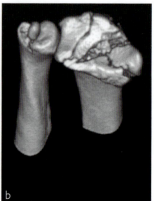

Fig 4.4-3a–c   The 2-D sagittal CT scans showed the palmar subluxation of the carpus with a palmar shearing fracture and a centrally impacted articular fragment of the scaphoid facet.

Fig 4.4-4a–b   The 3-D CT scans showed that the sigmoid notch and the ulnar corner of the lunate facet were not injured and remained in continuity with the metaphysis.

For this patient, a small ulnar styloid fracture was evident in addition to the radius injury, however, for the purposes of this chapter, only the distal radius is discussed. For further information on treating ulnar styloid fractures see chapter 3.1 Ulnar styloid—fracture treated with tension band wiring.

2   Indications

Shearing fractures

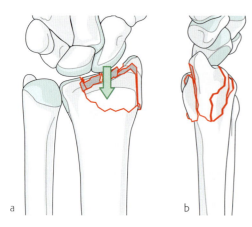

Fig 4.4-5a–b   Fractures are described as shearing when the opposite cortex remains intact. These partial intraarticular fractures can involve fragmentation and can occur on either the palmar (as in this case) or the dorsal side (see the alternative technique later in this chapter). Shearing fracture injuries result in joint incongruity and subluxation of the carpus and are best shown in CT scans. Most shearing fractures are unstable and displaced and for that reason require operative treatment to restore anatomy and stability. An intact opposite cortex allows a buttress plating technique to be used as the treatment of choice.

2 Indications (cont)

Associated median nerve compression

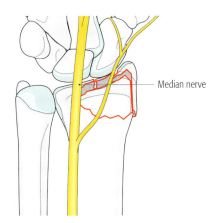

Median nerve

Fig 4.4-6   If there is dense sensory loss or other signs of median nerve compression, the median nerve should be decompressed.

Associated ulnar injuries

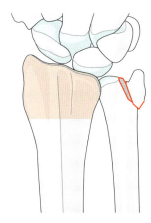

Fig 4.4-7   These injuries can also be accompanied by avulsion of the ulnar styloid and/or disruption of the distal radioulnar joint (DRUJ). If there is gross instability after the fixation of the radial fracture, it is recommended that the ulnar styloid and/or the triangular fibrocartilage disc (TFC) is reattached. This is not common in simple fractures but can occur in some high-energy injuries. The uninjured side should be tested as a reference for the injured side. However, it may not be possible to assess DRUJ stability until the fracture has been stabilized.

Choice of implant

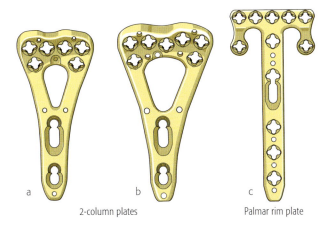

a   b   c

2-column plates   Palmar rim plate

Fig 4.4-8a–c   A variety of plate options are available to treat shearing fractures with buttress plating, and the size of the palmar rim fragment(s) will influence the choice of plate. Plates with variable angle (VA) locking screw options can be useful. For this patient, a 2-column palmar plate with a 7-hole head was selected.

Equipment

- VA locking compression plate (LCP) distal radius set
- VA LCP 2-column plate 2.4
- 1.1 mm or 1.2 mm K-wires
- Pointed reduction forceps
- Image intensifier

Patient preparation and positioning

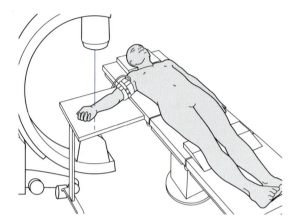

Fig 4.4-9   Position the patient supine and place the forearm on a hand table. Supinate the forearm. The position of the limb should allow complete imaging in the frontal and sagittal planes of the distal radius. A nonsterile pneumatic tourniquet is used. Prophylactic antibiotics are optional.

4   Surgical approach

Approach

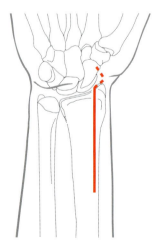

Fig 4.4-10   The surgical approach used was a modified Henry palmar approach (see Chapter 1.6 Modified Henry palmar approach to the distal radius).

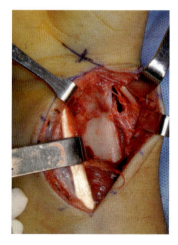

Fig 4.4-11   The modified Henry palmar approach was performed with the flexor carpi radialis and the flexor pollicis longus being separated ulnarly, protecting the median nerve and the radial artery separated radially. The pronator quadratus muscle was incised on its radial border and was stripped off the distal radius together with the periosteum. This made the fracture more visible.

5 Reduction

Hyperextend the wrist

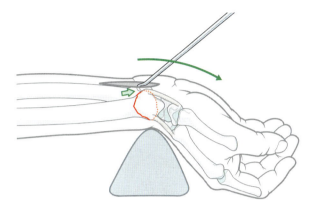

Fig 4.4-12 To assist in the approach and to help reduce the fracture, place a rolled towel or bolster under the wrist and hyperextend it. Perfect anatomical reduction can be achieved by direct manipulation of the distal fragment using a dental pick or a fine hook. Reduction can be maintained using a pointed reduction forceps.

6 Fixation

Contour the plate

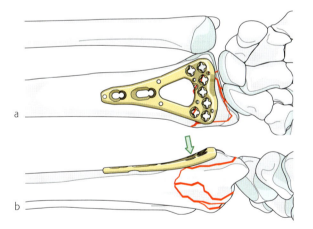

a

b

Fig 4.4-13a–b The distal end of the plate should end at the anatomical watershed zone of the distal radius (**a**). Once positioned, ensure that the plate is contoured so that its distal limb exerts even pressure over the fragment or fragments of the palmar rim of the radius (**b**).

Apply the plate in buttress mode

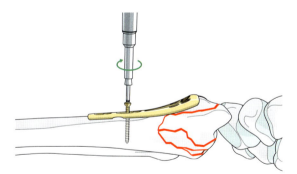

Fig 4.4-14 Attach the plate to the distal radial shaft using an appropriate cortex screw through the oblong plate hole. Before fully tightening it, check the plate position using intraoperative imaging, adjusting the position of the plate as necessary so as to provide an optimal buttress effect.

6 Fixation (cont)

Insert second screw

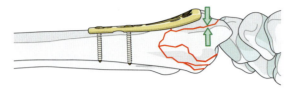

Fig 4.4-15 Now tighten the first screw and insert a second cortex screw. Check adequate buttress pressure on the palmar rim fragment(s).

Insert distal screws and complete the fixation

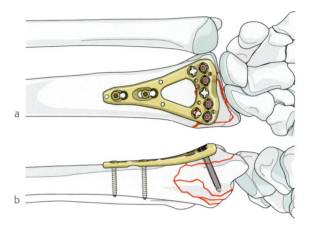

Fig 4.4-16a–b Secure the distal fragment(s) with at least two screws through the appropriate distal holes, as dictated by the fracture pattern. The screws must not penetrate the dorsal radial cortex. If a plate is selected with threaded holes in the distal limb, then locking head screws are used. Confirm reduction using image intensification.

Distal radioulnar joint assessment

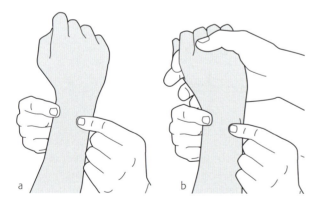

Fig 4.4-17a–b After fixation, the DRUJ should be assessed for both forearm rotation and stability. The methods for determining if DRUJ instability exists are shown in the fixation topic in chapter 4.1 Radial styloid—fracture treated with a radial column plate.

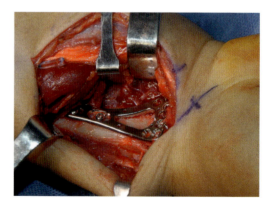

Fig 4.4-18 The VA LCP 2.4 was applied to the palmar aspect of the radius. Care was taken not to extend past the watershed line with the plate.

7 Rehabilitation

Aftercare, follow-up, and functional exercises

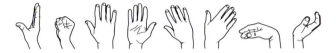

Fig 4.4-19 The patient should receive the standard postoperative rest, injury elevation, follow-up, removal of stitches, and immobilization as required. Following surgery, begin active controlled range of motion exercises. For further information see the rehabilitation topic in chapter 4.1 Radial styloid—fracture treated with a radial column plate.

8 Outcome

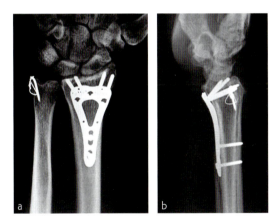

Fig 4.4-20a–b At the 12-month follow-up, the AP and lateral x-rays showed full healing in anatomical position.

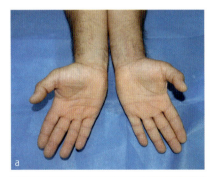

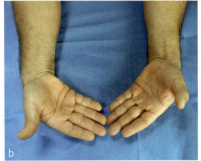

Fig 4.4-21a–b There was normal radial and ulnar deviation 12 months after the initial trauma.

8 Outcome (cont)

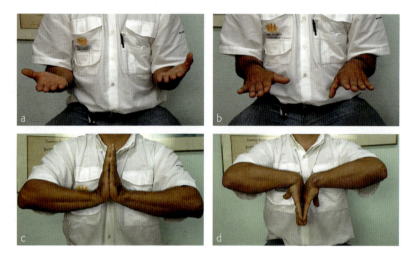

Fig 4.4-22a–d   By this stage, the patient had also obtained full wrist range of motion.

9 Alternative technique: case description

Dorsal shearing fracture treated with dorsal plates

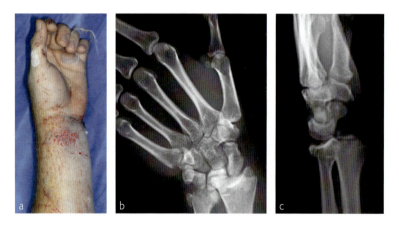

Fig 4.4-23a–c   Just as palmar shearing distal radial fractures can occur, so too can such fractures occur on the dorsal side. A 24-year-old engineer had a work-related motor vehicle accident sustaining gross deformity, severe pain and swelling, and multiple skin abrasions along the palmar aspect of his left wrist, thumb, and forearm. After wound cleaning and sedation, the patient was immobilized in a padded sugar-tong splint. Ten days after the injury, when swelling had subsided and infection was ruled out, he was taken to the operating room. New PA and lateral x-rays demonstrated a dorsal shearing articular fracture.

9 Alternative technique: case description (cont)

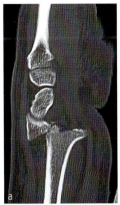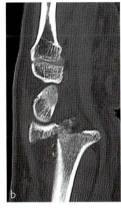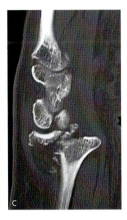

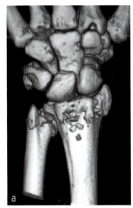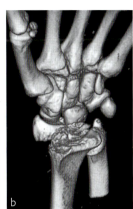

Fig 4.4-24a–c Three 2-D lateral view CT scans revealed the radial styloid and the dorsal rim of the distal radius were displaced with the proximal carpal row.

Fig 4.4-25a–b The 3-D CT scans further showed the multifragmentary dorsal shearing fracture in the left wrist.

Dorsal shearing fractures

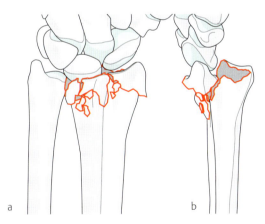

Fig 4.4-26a–b Dorsal shearing fractures are less common than palmar shearing fractures but are also often the result of high-energy trauma. They are typically multifragmentary fractures and associated with dorsal subluxation of the carpus. There can be a spectrum of injury types with variation in the size of the dorsal fragments.

Choice of implant

If the distal radial fragments are predominantly dorsal, they can be held with dorsally applied plates, but if there is a significant radial styloid fragment, it is stabilized more effectively with a radial plate.

9 Alternative technique: case description (cont)

Approach

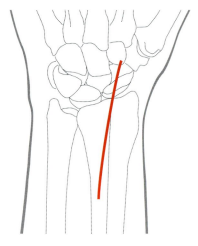

Fig 4.4-27 The surgical approach used was a dorsal approach (see chapter 1.8 Dorsal approach to the distal radius).

Arthrotomy

If direct vision of the articular surface is needed, a limited transverse radiocarpal arthrotomy is performed.

10 Alternative technique: reduction and fixation

Provisional reduction

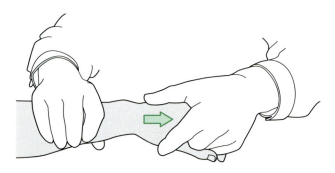

Fig 4.4.28 Reduction is achieved by applying longitudinal traction either manually or using finger traps. The reduction is maintained by a temporary splint. If definitive surgery is planned but cannot be performed within a reasonable time scale, a temporary external fixator may be helpful.

Provisional intermediate column fixation

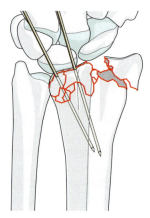

Fig 4.4-29 If the dorsal rim fragments are large enough, obtain provisional fixation with K-wires.

10 Alternative technique: reduction and fixation (cont)

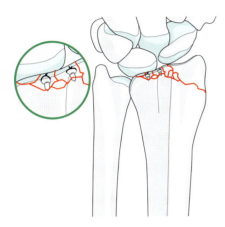

Fig 4.4-30 If the fragment are too small they can be held with suture anchors or transosseous sutures.

Provisional radial styloid fixation

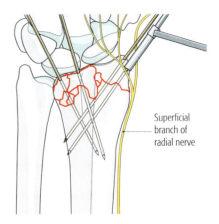

Superficial branch of radial nerve

Fig 4.4-31 The radial styloid fragments are reduced under direct vision with either a K-wire on the dorsoradial aspect or percutaneously. In the latter case, in order not to injure the sensory branch of the radial nerve, make a small incision over the tip of the radial styloid and use a protective drill guide to insert two K-wires. Confirm using image intensification.

Intermediate column fixation

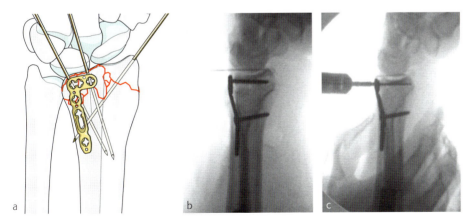

Fig 4.4-32a–c Following reduction of the dorsal rim fractures, the distal radius was supported by fixation of a VA L-plate 2.4.

The fixation procedure follows the usual steps of selecting, contouring, and applying the plate, and inserting proximal and distal screws. For further information on these steps see chapter 4.11 Distal radius—radiocarpal fracture dislocation treated with double plating.

10 Alternative technique: reduction and fixation (cont)

Radial column fixation

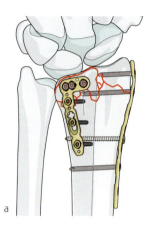
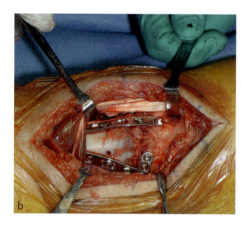
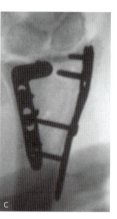

Fig 4.4-33a–c The radial column plate was placed underneath the first compartment and applied. Intraoperative imaging shows the completed double plate fixation.

The fixation procedure follows the usual steps of selecting, contouring, and applying the plate, stabilizing the radial column, inserting proximal and distal screws, and confirming screw placement with imaging or x-rays. For further information on these steps see chapter 4.11 Distal radius—radiocarpal fracture dislocation treated with double plating.

Palmar ligamentous avulsion reattachment

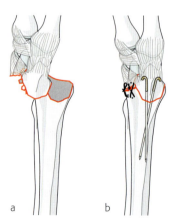

Fig 4.4-34a–b Dorsal carpal subluxation may be associated with avulsion of the palmar wrist capsule from the distal radius (**a**).

After dorsal fixation, check the carpal position and stability under image intensification. If there is carpal ulnar and/or palmar translation, consider an additional palmar approach to repair soft tissues. The capsule can be reattached using multiple suture anchors or transosseous sutures (**b**).

Additional external fixation

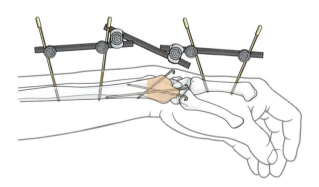

Fig 4.4-35 If the dorsal rim fragments are large enough, they may be held in place with a buttress plate. If they are too small, K-wires may be the definitive fixation, in which case, an external fixator should be applied.

10 Alternative technique: reduction and fixation (cont)

Outcome

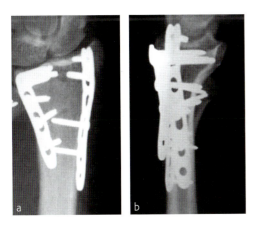

Fig 4.4-36a–b The x-rays at the 6-month follow-up show the reduction had been maintained until bone healing.

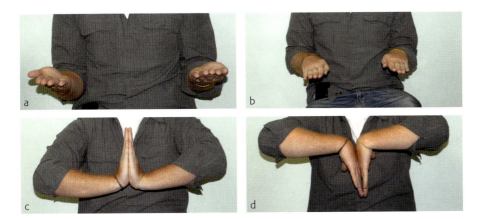

Fig 4.4-37a–d There was an excellent final functional result

Manual of Fracture Management—Wrist   Jesse B Jupiter, Douglas A Campbell, Fiesky Nuñez

4.5 Distal radius—dorsally displaced intraarticular fracture treated with double plating

1 Case description

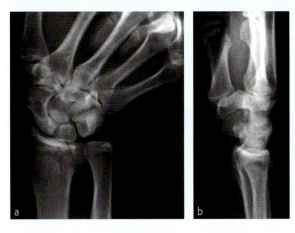

Fig 4.5-1a–b A 57-year-old man fell on his outstretched right hand while carrying groceries, sustaining a closed wrist injury. The x-rays indicated an intraarticular, dorsally displaced distal radial fracture.

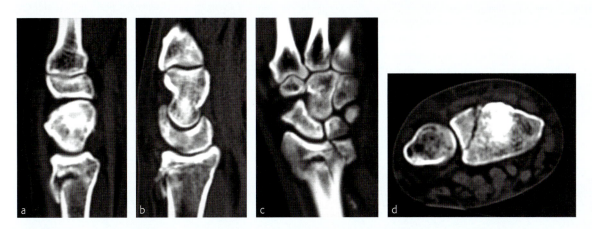

Fig 4.5-2a–d The 2-D CT images also showed a dorsal lunate facet component with impaction.

2 Indications

Complete intraarticular fractures

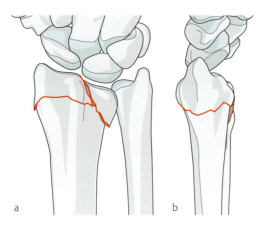

Fig 4.5-3a–b Complete intraarticular fractures of the distal radius occur when there is no part of the articular surface in continuity with the diaphysis. This case involves a complete intraarticular fracture with a dorsoulnar postero-medial articular fragment associated with metaphyseal displacement. As with all intraarticular fractures, it should be treated with anatomical reduction and absolute stability in order to minimize the risk of subsequent degenerative changes in the joint. Anatomical reduction and stabilization of these fractures is also essential because of the functional implications of the involvement of the distal radioulnar joint (DRUJ).

Dorsally displaced fractures may involve loss of radial length and a displaced coronal split in the lunate fossa. Optimum hold and stability is best obtained with separate plating of both the radial and intermediate columns. The fixation of small distal fragments is more secure with locking plates.

Principle of columns

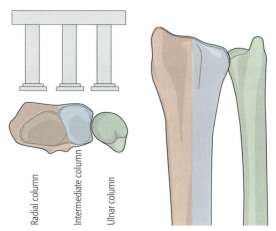

Fig 4.5-4 The distal forearm can be thought of in terms of three columns. The ulna forms one column (the ulnar column) while the radius can be separated into two (the intermediate column and the radial column). The 3-column principle helps in describing the location of wrist injuries and is further explained in the indications topic in chapter 1.8 Dorsal approach to the distal radius.

In dorsal double plating, understanding the principle of columns is important as the intermediate and radial columns are each stabilized with a separate plate. The radial column is stabilized by a plate placed radially, deep to the first extensor compartment. The intermediate column is stabilized with a separate precontoured plate on the dorsal aspect of the intermediate column.

2 Indications (cont)

Associated median nerve compression

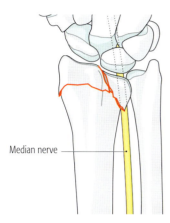

Median nerve

Fig 4.5-5 If there is dense sensory loss or other signs of median nerve compression, the median nerve should be decompressed.

Associated carpal injuries

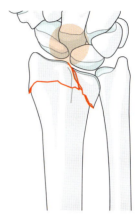

Fig 4.5-6 These injuries may be associated with shearing injuries of the articular cartilage, scaphoid fractures, and ruptures of the scapholunate ligament. Every patient should be assessed for these injuries.

Choice of implant

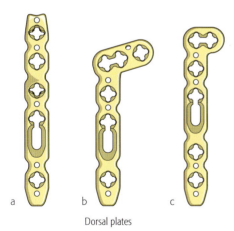

a   b   c

Dorsal plates

Fig 4.5-7a–c A selection of plates used for stabilizing the radial and intermediate columns is available. Plates with variable angle (VA) locking screw options can be useful. For this patient VA straight and L-plates were used, with the intermediate column being treated first.

3 Preoperative planning

Equipment

- VA locking compression plate (LCP) distal radius set
- VA LCP radial column plate 2.4
- VA LCP intermediate column plate 2.4
- 1.1 mm or 1.2 mm K-wires
- Image intensifier

Patient preparation and positioning

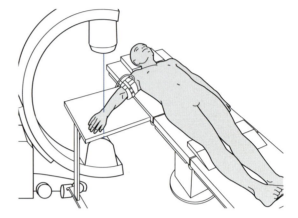

Fig 4.5-8 Position the patient supine and place the forearm on the hand table. Pronate the forearm. The position of the limb should allow complete imaging in the frontal and sagittal planes of the distal radius. A nonsterile pneumatic tourniquet is used. Prophylactic antibiotics are optional.

4 Surgical approach

Approach

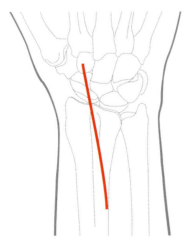

Fig 4.5-9 The surgical approach used was a dorsal approach (see chapter 1.8 Dorsal approach to the distal radius).

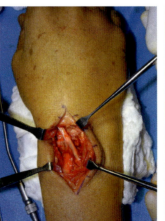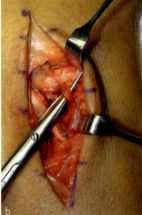

Fig 4.5-10a–b Following the dorsal approach, the extensor pollicis longus was elevated (**a**). The terminal branch of the posterior interosseous nerve was identified (**b**).

4 Surgical approach (cont)

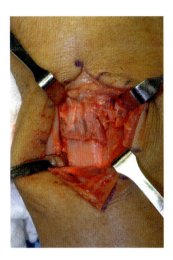

Fig 4.5-11   Through the dorsal exposure, the intermediate and radial column injuries were clearly visible.

5 Reduction

Provisional reduction

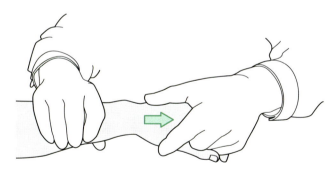

Fig 4.5-12   Reduction is achieved by applying longitudinal traction either manually or using finger traps. The reduction is maintained by a temporary splint. If definitive surgery is planned but cannot be performed within a reasonable time scale, a temporary external fixator may be helpful.

Provisional fixation

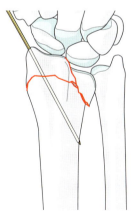

Fig 4.5-13   Insert a K-wire through the tip of the radial styloid to provisionally hold the fragments. Confirm using image intensification.

6 Fixation

Contour the plates

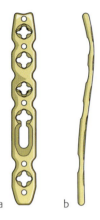

Fig 4.5-14a–b Plates used in treating radial and intermediate column injuries are available precontoured. However, some additional contouring may be necessary to accommodate the individual anatomy of the patient.

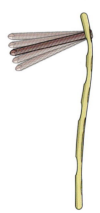

Fig 4.5-15 Variable angle locking plates enable precise positioning of the distal screws in desired directions because there is 30 degrees of freedom for each screw inside the plate hole in order to address the individual fracture patterns.

Pitfall: screw hole distortion

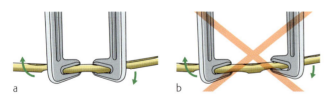

Fig 4.5-16a–b Avoid contouring the plate through the locking holes otherwise the locking head screw might no longer fit.

Fixation of intermediate column
Arthrotomy

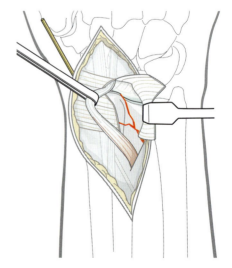

Fig 4.5-17 If direct vision of the articular surface is needed, a limited transverse radiocarpal arthrotomy is performed. The joint surface is now visible. Check the proximal carpal row for additional ligament injuries. The radial insertion of the triangular fibrocartilage complex can also be checked.

6 Fixation (cont)

Reduce the ulnar articular fragment

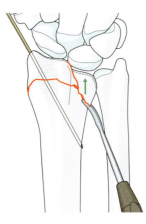

Fig 4.5-18 The intermediate column must now be restored. The ulnar fragment may be found impacted into the metaphysis. This must be levered up to the level of the joint. Anatomically reduce the entire radiocarpal joint under direct vision. Preliminary fixation with K-wires is an option.

Select and apply the plate

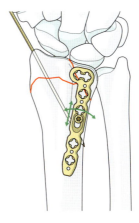

Fig 4.5-19 The appropriate plate is selected according to the fracture configuration. The plate should fit exactly the anatomy of the intermediate column and contoured if necessary. The plate is positioned so that it buttresses the intermediate column and supports the reconstructed radiocarpal joint surface. Fix the plate provisionally to the bone with a standard cortex screw inserted through the oblong plate hole. Before fully tightening it, check the plate position using intraoperative imaging, adjusting the position of the plate as necessary.

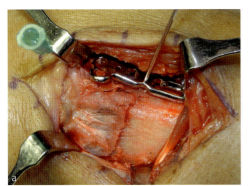
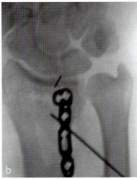
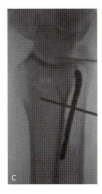

Fig 4.5-20a–c For this patient, following placement of a small needle into the radiocarpal joint for orientation, a VA L-plate 2.4 was positioned and held with a 1.2 mm K-wire (**a**). Intraoperative imaging confirmed the position of the plate and reduction of the intermediate column (**b–c**).

6 Fixation (cont)

Insert proximal screws

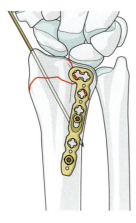

Fig 4.5-21 Insert proximal screws as necessary to complete the fixation of the intermediate column plate.

Insert distal screws

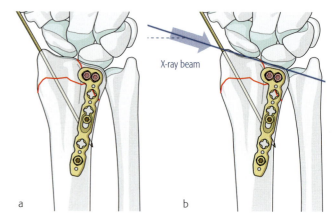

X-ray beam

a   b

Fig 4.5-22a–b Following insertion of the distal locking screws, angled lateral images are taken to confirm extraarticular placement. If the screws appear to enter the radiocarpal joint, they can be repositioned if a VA LCP has been used.

Fixation of radial column
Select and apply the plate

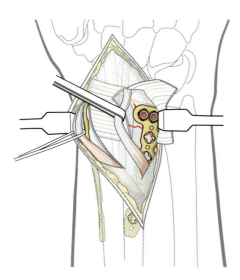

Fig 4.5-23 The appropriate plate is selected according to the fracture configuration and contoured if necessary. Slide the plate underneath the first compartment and apply it onto the radial column.

Stabilize the radial column

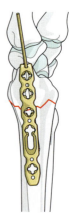

Fig 4.5-24 Ideally while applying the plate, the notch in the distal tip of the implant is placed against the temporary K-wire.

6 Fixation (cont)

Pitfall: incorrect placement

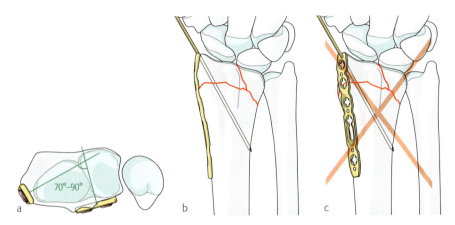

Fig 4.5-25a–c To optimally stabilize the radial styloid, the plates must be positioned correctly at 70–90 degrees to each other. Avoid placement of the radial plate on the dorsal aspect of the radial column, as it will not buttress the reduction adequately against axial shear forces.

Insert the first screw in the radial column plate

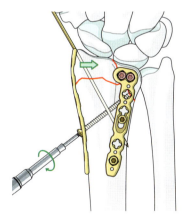

Fig 4.5-26 Insert a standard cortex screw into the oblong plate hole proximal to the fracture. The screw should engage the far cortex. The position of the plate may be adjusted before the screw is tightened. Tightening this screw will reduce the radial styloid.

Insert the first locking head screw

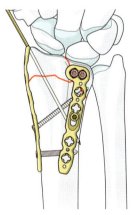

Fig 4.5-27 To prevent rotation of the plate during distal locking screw fixation, the plate should be secured to the bone by inserting the most proximal screw.

6   Fixation (cont)

Insert distal locking head screws and complete the fixation

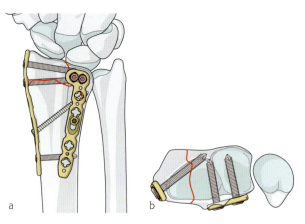

Fig 4.5-28a–b   If a K-wire was used, it is now removed. Distal locking head screw(s) are inserted to support the radial styloid. Confirm screw positioning using the image intensifier.

Distal radioulnar joint assessment

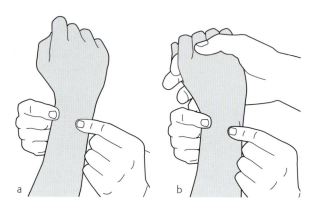

Fig 4.5-29a–b   After fixation, the DRUJ should be assessed for both forearm rotation and stability. The methods for determining if DRUJ instability exists are shown in the fixation topic in chapter 4.1 Radial styloid—fracture treated with a radial column plate.

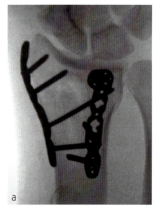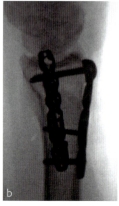

Fig 4.5-30a–b   Intraoperative view of the double plate fixation. The intraoperative image confirmed an anatomical reduction and stable internal fixation.

7 Rehabilitation

Aftercare, follow-up, and functional exercises

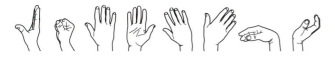

Fig 4.5-31 The patient should receive the standard postoperative rest, injury elevation, follow-up, removal of stitches, and immobilization as required. Following surgery, begin active controlled range of motion exercises. For further information see the rehabilitation topic in chapter 4.1 Radial styloid—fracture treated with a radial column plate.

8 Outcome

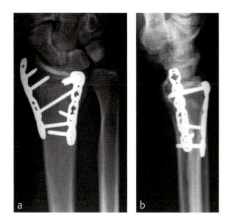

Fig 4.5-32a–b The 4-month follow-up x-rays showed complete fracture union.

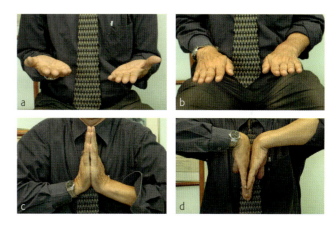

Fig 4.5-33a–d There was excellent pain-free motion and recovery.

8 Outcome (cont)

Video

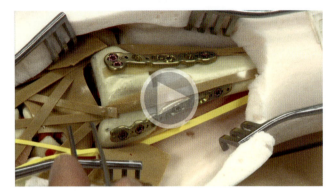

Video 4.5-1   This video demonstrates an intraarticular distal radial fracture treated using dorsal double plate fixation.

4.6 Distal radius—multifragmentary intraarticular fracture treated with a palmar plate

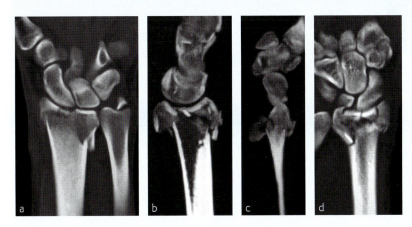

Fig 4.6-1a–d A 38-year-old engineer was injured while participating in a dirt bike competition. When he arrived at the emergency department he complained of pain in his nondominant left wrist, and there was evidence of edema and deformity. The x-rays and CT scans indicated extensive multifragmentation in both the intermediate and radial columns of the distal radius, and on the coronal plane, the articular component and central impaction fragments were apparent.

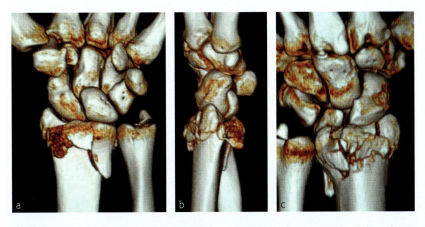

Fig 4.6-2a–c The 3-D CT scans demonstrated the palmar and dorsal multi-fragmentation as well as an ulnar styloid fracture.

---

1   Case description (cont)

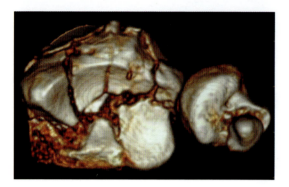

Fig 4.6-3   A view of the joint surface of the radius in the 3-D CT scan showed the severity of the articular component.

In addition to the obvious distal radial injuries there was also a fracture at the base of the ulnar styloid, so all three columns were involved. Treatment for this patient's ulnar styloid fracture has already been discussed in detail in chapter 3.1 Ulnar styloid—fracture treated with tension band wiring, so for the purposes of this chapter, only the multifragmentary distal radial fracture is discussed.

---

2   Indications

Multifragmentary complete intraarticular fractures

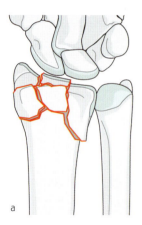 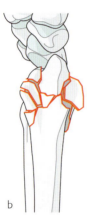

a   b

Fig 4.6-4a–b   Complete intraarticular fractures of the distal radius occur when there is no part of the articular surface in continuity with the diaphysis, and they require anatomical reduction except in low demand patients. When the fracture is multifragmentary it can be classified according to the extent of the metaphyseal fragmentation, varying from those involving fragmentation of the articular surface but with a simple metaphyseal fracture, as seen on the left hand of this patient, to those involving severe fragmentation in the metaphysis, or the most complex with fracture lines extending well into the diaphysis.

Plate fixation is appropriate for these fractures. As long as the articular surface is accurately reduced and is fixed in the correct position in relation to the radial shaft, it is not necessary to fix all the metaphyseal fragments and the plate can be used in a bridging mode.

2 Indications (cont)

Associated ulnar injuries

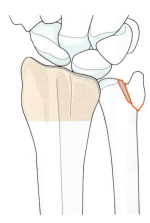

Fig 4.6-5 These injuries can also be accompanied by avulsion of the ulnar styloid and/or disruption of the distal radioulnar joint (DRUJ). If there is gross instability after the fixation of the radial fracture, it is recommended that the ulnar styloid and/or the triangular fibrocartilage (TFC) disc is reattached. This is not common in simple fractures but can occur in some high-energy injuries. The uninjured side should be tested as a reference for the injured side. However, it may not be possible to assess DRUJ stability until the fracture has been stabilized.

Imaging

It is not possible to make an accurate assessment of the details of these injuries without a CT scan.

Choice of implant

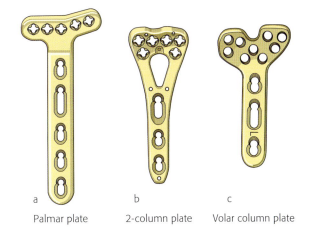

a   b   c

Palmar plate   2-column plate   Volar column plate

Fig 4.6-6a–c In most complete intraarticular fractures with multifragmentation of the articular surface, standard palmar locking plates are long enough to obtain adequate proximal hold. However, if there is multifragmentation involving a significant length of the metaphysis, standard palmar plates may be too short to provide adequate stabilization. Specially designed longer angular stable plates and plates with larger multiple-hole heads and variable angle (VA) locking screw options have been developed to help stabilize the distal and proximal fragments. For this patient, a volar column distal radius plate was selected.

3 Preoperative planning

Equipment

- VA locking compression plate (LCP) distal radius set
- VA LCP volar column plate 2.4
- 1.1 mm or 1.2 mm K-wires

Patient preparation and positioning

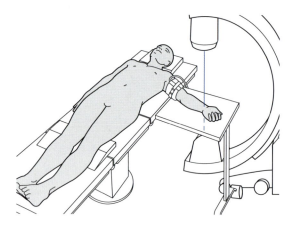

Fig 4.6-7 Position the patient supine and place the forearm on a hand table. Supinate the forearm. The position of the limb should allow complete imaging in the frontal and sagittal plane of the distal radius. A nonsterile pneumatic tourniquet is used. Prophylactic antibiotics are optional.

4 Surgical approach

Approach

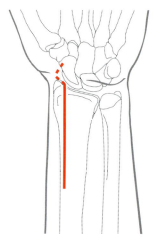

Fig 4.6-8 The surgical approach used was a modified Henry palmar approach (see chapter 1.6 Modified Henry palmar approach to the distal radius).

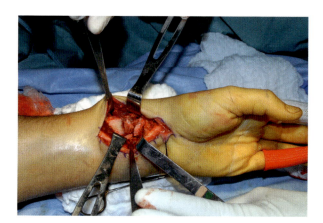

Fig 4.6-9 The radius was exposed through the modified Henry approach where severe fracture fragmentation became apparent.

5 Reduction

Provisional reduction

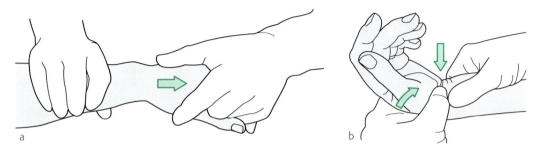

Fig 4.6-10a–b Reduction is achieved by applying longitudinal traction either manually or using finger traps. Manipulative reduction is used to provisionally hold the fragments. The reduction is maintained by a temporary splint. If definitive surgery is planned but cannot be performed within a reasonable time scale a temporary external fixator may be helpful.

6 Fixation

Select the plate

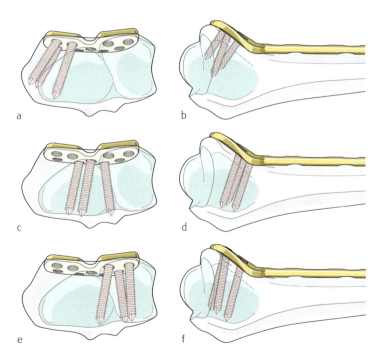

Fig 4.6-11a–f A volar column distal radius plate was used to stabilize the fracture in this case. Volar column plates (VCP) are precontoured for anatomical fit on the palmar aspect of the distal radius. Multiple locking screw holes in the head of the plate provide additional fixation of the radial and intermediate columns, with screw trajectories designed to address a wide variety of fracture types.

6 Fixation (cont)

Apply the plate and insert the first screw

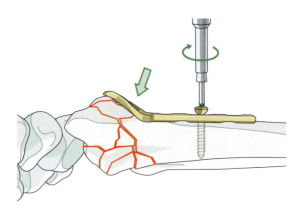

Fig 4.6-12 Apply the VCP to the bone so that the distal end of the plate ends at the anatomical watershed zone of the distal radius. Insert an appropriate cortex screw through the oblong plate hole into the proximal radial fragment. Select a screw that is long enough to engage both cortices. Before fully tightening it, check the plate position using intraoperative imaging, adjusting the position of the plate as necessary.

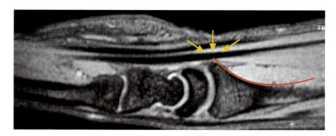

Fig 4.6-13 This sagittal view MRI shows how close the flexor tendons are to the radius (yellow arrows), making it clear that the plate should be placed proximally to the anatomical watershed zone to avoid tendon irritation and ruptures.

Insert the first distal screw

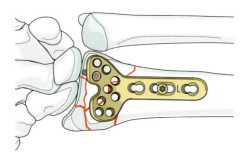

Fig 4.6-14 The initial distal screw should be placed through the ulnar sided screw holes to stabilize the intermediate column. This distal screw should be placed just in the subchondral bone to buttress the articular fragments and to avoid later displacement.

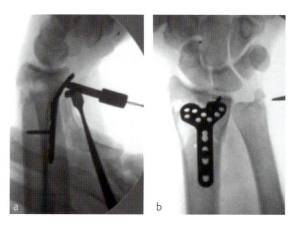

Fig 4.6-15a–b The intraoperative images show the plate being applied to the bone. Once the first screw was introduced through the proximal oblong plate hole, the image intensifier was used to evaluate the direction of the most ulnar distal screw.

6 Fixation (cont)

Insert additional distal screws

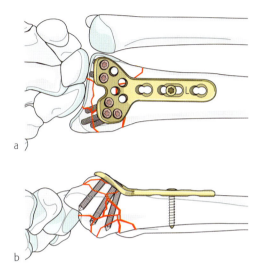

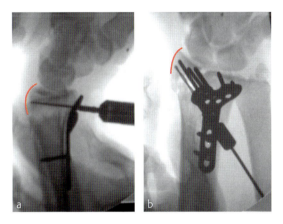

Fig 4.6-17a–b Precise measurement is required to avoid any screw tip protruding through the dorsal aspect of the radius (red line) to avoid tendon ruptures. Screws placed in the radial styloid should reach the tip of the radial styloid for the best purchase. This can be evaluated using the image intensifier.

Fig 4.6-16a–b Insert distal locking head screws to secure articular reduction.

Confirm screw positioning

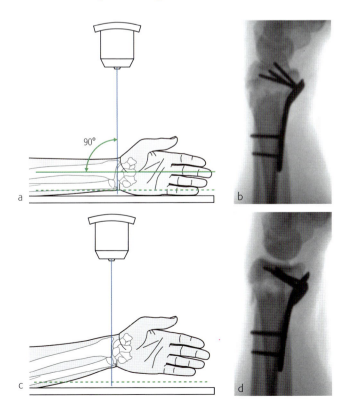

Fig 4.6-18a–d A sagittal image with the angle of the x-ray beam directed 20 degrees obliquely to the radius can confirm that the screw is not penetrating the radiocarpal joint. With this view, the subchondral positioning of the distal screws is accurately evaluated. If the screw is found to penetrate the articular surface, it must be removed and repositioned.

6 Fixation (cont)

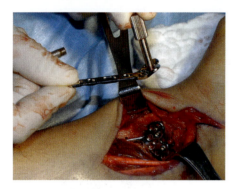

Fig 4.6-19 This intraoperative image demonstrates how placing the drill guide into the distal holes of the plate assists in evaluating the direction of the screws.

Insert proximal screws and complete the fixation

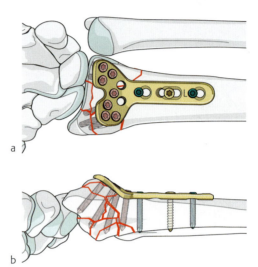

Fig 4.6-20a–b Insert further proximal screws as required and complete the fixation.

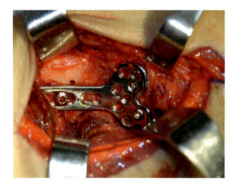

Fig 4.6-21 Further screws were inserted and the distal radius fixation later completed.

Distal radioulnar joint assessment

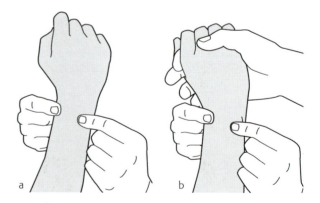

Fig 4.6-22a–b After fixation, the DRUJ should be assessed for both forearm rotation and stability. The methods for determining if DRUJ instability exists are shown in the fixation topic in chapter 4.1 Radial styloid—fracture treated with a radial column plate.

6 Fixation (cont)

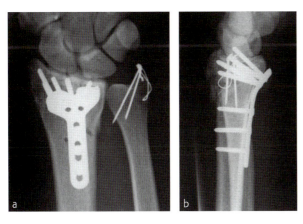

Fig 4.6-23a–b AP and lateral x-rays were taken 1 week after surgery to confirm perfect reduction of the fractures and correct location of implants.

7 Rehabilitation

Aftercare, follow-up, and functional exercises

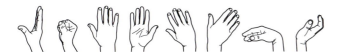

Fig 4.6-24 The patient should receive the standard postoperative rest, injury elevation, follow-up, removal of stitches, and immobilization as required. Following surgery, begin active controlled range of motion exercises. For further information see the rehabilitation topic in chapter 4.1 Radial styloid—fracture treated with a radial column plate.

8 Outcome

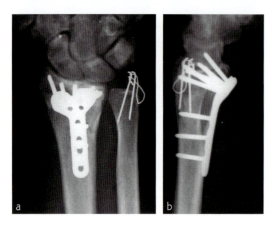

Fig 4.6-25a–b At the 1-year follow-up, there was an excellent radiological outcome.

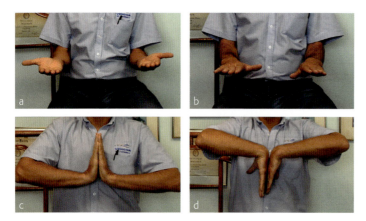

Fig 4.6-26a–d There was also an excellent functional outcome with no pain. The patient had returned to his normal work and motor bike sporting activities.

4.7 Distal radius—multifragmentary intraarticular fracture with defect treated with a palmar plate

1 Case description

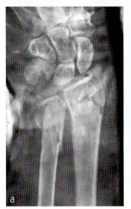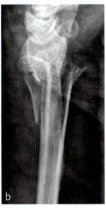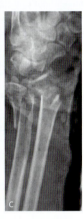

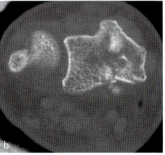

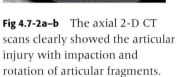

Fig 4.7-1a–c   A 57-year-old professional housekeeper tripped and fell onto her outstretched right wrist while walking a dog. She presented to the emergency department with a swollen wrist but with a normal neurovascular examination. The AP, lateral, and oblique x-rays demonstrated a multifragmentary complete intraarticular fracture of the distal radius with extension into the metaphysis as well as a complex fracture of the distal ulna extending into the ulnar head.

Fig 4.7-2a–b   The axial 2-D CT scans clearly showed the articular injury with impaction and rotation of articular fragments.

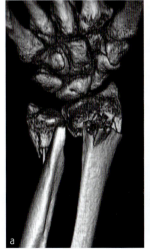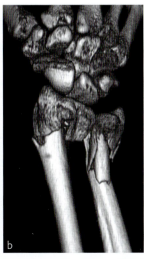

Fig 4.7-3a–b   The extension of the radial fracture into the distal diaphyseal-metaphyseal junction is shown in the 3-D CT scans.

For this patient, both the distal ulna and radius sustained multifragmentary fractures requiring open reduction and internal fixation. However, for the purposes of this chapter, only the distal radius is discussed. For further information on treating distal ulnar fractures see chapter 3.2 Ulna, head and neck—multifragmentary fracture treated with a hook plate.

309

2   Indications

Multifragmentary complete intraarticular fractures with metaphyseal defect

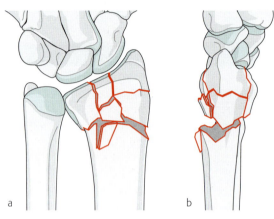

Fig 4.7-4a–b   In some instances, complete intraarticular fractures of the distal radius can involve severe fragmentation in the metaphysis resulting in a metaphyseal defect. There are often small articular fragments and impacted fragments. Anatomical reduction and stabilization of these intraarticular fractures is essential because of the functional implications of the involvement of the distal radioulnar joint (DRUJ). Plate fixation is appropriate provided the distal fragments are large enough to be held with screws. As long as the articular surface is accurately reduced and is fixed in the correct position in relation to the radial shaft it is not necessary to fix all the metaphyseal fragments.

Associated ulnar injuries

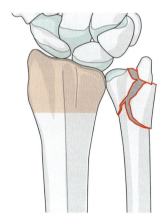

Fig 4.7-5   Head, neck, and multifragmentary fractures of the distal ulna often occur in combination with distal radial fractures. With these ulnar fractures there is instability and shortening, so the distal ulna hook plate can be used to hold the fracture. Attention should be paid to restoring correct rotation and length in relation to the radius. Complete dislocation of the radiocarpal joint is often associated with disruption of the distal radioulnar joint (DRUJ).

Imaging

It is not possible to make an accurate assessment of the details of these injuries without a CT scan.

2 Indications (cont)

Choice of implant

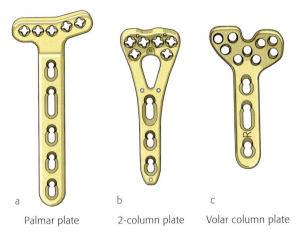

a Palmar plate

b 2-column plate

c Volar column plate

Fig 4.7-6a–c In most complete intraarticular fractures with multifragmentation of the articular surface, standard palmar locking plates are long enough to obtain adequate proximal hold. However, if there is multifragmentation involving a significant length of the metaphysis, standard palmar plates may be too short to provide adequate stabilization. Specially designed longer angular stable plates and plates with larger multiple-hole heads and variable angle (VA) locking screw options have been developed to help stabilize the distal and proximal fragments. For this patient, a 2-column palmar plate with the longer 3-hole shaft was selected.

3 Preoperative planning

Equipment

- VA locking compression plate (LCP) distal radius set
- VA LCP 2-column plate 2.4
- 1.1 mm or 1.2 mm K-wires
- Pointed reduction forceps
- Small external fixator for the distal radius
- Ball tip reduction forceps
- Laminar spreader
- Image intensifier

Patient preparation and positioning

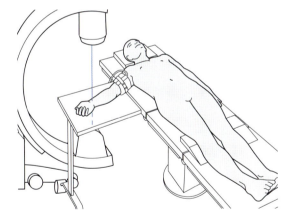

Fig 4.7-7 Position the patient supine and place the forearm on a hand table. Supinate the forearm. The position of the limb should allow complete imaging in the frontal and sagittal plane of the distal radius. A nonsterile pneumatic tourniquet is used. Prophylactic antibiotics are optional.

4 Surgical approach

Approach

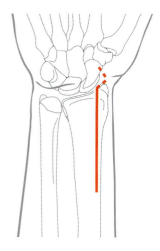

Fig 4.7-8 The surgical approach used was a modified Henry palmar approach (see chapter 1.6 Modified Henry palmar approach to the distal radius).

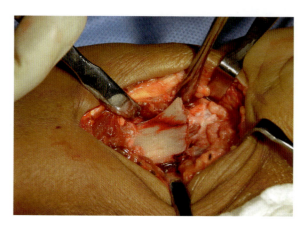

Fig 4.7-9 Through the modified Henry approach, the palmar fracture lines were exposed.

5 Reduction

Provisional reduction

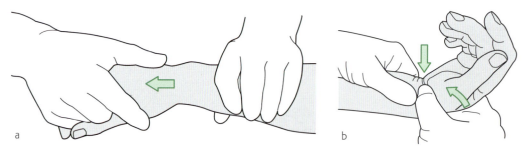

Fig 4.7-10a–b Reduction is achieved by applying longitudinal traction either manually or using finger traps. Manipulative reduction is used to provisionally hold the fragments. The reduction is maintained by a temporary splint. If definitive surgery is planned but cannot be performed within a reasonable time scale a temporary external fixator may be helpful.

5 Reduction (cont)

Provisional fixation with K-wires

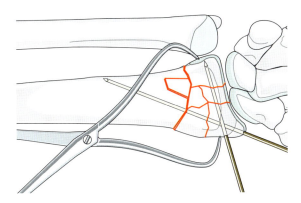

Fig 4.7-11 Insert a K-wire across the fracture, through the radial styloid, to provide provisional stabilization. The major articular fragments can be reduced with the aid of a pointed reduction forceps. Temporary fixation of the major articular fragments with K-wires is also an option. The aim is to achieve an accurate anatomical reduction of the articular fragments before the plate is applied.

Provisional reduction with an external fixator

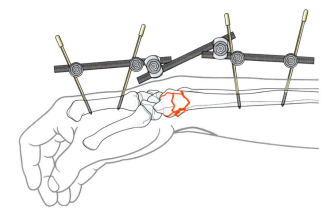

Fig 4.7-12 In cases of extensive metaphyseal and/or diaphyseal comminution, reduction can be achieved and maintained with the help of an external fixator.

Reduction with a spreader/manual traction

In cases of moderate fragmentation on the dorsal and palmar cortex, it is difficult to maintain temporary reduction with K-wires. Reduction with the help of a spreader and/or manual traction is then recommended.

5 Reduction (cont)

Reduction using a ball tip reduction forceps

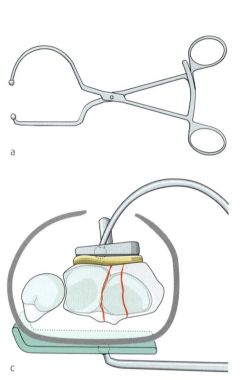

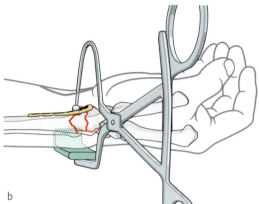

Fig 4.7-13a–c An alternate method to ensure reduction is by using a ball tip reduction forceps (**a**). Using a bolster or towel to assist with flexing the wrist can sometimes make it difficult to access the distal segments of the radius, yet lying the wrist flat on the table can make access easier but fracture reduction more difficult. With the ball tip reduction forceps, the thick rubber on the dorsal side helps to reduce the dorsal aspect of the fracture without putting stress on the tendons or the skin (**b–c**).

6 Fixation

Select and apply the plate and insert distal screws

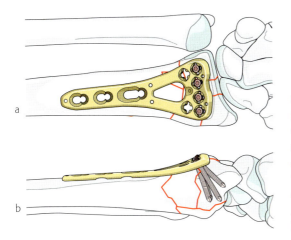

Fig 4.7-14a–b The locking plate is first positioned distally on the flat reduced palmar surface of the distal radius at the anatomical watershed zone and fixed with distal locking screws parallel to the articular surface with at least one but preferably two screw(s) in each articular fragment, depending on the quality of bone stock. The first screw inserted is the ulnar one and its position should be checked under image intensification with the hand elevated 20–30 degrees off the table, in lunate facet view. Once the articular block is securely held to the plate any K-wire(s) can be removed.

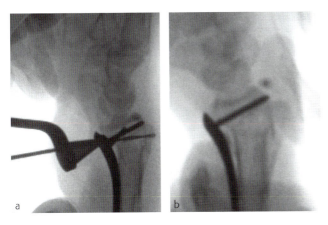

Fig 4.7-15a–b Intraoperative images confirmed the placement of the plate and preliminary screw placement.

6 Fixation (cont)

Determine correct bone length

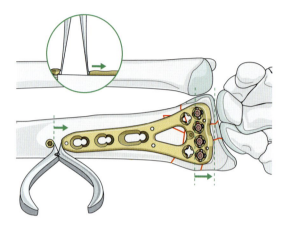

Fig 4.7-16 The correct length of the radius in relation to the ulna should be established preoperatively by taking x-rays of the opposite wrist. The length of the radius in relation to the ulna is then achieved by inserting a unicortical screw, just proximal of the proximal end of the plate, and then using a spreader as illustrated to move the plate gently distally.

Insert first proximal screw

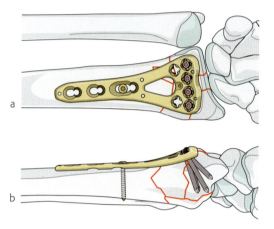

Fig 4.7-17a–b Once the correct length is achieved, the plate is provisionally fixed proximally with an appropriate cortex screw through the oblong hole.

Insert proximal locking screws and complete the fixation

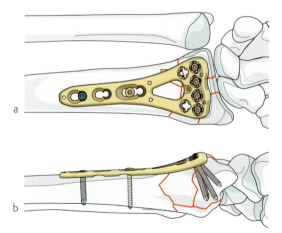

Fig 4.7-18a–b The relationship of the radius to the distal ulna is checked under image intensification before the plate is fixed with additional proximal locking screws.

6   Fixation (cont)

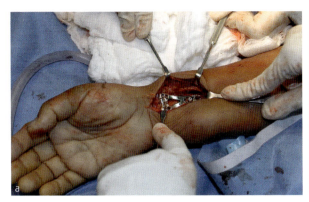
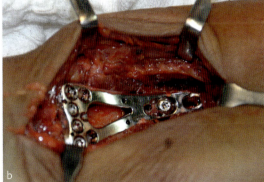

Fig 4.7-19a–b   Two views of the VA LCP palmar plate 2.4 in position after placement of the remaining screws.

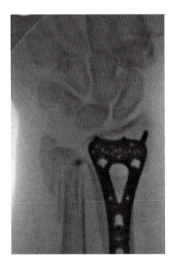

Fig 4.7-20   Intraoperative image following fixation of the distal radius.

Distal radioulnar joint assessment

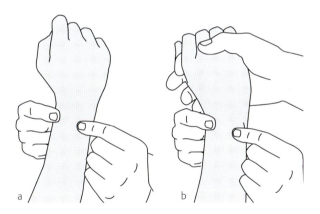

Fig 4.7-21a–b   After fixation, the DRUJ should be assessed for both forearm rotation and stability. The methods for determining if DRUJ instability exists are shown in the fixation topic in chapter 4.1 Radial styloid—fracture treated with a radial column plate.

7 Rehabilitation

Aftercare, follow-up, and functional exercises

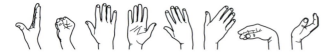

Fig 4.7-22 The patient should receive the standard postoperative rest, injury elevation, follow-up, removal of stitches, and immobilization as required. Following surgery, begin active controlled range of motion exercises. For further information see the rehabilitation topic in chapter 4.1 Radial styloid—fracture treated with a radial column plate.

8 Outcome

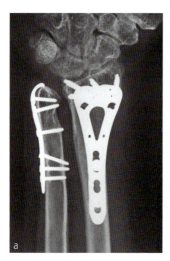
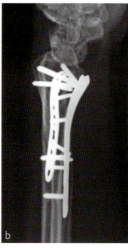

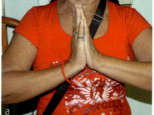
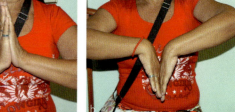
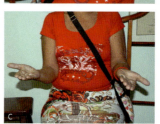

Fig 4.7-23a–b At the 6-month follow-up, the AP and lateral x-rays demonstrated full healing in an anatomical position.

Fig 4.7-24a–c By this stage, nearly full wrist and forearm motion had been achieved.

4.8 Distal radius—multifragmentary intraarticular fracture treated with triple plating

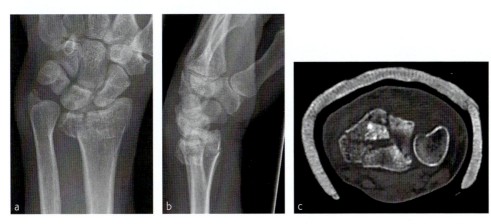

Fig 4.8-1a–c A 48-year-old office manager fell onto her dominant outstretched left hand when she tripped over a box in her office. She sustained a multifragmentary intraarticular fracture of the left distal radius. The PA and lateral x-rays revealed the complex nature of the distal radial fracture. Axial 2-D CT scans further demonstrated the involvement of the articular surfaces of both columns of the distal radius and the articular surface of the distal radioulnar joint.

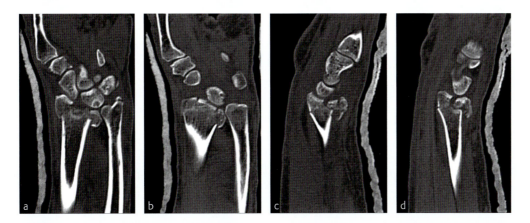

Fig 4.8-2a–d Additional sagittal and coronal 2-D CT scans revealed the impacted and displaced intraarticular component of the radial fracture in both radial and intermediate columns (**a**), as well as the comminuted nature of the articular fragments (**b**), the palmar displacement of the lunate facet component (**c**), and the impacted and unstable nature of the scaphoid facet component (**d**).

2   Indications

Complete intraarticular fractures with impaction

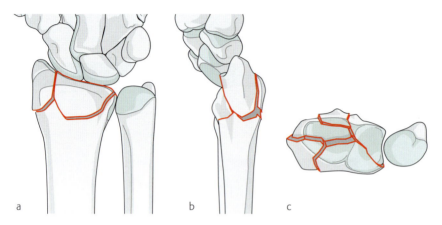

a   b   c

Fig 4.8-3a–c   A strong force or fall can be enough to cause a complete intraarticular fracture of the distal radius with no part of the articular surface in continuity with the diaphysis. Multifragmentation can result, as can fracture lines extending into the diaphysis. Additionally, the injury can involve impaction, which can occur in the more osteoporotic bone of an elderly patient or in younger patients typically as a result of high-energy trauma. As these are intraarticular fractures, where possible, they should be treated with anatomical reduction and absolute stability to minimize the risk of subsequent degenerative changes in the joint. Use of CT scans can be helpful for treatment decisions.

2   Indications (cont)

Principle of columns

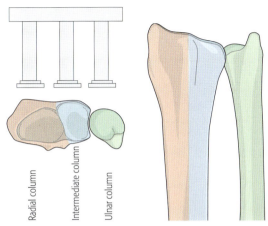

Fig 4.8-4   The distal forearm can be thought of in terms of three columns. The ulna forms one column (the ulnar column) while the radius can be separated into two (the intermediate column and the radial column). The 3-column principle helps in describing the location of wrist injuries and is further explained in the indications topic in chapter 1.8 Dorsal approach to the distal radius.

In injury types similar to this patient, understanding of the 3-column principle is particularly helpful in preparing a plan for surgical reduction and stabilization and will assist in interpretation of the imaging. It must be remembered that the intermediate column provides articular surfaces for both the radiocarpal and the distal radioulnar joints, so injuries to this column demand attention to reconstruct both components.

When facing injuries of this nature, open reduction and a combination of palmar and dorsal internal fixation are likely to be required. The rationale for using both palmar and dorsal approaches includes: the displaced palmoulnar fragment (intermediate column) and the rotated radial styloid (radial column) requiring a palmar approach; and the displaced and unstable dorsal fragment with central impaction (intermediate column) requiring a dorsal approach and arthrotomy. Appreciation of injuries to each column assists in planning the order of fixation.

2 Indications (cont)

Associated median nerve compression

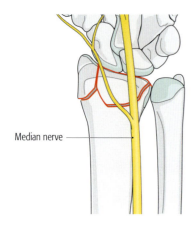

Median nerve

Fig 4.8-5 If there is dense sensory loss, or other signs of median nerve compression, the median nerve should be decompressed from the level of the fracture into the palm, releasing the carpal tunnel.

Choice of implant

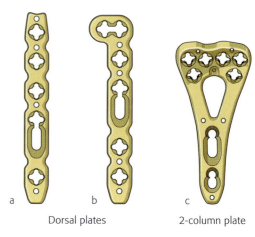

a   b   c

Dorsal plates   2-column plate

Fig 4.8-6a–c This case involves treatment of both the dorsal and palmar aspect, and so specific palmar and dorsal plates were selected including variable angle locking compression plate (VA LCP) dorsal distal radius plates and a VA LCP 2-column plate on the palmar side.

3 Preoperative planning

Equipment

- VA LCP distal radius set
- VA LCP 2-column plate 2.4
- VA LCP radial column plate 2.4
- VA LCP intermediate column plate 2.4
- 1.1 mm or 1.2 mm K-wires
- Image intensifier

Patient preparation and positioning

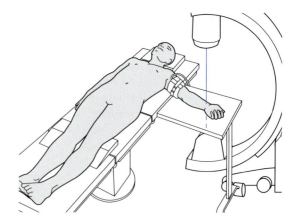

Fig 4.8-7 Position the patient supine and place the forearm on a hand table. The palmar approach will require the forearm to be placed in supination. A dorsal approach requires the forearm to be pronated. The position of the limb should allow complete imaging in the frontal and sagittal plane of the distal radius. A nonsterile pneumatic tourniquet is used. Prophylactic antibiotics are optional.

4 Surgical approach

Palmar and dorsal approaches

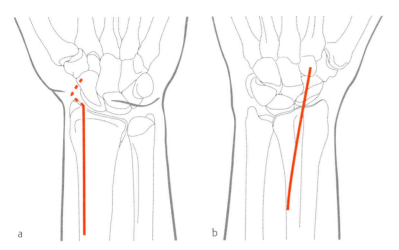

Fig 4.8-8a–b The initial surgical approach was a modified Henry palmar approach (see chapter 1.6 Modified Henry palmar approach to the distal radius). Subsequently, a dorsal approach was required to reduce and stabilize the dorsal components with dorsal implants and to perform an arthrotomy to assess articular reduction and to inspect the integrity of the intrinsic ligaments (see chapter 1.8 Dorsal approach to the distal radius).

5 Reduction and fixation

Provisional reduction

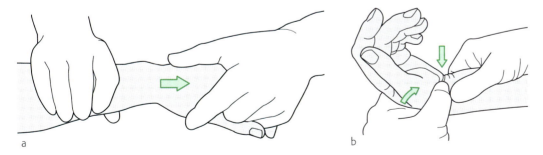

Fig 4.8-9a–b Reduction is achieved by applying longitudinal traction either manually or using finger traps. Manipulative reduction is used to provisionally hold the fragments. The reduction is maintained by a temporary splint. If definitive surgery is planned but cannot be performed within a reasonable time scale a temporary external fixator may be helpful.

Reduction is achieved by first recreating a stable palmar cortex so that the dorsal and articular fractures can be reduced against it in buttress mode.

5   Reduction and fixation (cont)

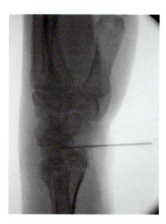

Fig 4.8-10   A hypodermic needle was placed into the radiolunate joint under image intensification to accurately define the distal limit of the distal radius for placement of the implant.

Reduction using the plate

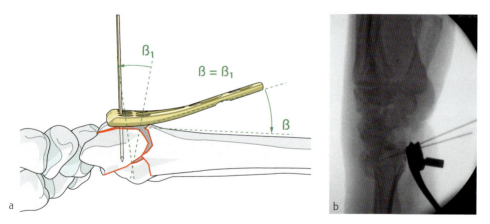

Fig 4.8-11a–b   Select and apply the palmar plate to the distal fragment (**a**). Insert temporary K-wires to stabilize the implant and to secure the correct position for implant placement. The nominal angle drill guide block is used to prevent inadvertent intraarticular screw penetration. Confirm using image intensification. A VA LCP 2-column plate was applied to the palmar surface of the distal radius under image intensification (**b**).

5 Reduction and fixation (cont)

Insert distal screws

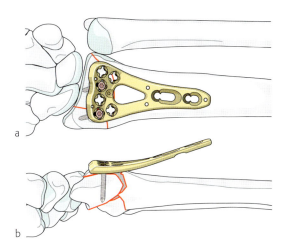

Fig 4.8-12a–b Short nominal angle locking screws are inserted into the palmar fragments only.

Insert proximal screws

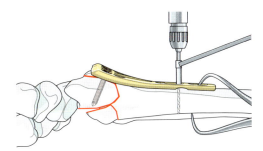

Fig 4.8-14 Once satisfactory reduction is confirmed, insert an appropriate cortex screw through the oblong plate hole.

Apply the plate to the shaft

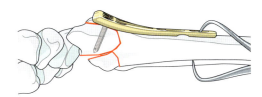

Fig 4.8-13 The implant is then used to reduce the fragments by pushing it onto the surface of the radius. Bring the plate onto the shaft and hold it with a forceps. Check correct placement with imaging and adjust the position of the distal fragment if necessary by moving the plate.

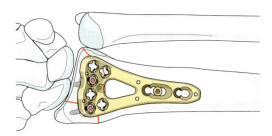

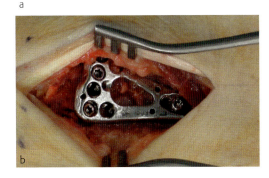

Fig 4.8-15a–b Using the palmar surgical approach, fixation of the palmar fragments of the intermediate column (lunate facet) was achieved using the VA LCP 2-column plate 2.4 with short locking screws. The palmar buttress was then reestablished.

5 Reduction and fixation (cont)

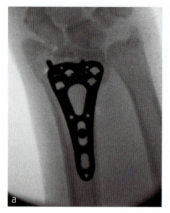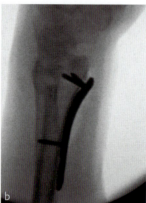

Fig 4.8-16a–b The procedure restores the palmar buttress that had been lost due to the fracture pattern. Intraoperative images confirm the reduction and stabilization of the displaced palmar fragments of the intermediate column.

It must be appreciated that neither the dorsal fragments of the intermediate column nor the fragments of the radial column have yet been reduced or stabilized. However, the restoration of an intact and stable palmar buttress allows these components of the fracture to be treated.

Dorsal plates fixation

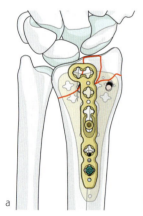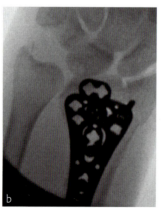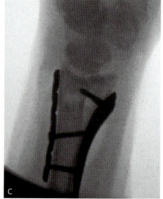

Fig 4.8-17a–c The dorsal surgical approach allows placement of VA LCP dorsal distal radius plates. Initially, the dorsal fragments of the intermediate column (and therefore also the distal radioulnar joint) were reduced by buttressing against the newly stabilized palmar surface/implant. The intermediate column can then be reduced and stabilized. The lunate facet of the distal radius and the distal radioulnar joint surfaces were restored.

5 Reduction and fixation (cont)

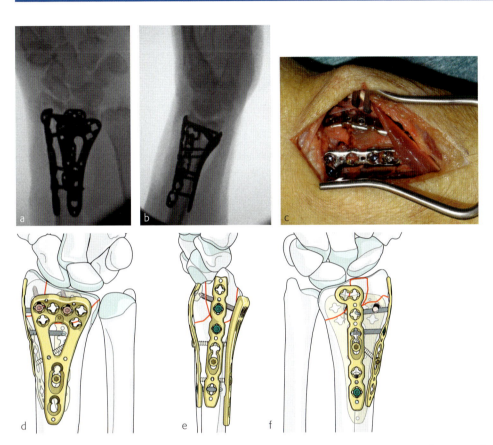

Fig 4.8-18a–f   Finally, the radial column is stabilized by the application of a radial VA LCP dorsal distal radius plate that also acts in buttress mode, this time buttressing against the reduced and stabilized intermediate column. The total combination of plates provides perfect reduction of all fragments and stable fixation. Intraoperative images and illustrations show the completed triple plating of the distal radial fracture. For further information on the steps for dorsal plating see chapter 4.5 Distal radius—dorsally displaced intraarticular fracture treated with double plating.

6 Rehabilitation

Aftercare, follow-up, and functional exercises

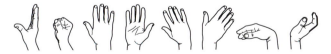

Fig 4.8-19   The patient should receive the standard postoperative rest, injury elevation, follow-up, removal of stitches, and immobilization as required. Following surgery, begin active controlled range of motion exercises. For further information see the rehabilitation topic in chapter 4.1 Radial styloid—fracture treated with a radial column plate.

7   Outcome

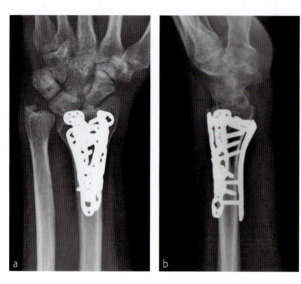

Fig 4.8-20a–b   At the 2-year follow-up, x-rays confirmed the fractures had healed anatomically.

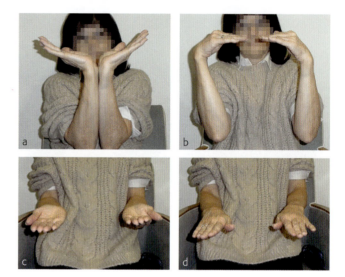

Fig 4.8-21a–d   The patient returned to normal function with no pain and a minor degree of restriction of flexion.

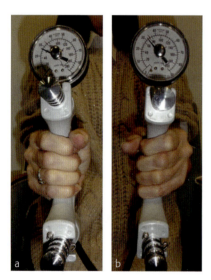

Fig 4.8-22a–b   The injured side (the dominant left hand) was now demonstrating greater grip strength than the uninjured nondominant side.

4.9 Distal radius—multifragmentary intraarticular fracture with associated scaphoid fracture treated with triple plating and screw

1 Case description

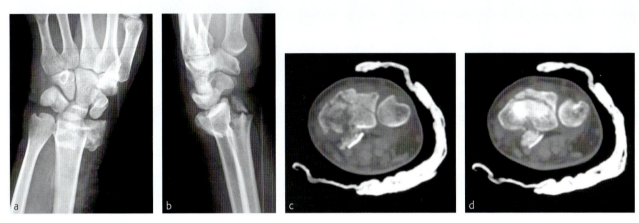

Fig 4.9-1a–d A 32-year-old salesman fell onto his outstretched left hand while running during a soccer match. He sustained a multifragmentary intraarticular distal radial fracture and an associated fracture of the proximal pole of the scaphoid. The PA and lateral x-rays of the left hand revealed the complex nature of the fractures in the radius and the scaphoid. Axial 2-D CT scans further demonstrated the major articular involvement of the distal radius scaphoid facet.

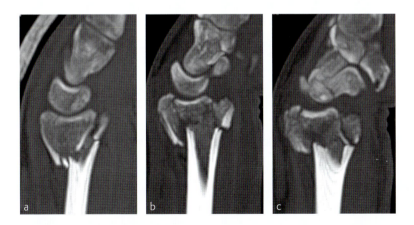

Fig 4.9-2a–c Additional sagittal 2-D CT scans made clear the distal radial and scaphoid fractures, showing the dorsal displacement (**a**), the centrally impacted intraarticular component of the radial fracture (**b**), and the proximal pole fracture of the scaphoid (**c**).

1 Case description (cont)

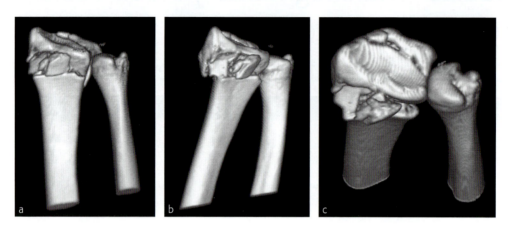

Fig 4.9-3a–c The 3-D CT images identified both palmar and dorsal metaphyseal aspects of the radial fracture and the multifragmentation of the articular surface.

2 Indications

Complete intraarticular fractures with associated carpal injuries

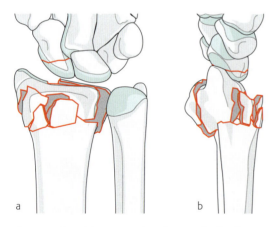

Fig 4.9-4a–b When complete intraarticular fractures of the distal radius occur, multifragmentation can often result, as can fracture lines extending into the diaphysis, and treatment must involve anatomical reduction and stabilization. Yet any patient who suffers high-energy impact onto an outstretched hand can also sustain intercarpal ligament injuries and carpal fractures. These can easily be missed on initial clinical assessment. Use of CT scans can be helpful for treatment decisions.

For injuries described above, open reduction and a combination of palmar and dorsal internal fixation may be required. The rationale for using both palmar and dorsal approaches includes: the hyperextended palmoulnar fragment (intermediate column) and the rotated radial styloid (radial column) requiring a palmar approach; and a displaced dorsal fragment and the impacted central articular fragment (intermediate column) requiring a dorsal approach and arthrotomy, and in this case a dorsal approach to treat the scaphoid proximal pole fracture.

4 Distal radius

4.9 Distal radius—multifragmentary intraarticular fracture with associated scaphoid fracture treated with triple plating and screw

2 Indications (cont)

Associated median nerve compression

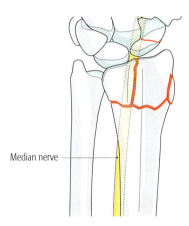

Median nerve

Fig 4.9-5 If there is dense sensory loss, or other signs of median nerve compression, the median nerve should be decompressed.

Anatomical and vascularity considerations

The scaphoid's unique anatomy and vascularity are critically important in cases involving the proximal pole. Refer to the indications topic in chapter 2.1 Scaphoid—nondisplaced fracture treated percutaneously with a headless compression screw for more information.

Associated scaphoid injuries

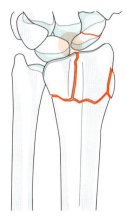

Fig 4.9-6 With high-energy distal radial injuries of this nature, associated carpal ligament injuries and fractures including the scaphoid can occur. The scaphoid proximal pole relies largely on a retrograde blood flow and so it relies on distal-to-proximal intraosseous blood supply for healing. This makes these fractures highly prone to avascular bone necrosis, delayed union, and nonunion. If the proximal fragment is large enough, a 2.4 mm or 3.0 mm implant using antegrade insertion is advisable.

Choice of implant

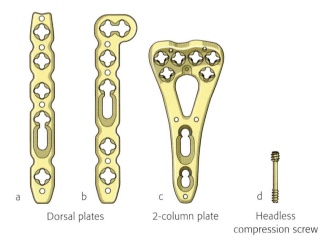

a	b	c	d
Dorsal plates		2-column plate	Headless compression screw

Fig 4.9-7a–d This case involves treatment of both the dorsal and palmar aspect, and so specific palmar and dorsal plates were selected including variable angle locking compression plate (VA LCP) dorsal distal radius plates and a VA LCP 2-column plate on the palmar side. A 3.0 mm headless compression screw was used to treat the scaphoid fracture.

3   **Preoperative planning**

Equipment

- VA LCP distal radius set
- VA LCP 2-column plate 2.4
- VA LCP radial column plate 2.4
- VA LCP intermediate column plate 2.4
- 1.1 mm or 1.2 mm K-wires
- 2.4 mm or 3.0 mm headless compression screw
- Pointed reduction forceps
- Image intensifier

Patient preparation and positioning

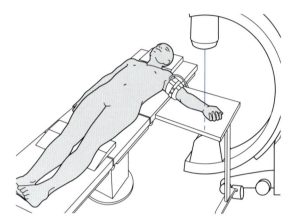

Fig 4.9-8   Position the patient supine and place the forearm on a hand table. As the first step involves a palmar approach, supinate the forearm. If a dorsal approach is also required, pronate the forearm at that stage. The position of the limb should allow complete imaging in the frontal and sagittal plane of the distal radius. A nonsterile pneumatic tourniquet is used. Prophylactic antibiotics are optional.

4   **Surgical approach**

Palmar and dorsal approaches

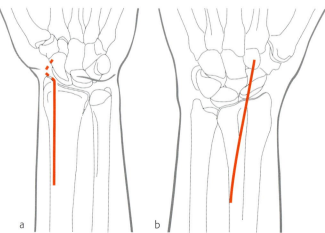

Fig 4.9-9a–b   The surgical approach initially used was a modified Henry palmar approach (see chapter 1.6 Modified Henry palmar approach to the distal radius). Later, a dorsal approach was required to apply dorsal plating and to treat the scaphoid fracture (see chapter 1.8 Dorsal approach to the distal radius).

4 Distal radius

4.9 Distal radius—multifragmentary intraarticular fracture with associated scaphoid fracture treated with triple plating and screw

5 Reduction

Provisional reduction

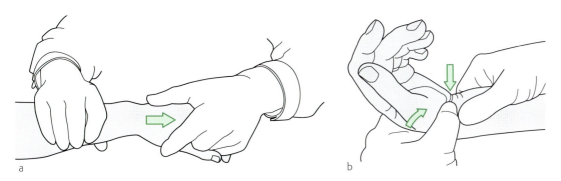

Fig 4.9-10a–b Reduction is achieved by applying longitudinal traction either manually or using finger traps. Manipulative reduction is used to provisionally hold the fragments. The reduction is maintained by a temporary splint. If definitive surgery is planned but cannot be performed within a reasonable time scale a temporary external fixator may be helpful.

Provisional fixation with K-wires

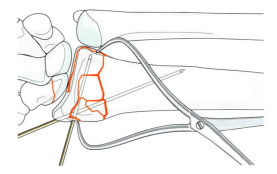

Fig 4.9-11 Insert a K-wire across the fracture through the radial styloid to provide provisional stabilization. The major articular fragments can be reduced with the aid of a pointed reduction forceps. Temporary fixation of the major articular fragments with K-wires is also an option. The aim is to achieve as accurate an anatomical reduction as possible of the articular fragments before the plate is applied.

Alternatively, use of a pointed reduction forceps or an external fixator to achieve reduction may be required.

6 Fixation

Palmar plate fixation

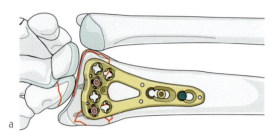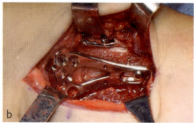

Fig 4.9-12a–b Using a palmar approach, fixation of the distal radial fragments was first attempted using a VA LCP 2-column plate 2.4.

The fixation procedure follows the usual steps of selecting and applying the plate, inserting distal screws, determining correct bone length, inserting proximal screws, and intraoperative imaging. For further information on these steps see chapter 4.7 Distal radius—multifragmentary intraarticular fracture treated with a palmar plate.

Dorsal plate fixation

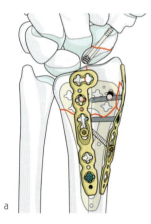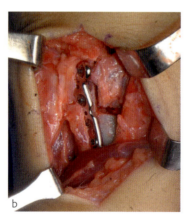

Fig 4.9-13a–b Unfortunately, the dorsal fragments were not reduced solely with the palmar plate, so additional dorsal implants were required. These fragments were then stabilized using VA LCP dorsal distal radius plates, one in the radial column, which was able to be inserted through the existing palmar approach, and the other in the intermediate column using a dorsal L-plate to buttress the fragments (but with no distal screws inserted into the head of the plate), and where a new dorsal approach was required. The total combination of plates provided perfect reduction of all fragments and stable fixation. For further information on the steps for dorsal plating see chapter 4.5 Distal radius—dorsally displaced intraarticular fracture treated with double plating.

4 Distal radius

4.9 Distal radius—multifragmentary intraarticular fracture with associated scaphoid fracture treated with triple plating and screw

6   Fixation (cont)

Scaphoid reduction and fixation

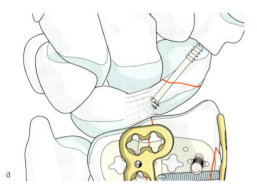
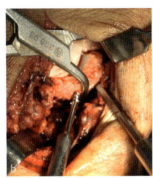

Fig 4.9-14a–b   Following reduction and insertion of a guide wire into the scaphoid, the scaphoid proximal pole fracture fixation was achieved using a 3.0 mm headless compression screw. For further information on treating scaphoid proximal pole fractures see chapter 2.4 Scaphoid, proximal pole—fracture treated with a headless compression screw.

6 Fixation (cont)

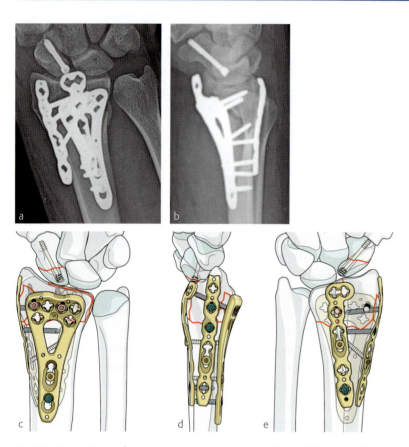

Fig 4.9-15a–e   Immediate postoperative x-rays (**a–b**) and illustrated versions (**c–e**) show the completed triple plating of the distal radial fracture and the internal screw fixation of the scaphoid.

7 Rehabilitation

Aftercare, follow-up, and functional exercises

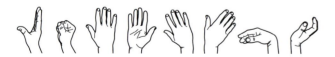

Fig 4.9-16   The patient should receive the standard postoperative rest, injury elevation, follow-up, removal of stitches, and immobilization as required. Following surgery, begin active controlled range of motion exercises. For further information see the rehabilitation topic in chapter 4.1 Radial styloid—fracture treated with a radial column plate.

4 Distal radius

4.9 Distal radius—multifragmentary intraarticular fracture with associated scaphoid fracture treated with triple plating and screw

8   Outcome

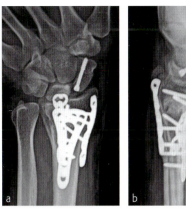
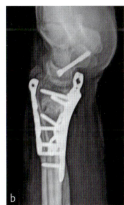

Fig 4.9-17a–b   At the 20-month follow-up, x-rays were taken with ulnar deviation of the wrist, and lateral view. The fractures were shown to have healed in near anatomical position.

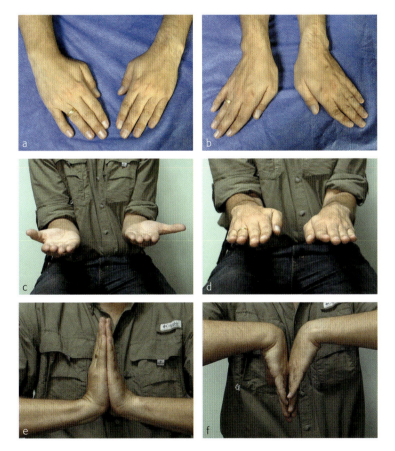

Fig 4.9-18a–f   The patient could perform near full wrist and forearm range of motion and there had been an excellent functional result.

8 Outcome (cont)

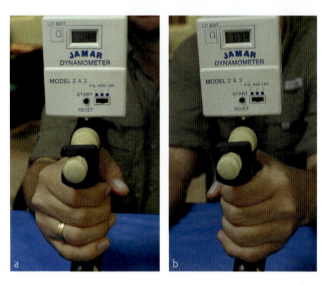

Fig 4.9-19a–b Excellent grip strength had returned when compared with the uninjured side.

4.10 Distal radius—displaced intraarticular fracture treated with a bridge plate

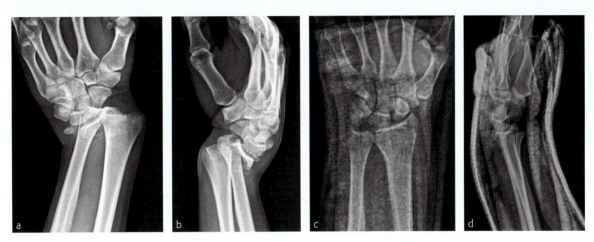

Fig 4.10-1a–d   A 29-year-old professional motorcyclist was involved in a high-speed crash while competing, sustaining an isolated right wrist injury. Upon admission to the emergency department he had median nerve dysfunction, which resolved with longitudinal traction using finger traps and closed reduction. The initial oblique and lateral x-rays demonstrated marked dorsal displacement of the articular surface with fragments that were small and close to the joint (**a–b**). Later AP and lateral x-rays were taken following plaster splint application, yet while the median nerve symptoms were resolved and reduction improved, the reduction remained unsatisfactory (**c–d**).

Given the unstable fracture pattern in and around the articular surface, and the proximity of the fractures to the joint, it was decided that internal fixation was indicated using a bridging plate technique. (Note: some additional intraoperative images from a 46-year-old woman with a similar fracture have been used in this case for further illustrative support).

2   Indications

Intraarticular wrist fractures requiring bridge plating

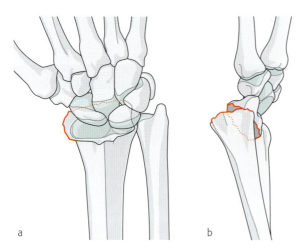

Fig 4.10-2a–b   The patient in this case had suffered displacement of the articular surface with fragmentation that was small and close to the joint. In some intraarticular distal radial fractures, the use of an extended surgical approach and a longer plate that bridges (or spans) the entire joint must be considered. The current indications for using this treatment technique include:

- Extremely fragmented intraarticular fractures in which fragment specific fixation may be unattainable due to the small size of the fragments
- Distal fractures that are so close to the joint that fixation with plates becomes extremely difficult or impossible
- High-energy injuries in polytraumatized patients where early weightbearing on the upper extremities is deemed necessary to help mobilize the patient in the early postoperative period, or where weightbearing was thought not as reliable when using other constructs
- Patients with osteoporotic fractures with significant fragmentation that might lead to collapse of the fracture if the compressive forces at the wrist are not properly neutralized
- High-energy multifragmentary fractures with extension into the metaphyseal-diaphyseal region of the distal radius in which distal fixation with diaphyseal/metaphyseal plates may be tenuous or impossible.

By spanning the wrist joint, the bridge plate acts as a bridging internal fixator and as a temporary method of fixation. It requires removal about 8–12 weeks after placement. The dorsal bridge plate provides both internal distraction and buttress support to the dorsal part of the fracture. Unlike external fixation, the bridge plate can be left in place without the risk of pin loosening or infection.

Contraindications of bridge plating

Relative contraindications of bridge plating include fractures in young individuals that are amenable to palmar plating or fragment specific fixation. It is also important to remember that bridge plating requires a second surgery for implant removal and carries the additional risks of wrist stiffness and extensor tendon irritation.

2 Indications (cont)

Choice of implant

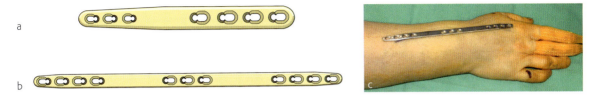

Fig 4.10-3a–c A number of implants are available to function as a bridge plate including a standard limited contact dynamic compression plate (LC-DCP), the specialized plates for distal radius total arthrodesis, or specifically designed plates using 2.7 mm screws. Plate selection is based on the size of the patient and the proximal extent of fragmentation along the distal radius. Lay the plate on the skin over the radial diaphysis to the metadiaphysis of the second or third metacarpal and use the image intensifier to ensure that a minimum of three cortex screws can be placed both proximal to the fracture and distal into the metacarpal. Plates can be precontoured with a bend or simply inserted straight. A straight plate 2.7 was used for this patient.

Imaging

It is not possible to make an accurate assessment of the details of these injuries without a CT scan. Image intensification is required throughout the procedure.

3 Preoperative planning

Equipment

- Bridge plate 2.7
- 1.1 or 1.2 mm K-wires
- Finger trap traction system
- Image intensifier

Patient preparation and positioning

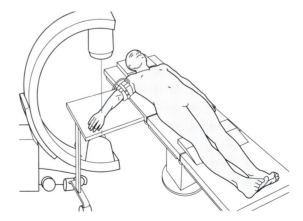

Fig 4.10-4 Position the patient supine and place the forearm on the hand table. Pronate the forearm. The position of the limb should allow complete imaging in the frontal and sagittal plane of the distal radius. A nonsterile pneumatic tourniquet is used. Prophylactic antibiotics are optional. For this patient the hand was supported with a rolled towel.

4 Closed reduction

Provisional reduction

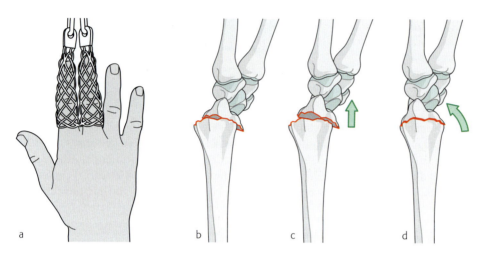

Fig 4.10-5a–d   In this injury type, reduction is required prior to performing the surgical approach. A closed reduction maneuver is performed that involves a combination of longitudinal traction and palmar translation to restore radial length, radial inclination, and palmar angulation. Reduction is achieved by applying longitudinal traction using finger traps to the index and middle fingers (**a–b**). Using the image intensifier for guidance, radial length is restored (**c**). Longitudinal traction is also used to assist in the reduction of the articular surface (**d**). This maneuver will determine the integrity of the palmoulnar corner of the radius. Finally, pronate the hand to correct the supination deformity.

Determine plate positioning

The first step in considering the surgical approach is to decide which metacarpal (either the second or third) will be used for plate fixation. Note that a minimum of three screws should be able to be placed in the metacarpal. The determining factor is the position that provides best reduction.

The method for determining which metacarpal to use is as follows:
1. Provisionally reduce the fracture
2. Place the plate onto the dorsal surface of the wrist
3. Using the image intensifier, make small adjustments in radial-ulnar deviation allowing the optimal plate location to be determined over either the second or third metacarpal
   Once this important step is accomplished the incisions are made.

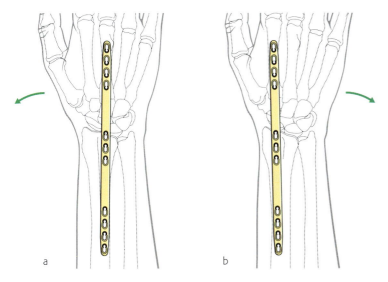

Fig 4.10-6a–b   When the third metacarpal is selected, the carpus is in slight radial deviation and the plate lies obliquely over the radius with the proximal end of the plate on the ulnar side of the diaphysis (**a**).

When the second metacarpal is selected, the carpus is in slight ulnar deviation and the plate lies obliquely over the radius with the proximal end of the plate on the radial side of the diaphysis (**b**). This allows better correction of radial height and inclination, however, the decision always depends on fracture alignment as seen via image intensification.

It is acceptable for the plate to lie obliquely on the radial shaft as long as the screws engage both cortices.

5   Surgical approach (cont)

Approach

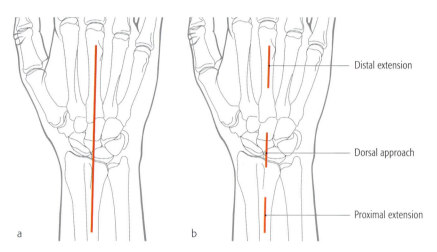

Distal extension

Dorsal approach

Proximal extension

a   b

Fig 4.10-7a–b   The surgical approach used was an extended dorsal approach (**a**) (see chapter 1.9 Extended dorsal approach to the distal radius). In most cases, this technique requires three incisions (**b**). For this patient, a three-incision technique was used involving a dorsal approach with both proximal and distal additional incisions.

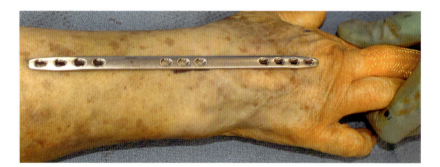

Fig 4.10-8   The plate is placed on the dorsal surface and assists in determining which metacarpal should be used for fixation. This technique is fully explained in the approach chapter 1.9 Extended dorsal approach to the distal radius.

6 Open reduction

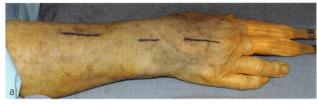

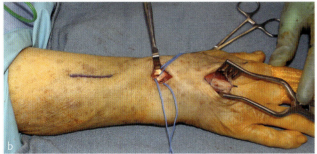

Fig 4.10-9a–b Alignment along the third metacarpal was chosen as providing the best reduction and three incision lines were drawn (**a**). The first 3 cm incision was made at the base of the third metacarpal and continued over the shaft. The second incision of 2 cm was then made directly over Lister tubercle (**b**). The extensor pollicis longus (EPL) was released and retracted ulnarly. Mobilizing the EPL helped with plate insertion and reduction of the articular surface and assisted with sliding the plate under the second compartment tendons. While the third (most proximal) incision line was drawn, it was not made until after plate insertion.

7 Fixation

Determine plate insertion direction

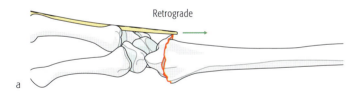

Retrograde

a

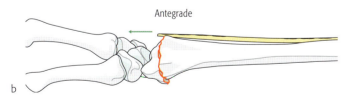

Antegrade

b

Fig 4.10-10a–b Consider the direction of the fracture displacement before inserting the plate to help avoid catching the plate on fracture fragments as it is advanced. With reduction achieved by traction applied through the finger traps, the plate is placed under the second dorsal compartment through either retrograde or antegrade insertion. Retrograde insertion is recommended in dorsal displacement of fragments (**a**). Antegrade insertion is recommended in palmar displacement of fragments (**b**). The plate is inserted underneath the tendons and muscle bellies and advanced in the chosen direction.

7 Fixation (cont)

Apply the drill guide

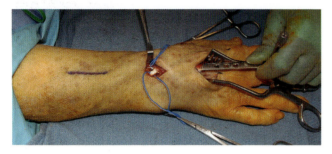

Fig 4.10-11 The drill guide can be screwed into one of the distal holes of the plate so it can be used as a handle to facilitate the sliding of the plate.

Insert the plate

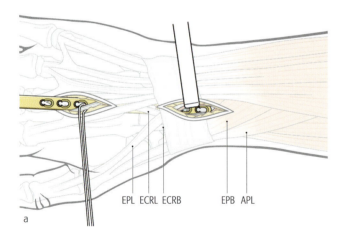

EPL ECRL ECRB   EPB APL

a

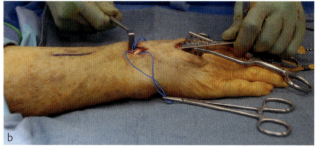

b

Fig 4.10-12a–b The plate is passed proximally under the second compartment tendons. The middle incision is recommended to avoid any damage to the EPL. The intraoperative image shows the plate insertion in retrograde fashion.

7 Fixation (cont)

Make the proximal incision

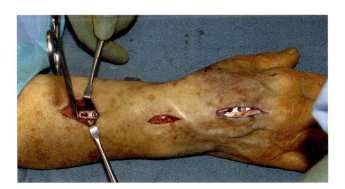

Fig 4.10-13 A 3 cm radial shaft incision is made over the dorsal aspect of the radius just proximal to the muscle bellies of the abductor pollicis longus (APL) and the extensor pollicis brevis (EPB), in line with the extensor carpi radialis longus (ECRL) and extensor carpi radialis brevis (ECRB) tendons. This incision was previously marked during initial imaging with the plate over the dorsal surface but confirmatory images can be taken before incision.

The exact location of the incision may depend on whether the plate will attach distally at the second or third meta-carpal. As this plate was attached to the third metacarpal, the interval between the first and second compartments was developed and the diaphysis of the radius exposed. Care was taken to avoid injury to the superficial branch of the radial nerve. Retract the first compartment muscles ulnarly and the second compartment radially. The proximal holes of the plate should be visible at this point.

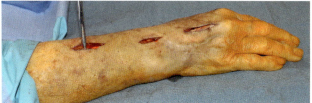

Fig 4.10-14 An optional toothed forceps can be placed in the shaft to prevent the plate from moving too ulnarly or radially. During drilling, the universal drill guide can also help stabilize the plate's position as required.

Insert distal screws

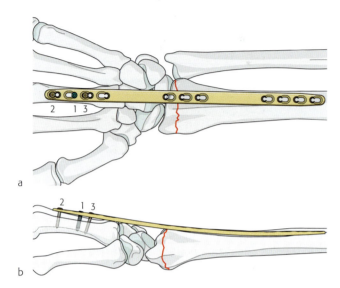

a

b

Fig 4.10-15a–b   The metacarpal shaft is narrow and does not tolerate lateral shifting of the plate. For this reason, it is recommended to insert the three metacarpal screws first (with recommended sequence of screw insertion shown). Care must be taken to center the plate to ensure all screws engage both cortices.

It is recommended to use at least one locking screw in both the metacarpal and the radius. This allows the plate to be used as an internal fixator. The use of locking screws in the metacarpal is also beneficial because the screw heads lie flush with the plate and avoid extensor tendon irritation.

Insert proximal screws

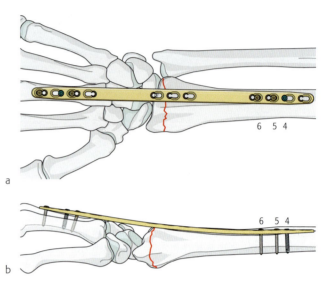

a

b

Fig 4.10-16a–b   Before securing the plate proximally, confirm that full passive motion of all digits is possible. If full finger flexion is not possible, plate impingement of the extensor tendons is the likely cause, and these must be released.

Fix the plate to the radius with three or four screws proximal to the fracture. Once radial shaft fixation is completed, appropriate length and reduction of the fracture should be achieved with no more than 5 mm of distraction at the radiocarpal joint.

Reduce the articular surface

With the plate in its final position and radial length restored, the surgeon can now focus on reduction of the articular surface.

7 Fixation (cont)

Option: bone grafting

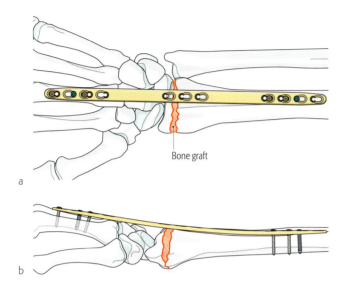

Fig 4.10-17a–b Any metaphyseal voids can be filled by using bone graft inserted through the middle incision. The primary objectives of bone grafting are to take advantage of the mechanical effect of buttressing the articular fragments and to accelerate the process of healing.

Option: screw insertion

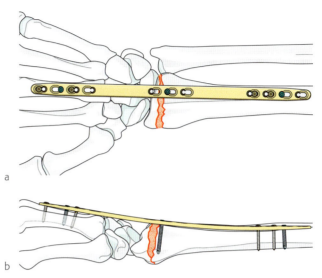

Fig 4.10-18a–b Further buttressing of the lunate facet can be provided by a 3.5 mm locking screw inserted through the mid-portion of the plate just under the subchondral bone of the lunate facet. Alternatively, a 2.7 mm cortex screw can be used but must engage both cortices.

Option: K-wire insertion

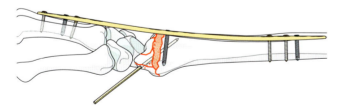

Fig 4.10-19 Some fragments that require reduction might be too small for screw purchase. In this instance, 1.1 or 1.2 mm K-wires should be used to reduce and stabilize these fragments. This is often the case with radial styloid and intermediate column fragments.

Additional palmar plating

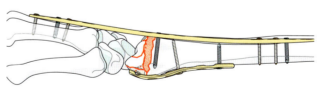

Fig 4.10-20 Some displaced palmar lunate facet fragments cannot be reduced solely by ligamentotaxis or dorsal bridge plating. In these cases, an additional palmar approach is recommended, and a small buttress plate is used for supplemental fixation of the fragment.

7 Fixation (cont)

Distal radioulnar joint assessment

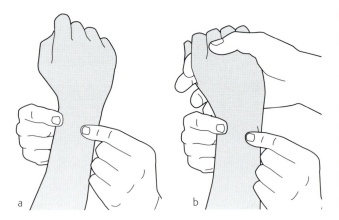

Fig 4.10-21a–b After fixation, the DRUJ should be assessed for both forearm rotation and stability. The methods for determining if DRUJ instability exists are shown in the fixation topic in chapter 4.1 Radial styloid—fracture treated with a radial column plate.

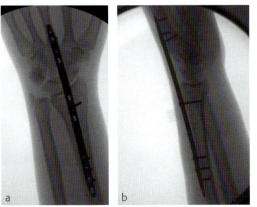

Fig 4.10-22a–b Following fixation of the bridging plate onto the patient's third metacarpal, and with a screw supporting the lunate facet through the midsection of the plate, intraoperative images were used to confirm good alignment and reduction of the radial fracture.

8 Rehabilitation

Aftercare

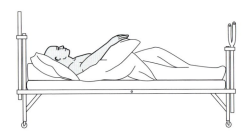

Fig 4.10-23 While the patient is in bed, use pillows to keep the hand elevated above the level of the heart to reduce swelling.

Follow-up

See the patient after 2–5 days to change the dressing. After 10 days, remove the sutures and confirm with x-rays that no secondary displacement has occurred.

8 Rehabilitation (cont)

Immobilization

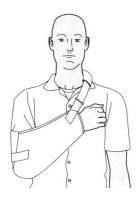

Fig 4.10-24 The type and duration of postoperative immobilization depends on a number of factors including the quality of the internal fixation as well as patient activity and reliability. It may be necessary to rest the wrist for several weeks in a plaster or removable splint.

Functional exercises and patient mobilization

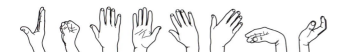

Fig 4.10-25 Following surgery, begin active controlled range of motion exercises. Weightbearing is permitted on the forearm and elbow after surgery. Additionally, after the patient is stabilized, a platform crutch can be used. Three to 4 weeks following the surgery, the platform is removed and weightbearing is allowed through the hand grip of regular crutches. It is recommended to restrict lifting and carrying to no more than 5 kg until the fracture has healed.

The protocol will be different when there is associated DRUJ instability. A long arm splint is applied for 3 weeks following surgery, after which DRUJ stability and active supination of the forearm is assessed. If the patient's arm can be fully supinated, splinting is discontinued. Axial loading through the extremity is allowed for transfers and all weightbearing needs. However, if supination is difficult or if the DRUJ required reconstruction, then a removable long arm splint is provided. If the DRUJ was transfixed with K-wires, then the wires are removed after 6 weeks and DRUJ stability is reassessed.

Implant removal

The K-wires may be removed at approximately 6 weeks, but the plate is left in place until bone healing has been radiologically confirmed, usually between 3–4 months. At time of removal, extensor tenolysis is recommended followed by an active rehabilitation program.

9 Outcome

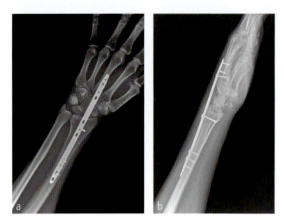

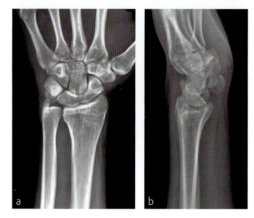

Fig 4.10-26a–b At the 2-week follow-up the postoperative images of the bridging plate showed maintained alignment and reduction. The bridging plate was removed 12 weeks after surgery.

Fig 4.10-27a–b At a further follow-up 5 months after plate removal, PA and lateral x-rays showed healing of the fracture and perfect congruency and alignment of the joint.

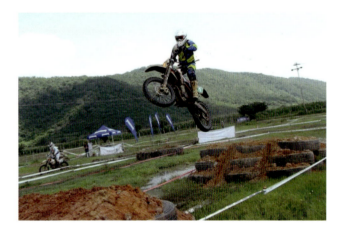

Fig 4.10-28 The patient had achieved a near full range of motion and was able to recontinue his motorbike riding activities without difficulties.

10 Alternative technique

Using a 2-incision technique

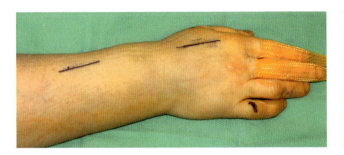

Fig 4.10-29   As an alternative, the approach can be made using proximal and distal incisions only. The 2-incision approach might be considered when there is gross comminution and multiple small bone fragments. After closed reduction, use the image intensifier to determine which metacarpal to use for fixation. With the plate sitting on the skin, mark the skin at the level of the proximal and distal screw holes. Make a 3 cm distal incision and insert the plate.

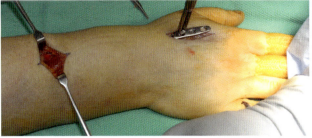

Fig 4.10-30   Insert a drill guide into one of the distal screw holes for use as a handle. Once the plate has been inserted and is in position over the radius proximal to the fracture, a second incision measuring approximately 3 cm is made over the dorsal aspect of the radius just proximal to the muscle bellies of the APL and EPB, in line with the ECRL and ECRB tendons.

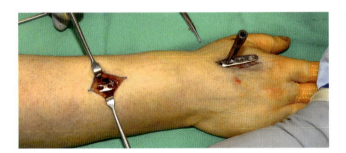

Fig 4.10-31   By blunt dissection, the interval between the ECRL/ECRB and the APL/EPB is developed, and the plate can be seen over the diaphysis of the radius. Care must be taken to avoid injury to the superficial branch of the radial nerve.

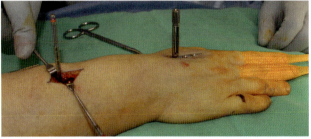

Fig 4.10-32   A drill guide, used as a second handle, is inserted into one of the proximal holes of the plate to facilitate the alignment of the plate over the radius. Fixation is completed in the standard way.

4.11 Distal radius—radiocarpal fracture dislocation treated with double plating

1 Case description

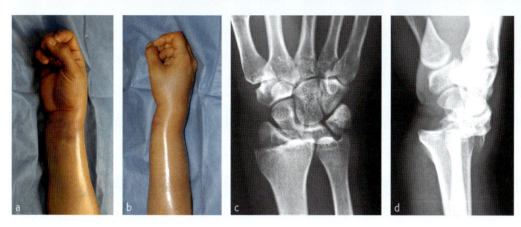

Fig 4.11-1a–d   A 30-year-old building supervisor was seen in the emergency department in severe pain 2 hours after falling from a height. On clinical examination there was evidence of gross deformity and swelling of the hand and wrist extending to the forearm (**a–b**). The PA and lateral x-rays revealed a complex radiocarpal fracture dislocation of his right wrist (**c–d**).

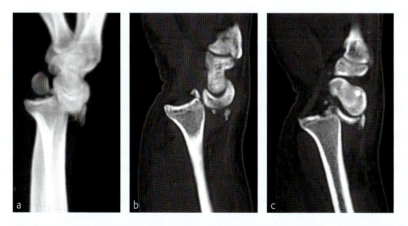

Fig 4.11-2a–c   Sagittal 2-D CT scans demonstrated complete dislocation dorsally of the carpus as well as a small shearing fracture of the dorsal aspect of the distal radius.

1   Case description (cont)

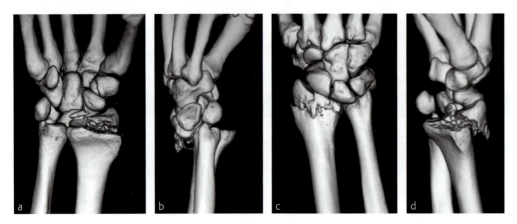

Fig 4.11-3a–d   Multiple 3-D CT scans show the dorsal shearing fracture fragments but the palmar rim of the radius was still intact.

2   Indications

Radiocarpal fracture dislocations

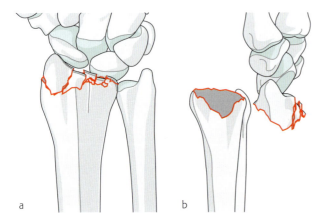

Fig 4.11-4a–b   Radiocarpal fracture dislocations are the result of higher-energy trauma, can have associated soft-tissue injuries, and are often found in polytrauma cases. The injury is characterized by multifragmentary dorsal rim fractures and dorsal dislocation of the carpus. In these fractures, the fracture of the dorsal rim is associated with a radial styloid fracture as well, with greater marked instability. As these are partial intraarticular injuries, with an existing or a high risk of later radiocarpal subluxation, they should normally be treated with open reduction and internal fixation.

If the distal radial fragments are predominantly dorsal, reduction and fixation is performed using dorsally applied plates but if there is a significant radial styloid fragment this is helped more effectively with a radial column plate. Large fragments can be treated with plating or even lag screws while smaller fragments may require fixation with K-wires or suture anchors, although reduction and stabilization by external fixation may be needed initially because of marked swelling.

2 Indications (cont)

Initial assessment

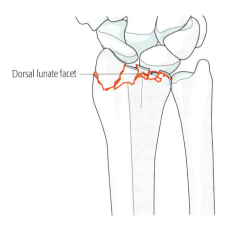

Dorsal lunate facet

Fig 4.11-5 Under direct vision, approach the radial styloid and dorsal lunate facet fragments. Usually the dorsal capsule is torn, but if it is intact, a dorsal arthrotomy is made parallel to the dorsal rim to inspect the articular surface and look for any associated carpal injuries.

Associated carpal injuries

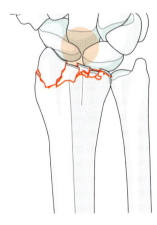

Fig 4.11-7 These injuries may be associated with shearing injuries of the articular cartilage, scaphoid fractures, and ruptures of the scapholunate ligament. Every patient should be assessed for these injuries.

Median nerve compression

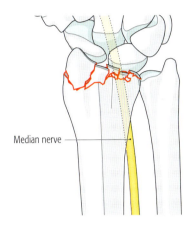

Median nerve

Fig 4.11-6 If there is dense sensory loss or other signs of median nerve compression, the median nerve should be decompressed.

Imaging

Using CT scans can be helpful for treatment decisions with this injury.

Choice of implant

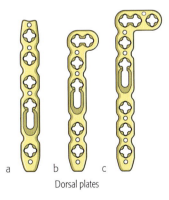

Dorsal plates

Fig 4.11-8a–c A selection of plates can be used to stabilize dorsal radiocarpal fracture dislocations by stabilizing the radial and intermediate columns. Plates with variable angle (VA) locking screw options can be useful. For this patient, VA straight and L-plates were used, with the intermediate column being treated first.

3 Preoperative planning

Equipment

- VA locking compression plate (LCP) distal radius set
- VA LCP radial column plate 2.4
- VA LCP intermediate column plate 2.4
- 1.1 mm or 1.2 mm K-wires
- Image intensifier

Patient preparation and positioning

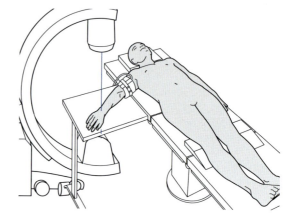

Fig 4.11-9 Position the patient supine and place the forearm on the hand table. Pronate the forearm. The position of the limb should allow complete imaging in the frontal and sagittal plane of the distal radius. A nonsterile pneumatic tourniquet is used. Prophylactic antibiotics are optional.

4 Surgical approach

Approach

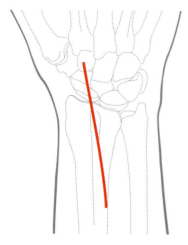

Fig 4.11-10 The surgical approach used was a dorsal approach (see chapter 1.8 Dorsal approach to the distal radius).

4 Surgical approach (cont)

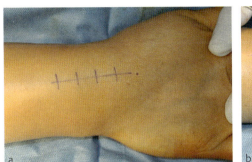
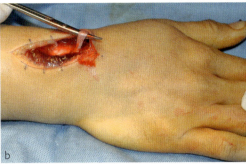

Fig 4.11-11a–b   The dorsal surgical approach was marked. After the incision, the extensor pollicis longus was elevated from the extensor retinaculum.

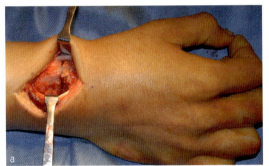
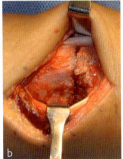

Fig 4.11-12a–b   The small dorsal rim fractures then became visible. The approach allowed access to both the radial and intermediate columns.

Arthrotomy

If direct vision of the articular surface is needed, a limited transverse radiocarpal arthrotomy is performed.

5 Reduction

Provisional reduction

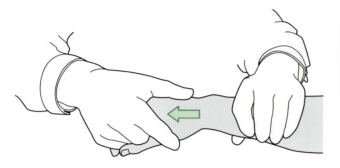

Fig 4.11-13 Reduction is achieved by applying longitudinal traction either manually or using finger traps. The reduction is maintained by a temporary splint. If definitive surgery is planned but cannot be performed within a reasonable time scale a temporary external fixator may be helpful.

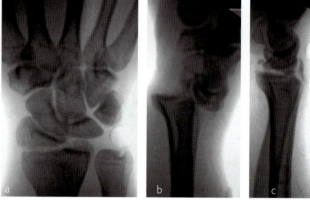

Fig 4.11-14a–c Intraoperative reduction was checked using the image intensifier.

Provisional fixation

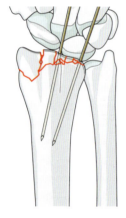

Fig 4.11-15 If the dorsal rim fragments are large enough, obtain provisional fixation with K-wires.

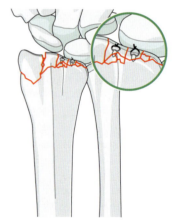

Fig 4.11-16 If they are too small they can be held with suture anchors or transosseous sutures.

5   Reduction (cont)

Provisional radial styloid fixation

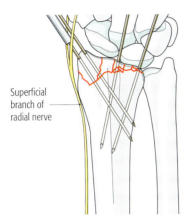

Superficial branch of radial nerve

Fig 4.11-17   The radial styloid fragments are reduced under direct vision with either a K-wire on the dorsoradial aspect or percutaneously. In the latter case, in order not to injure the sensory branch of the radial nerve, make a small incision over the tip of the radial styloid and use a protective drill guide to insert two K-wires. Confirm using image intensification.

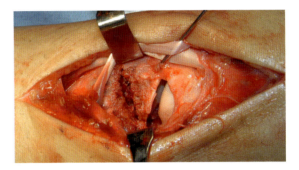

Fig 4.11-18   The radial styloid fracture component was reduced and held with a K-wire. A dorsal wrist arthrotomy had been performed for direct vision of the articular reduction.

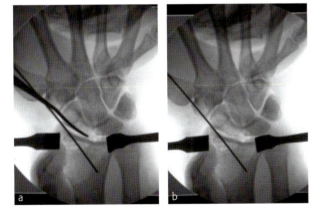

Fig 4.11-19a–b   The articular reduction was confirmed using intraoperative imaging.

6 Fixation

Contour the plate

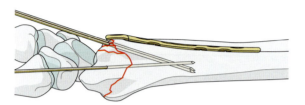

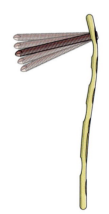

Fig 4.11-20 Plates used in treating radial and intermediate column injuries are available precontoured. However, because of the shape of the dorsal distal metaphysis, the plate may need to be contoured to fit the bone surface and the proximal limb may require some torsional adaptation. If the distal transverse limb of the plate does not exert sufficient compression on the distal fragments, remove the plate and overbend the transverse distal limb.

Fig 4.11-21 Variable angle locking plates enable precise positioning of the distal screws in desired directions because there is 30 degrees of freedom for each screw inside the plate hole to address the individual fracture patterns.

Pitfall: screw hole distortion

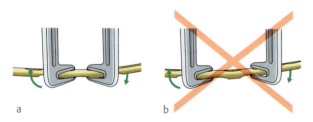

a   b

Fig 4.11-22a–b Avoid contouring the plate through the locking holes otherwise the locking head screw might no longer fit.

Fixation of intermediate column
Select and apply the plate

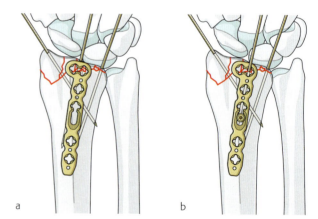

a   b

Fig 4.11-23a–b The appropriate plate is selected according to the fracture configuration. The plate should be applied as distally as possible over the dorsal rim fragments (**a**). If the provisional K-wires conflict with the optimal plate position, the plate can be slipped over the wires, or the wires can be repositioned (**b**).

6 Fixation (cont)

Insert proximal screws

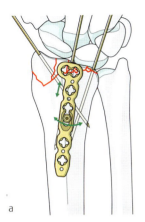
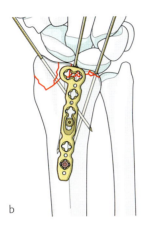

a   b

Fig 4.11-24a–b Fix the plate provisionally to the bone with a standard cortex screw inserted through the oblong plate hole (**a**). Before fully tightening it, check the plate position using intraoperative imaging, adjusting the position of the plate as necessary. Once the plate position is satisfactory, it should be secured with a locking screw in the proximal screw holes (**b**).

Insert distal screws

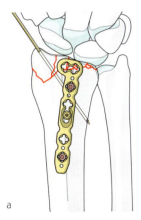
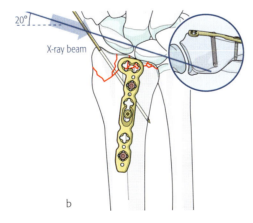

20°

X-ray beam

a   b

Fig 4.11-25a–b Screws are inserted through the distal plate holes before or after removal of the K-wire(s), as appropriate (**a**). With image intensification, confirm that the distal screws have not penetrated the articular surface. To have a view in line with the articular surface, the beam should be angled 20 degrees from the true lateral (**b**).

Fixation of radial column
Select and apply the plate

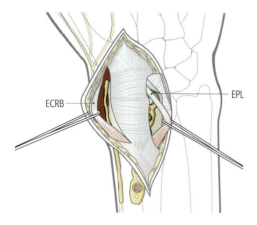

Fig 4.5-26   The appropriate plate is selected according to the fracture configuration and contoured if necessary. Slide the plate underneath the first compartment and apply it onto the radial column. Extensor carpi radialis brevis (ECRB); extensor pollicis longus (EPL).

Stabilize the radial column

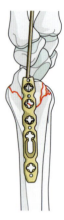

Fig 4.11-27   Ideally, while applying the plate the notch in the distal tip of the implant is placed against the temporary K-wire.

Pitfall: incorrect placement

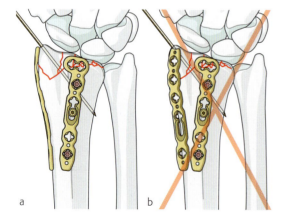

Fig 4.11-28a–b   Avoid placement of the radial plate on the dorsal aspect of the radial column as it will not buttress the reduction adequately against axial shear forces.

Insert the first screw in the radial column plate

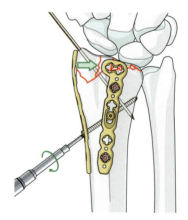

Fig 4.11-29   Insert a standard cortex screw through the oblong plate hole proximal to the fracture. The screw should engage the far cortex. The position of the plate may be adjusted before the screw is tightened. Tightening this screw will reduce the radial styloid.

6 Fixation (cont)

Insert first locking head screw

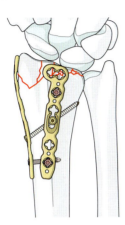

Fig 4.11-30 To prevent rotation of the plate during distal locking screw fixation, the plate should be secured to the bone by inserting the most proximal screw.

Insert distal locking head screws

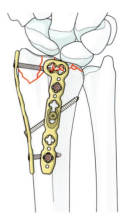

Fig 4.11-31 If a K-wire was used, it is now removed. Distal locking head screw(s) are inserted to support the radial styloid. Using VA screws allow optimal direction of fixation. The position of the most distal screw should be just under the subchondral bone.

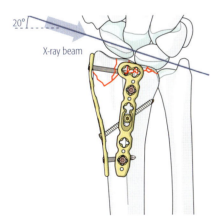

Fig 4.11-32 Confirm that the screw does not protrude into the joint under direct vision and using an image intensifier, with the beam angled 20 degrees from the true lateral. This projection will profile the radial articular surface and visualize any encroachment of the screw into the joint.

Pitfall: penetration of sigmoid notch

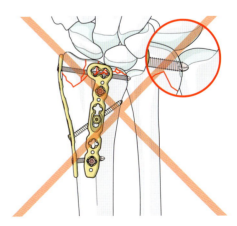

Fig 4.11-33 Beware of the tip of the screw penetrating into the sigmoid notch. It is safer to leave the screw a little short and it should not be drilled into the opposite cortex.

6   Fixation (cont)

Complete the fixation

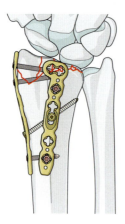

Fig 4.11-34   If necessary, insert additional screws and complete the fixation.

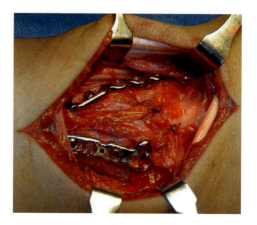

Fig 4.11-35   The definitive fixation was achieved using a radial column plate and a dorsal L-plate 2.4.

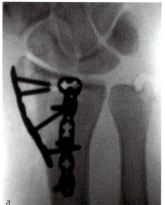
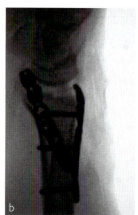

Fig 4.11-36a–b   Intraoperative imaging confirmed the plate position and the anatomical reduction of the fracture dislocation.

Palmar ligamentous avulsion reattachment

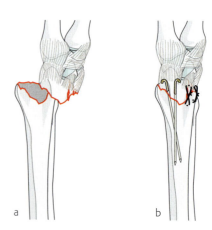

Fig 4.11-37a–b   Radiocarpal fracture dislocations may be associated with avulsion of the palmar wrist capsule from the distal radius. After dorsal fixation, check the carpal position and stability under image intensification. If there is carpal ulnar and/or palmar translation, consider an additional palmar approach to repair soft tissues. The capsule can be reattached using multiple suture anchors or transosseous sutures.

6 Fixation (cont)

Additional external fixation

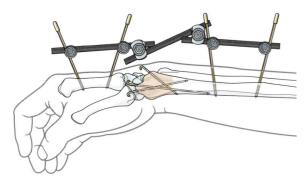

Fig 4.11-38 If the dorsal rim fragments are large enough, they may be held in place with a buttress plate. If they are too small, K-wires may be the definitive fixation, in which case, a neutralization external fixation should be applied.

7 Rehabilitation

Aftercare, follow-up, and functional exercises

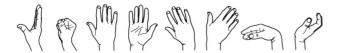

Fig 4.11-39 The patient should receive the standard postoperative rest, injury elevation, follow-up, removal of stitches, and immobilization as required. Following surgery, begin active controlled range of motion exercises. For further information see the rehabilitation topic in chapter 4.1 Radial styloid—fracture treated with a radial column plate.

8 Outcome

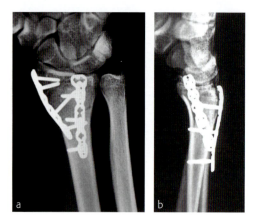

Fig 4.11-40a–b The follow-up x-rays at 6 weeks showed there was maintained reduction and early bone healing.

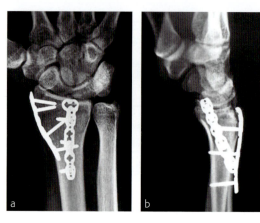

Fig 4.11-41a–b The 12-month follow-up x-rays showed good healing.

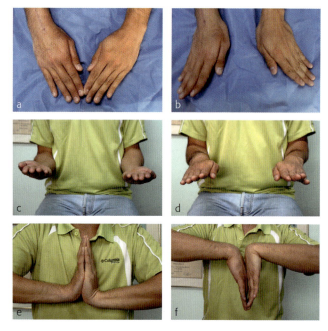

Fig 4.11-42a–f The patient had close to normal range of motion compared with the uninjured side.

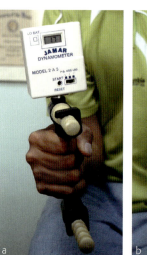
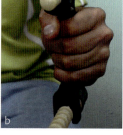

Fig 4.11-43a–b There was an excellent overall functional result.

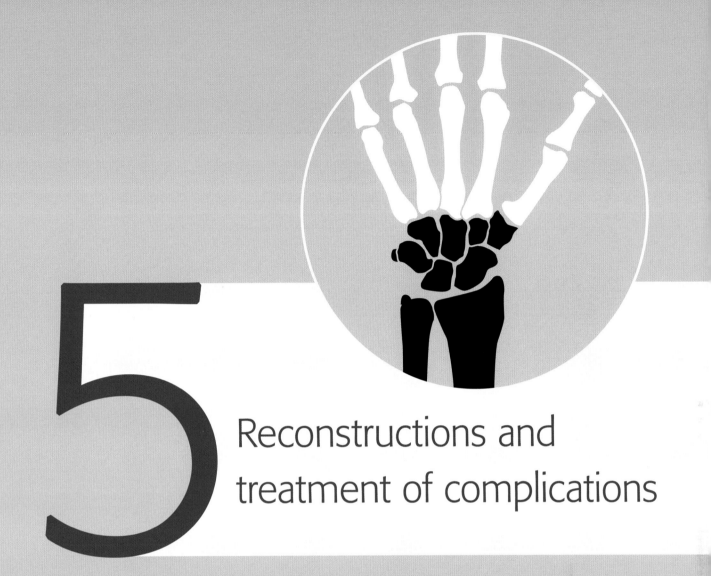

5

Reconstructions and treatment of complications

5.1 Distal radius—dorsal extraarticular malunion treated with osteotomy and double plating

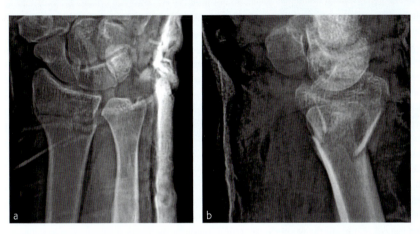

Fig 5.1-1a–b A 54-year-old man suffered a dorsally displaced distal radial fracture of the right hand with a small dorsal lunate intraarticular component, for which he received nonoperative treatment. The PA and lateral x-rays taken in the plaster cast showed the initial displaced fracture.

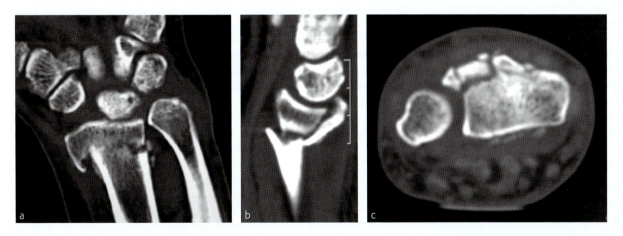

Fig 5.1-2a–c At the 4-month follow-up after the injury, 2-D CT scans showed a marked deformity existed while also indicating immature callus.

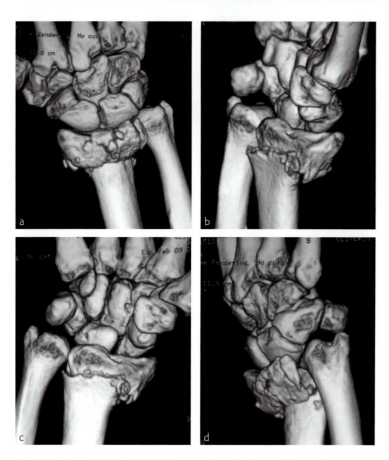

Fig 5.1-3a–d   Additional 3-D CT scans clearly showed the evident deformity. The deformity involved considerable shortening of the radius, loss of the wrist's normal radial and palmar inclination, and dorsal displacement of the distal fragment with dorsal fragmentation.

2 Indications

Dorsal extraarticular radius malunion

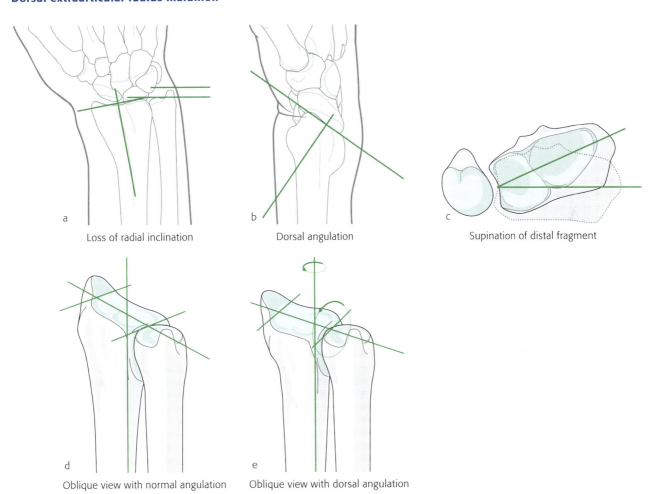

a — Loss of radial inclination
b — Dorsal angulation
c — Supination of distal fragment
d — Oblique view with normal angulation
e — Oblique view with dorsal angulation

Fig 5.1-4a–e Malunion is a common complication of distal radial fractures and occurs when the healed distal radius deviates from its original anatomical alignment. The most common deformity type involves dorsal extraarticular angulation, with radial shortening and supination of the distal fragment. The alteration of radial orientation can modify the loads transmitted in the carpus and the distal radioulnar joint (DRUJ), possibly causing them to change and adapt, and greatly increasing the risk of developing posttraumatic osteoarthritis.

Corrective osteotomy for malunion

A corrective osteotomy, involving bone lengthening or shortening or to change alignment, can often be chosen to treat a malunited distal radial fracture. When considering this, the following two questions must be answered:
- How much deformity can actually be tolerated?
- When is the optimal time to perform an osteotomy?

The question of how much deformity can be tolerated is not always easy to answer as it can be difficult to quantify an acceptable malalignment and depends on the needs of the individual. While some patients remain symptom free despite the deformity, others can present with pain or functional limitation. The extent of disability may depend on the amount of radial shortening, the loss of radial inclination, the amount of dorsal angulation, and any DRUJ instability.

2 Indications (cont)

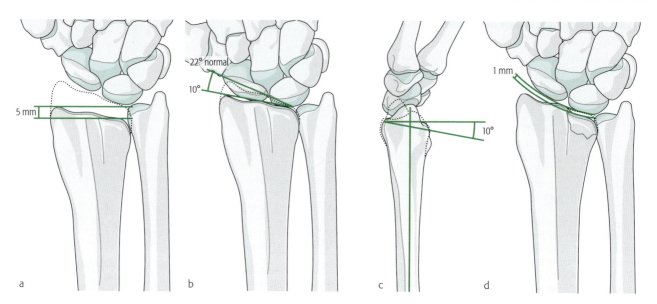

a   b   c   d

Fig 5.1-5a–d How much deformity in the distal radius can be accepted? While evidence of adaptive carpal instability (change in capitolunate or scapholunate alignment) is increasingly seen as an accurate predictor of outcome, as a general guide, the following measurements have been recognized as providing acceptable levels of dorsal deformity:
a Not greater than 5 mm of radial shortening
b Not less than 10 degrees of radial inclination
c Not greater than 10 degrees of dorsal angulation
d Not greater than 1 mm of step-off of the articular surface.

As for the most optimal time to perform the osteotomy, it is recommended to operate when the soft tissues demonstrate absence of trophic changes, when the x-rays reveal limited or no appearance of low bone density (osteopenia), and when wrist mobility is adequate. Regardless, there are advantages to early operative treatment such as decreased likelihood of deformity or when the correction is through an immaturely healed fracture site, which is always easier. This early approach can limit the problem of soft-tissue contractures and can minimize the economic and social impact to the patient.

Besides unacceptable deformities of the distal radius, other indications for corrective osteotomy are carpal malalignment, incongruence of the DRUJ, decreased range of motion, decreased grip strength, the presence of pain with motion and activity, and an unacceptable clinical appearance by the patient.

Imaging

When dealing with malunions, the correct length of the radius in relation to the ulna should always be established preoperatively by taking x-rays of the opposite wrist.

3 Preoperative planning

Equipment

- Variable angle (VA) locking compression plate (LCP) distal radius set
- VA LCP radial column plate 2.4
- VA LCP intermediate column plate 2.4
- 2.7 mm Schanz pins or 1.4 mm to 1.6 mm K-wires
- Conical drill guide
- Goniometer
- Osteotome
- Autogenous bone graft or bone substitute
- Small external fixation set
- Laminar spreader
- Image intensifier

Patient preparation and positioning

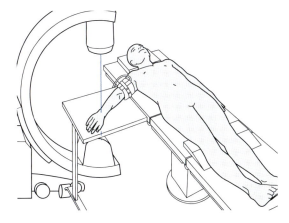

Fig 5.1-6   Position the patient supine and place the forearm on the hand table. Pronate the forearm. The position of the limb should allow complete imaging in the frontal and sagittal plane of the distal radius. A nonsterile pneumatic tourniquet is used. Prophylactic antibiotics are optional.

4 Surgical approach

Approach

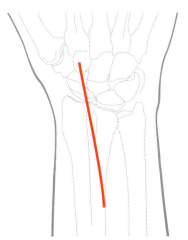

Fig 5.1-7   The surgical approach used was a dorsal approach (see chapter 1.8 Dorsal approach to the distal radius).

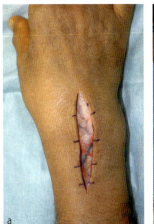
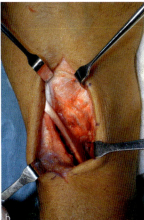

Fig 5.1-8a–b   During the approach, the extensor pollicis longus (EPL) was elevated from the third extensor compartment and protected.

5 Reduction and fixation

Plan the osteotomy

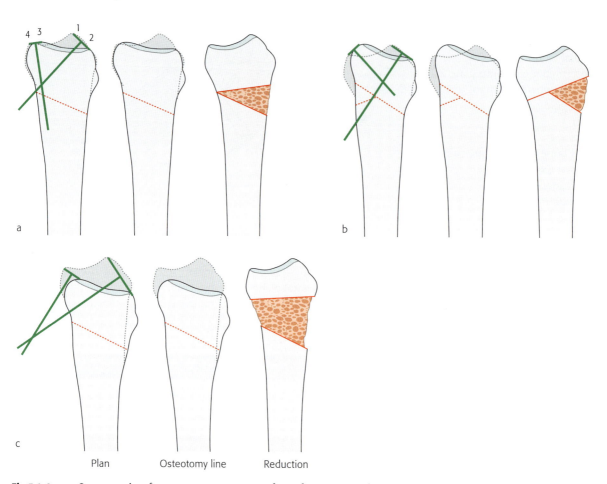

| Plan | Osteotomy line | Reduction |

Fig 5.1-9a–c In preparing for an osteotomy procedure three types of osteotomies can be considered:
a Incomplete (opening wedge)
b Rocking
c Complete (full thickness interpositional).

To determine the type of osteotomy required, superimpose the x-ray of the deformity side onto the x-ray of the uninjured side. In the sagittal view, draw a line between the most dorsal point of the normal x-ray (**1**) to the dorsal point of the malunion (**2**). Create a perpendicular line at the center of the line. This is followed by a line drawn from the most palmar aspect of the normal side (**3**) to the most palmar aspect of the malunion side (**4**) and a perpendicular line is drawn in the middle of this line to connect to the perpendicular line drawn from the dorsal side. Where these two perpendicular lines intersect will define what type of osteotomy will be required.

In some instances, the perpendicular lines intersect directly on or near the palmar cortex (but still within the radius), which demonstrates that the osteotomy once created does not need lengthening of the distal fragment and requires an incomplete osteotomy or a rocking method osteotomy.

However, If the lines intersect beyond the palmar cortex, as with this patient, it indicates that following the osteotomy of the malunion the distal fragment will require lengthening, creating a defect of both the dorsal and palmar aspects of the distal radius. A complete osteotomy will therefore be required (**c**).

5 Reduction and fixation (cont)

Determine degree of deformity

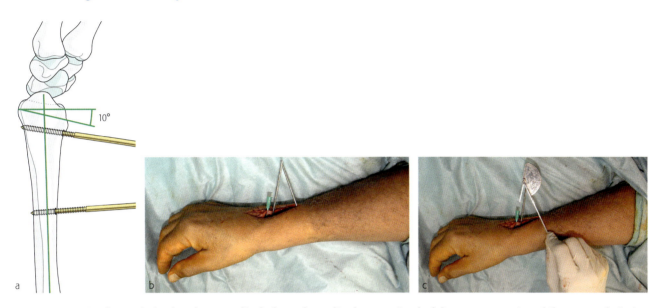

Fig 5.1-10a–c A Schanz pin is placed perpendicularly to the radius but proximal of the osteotomy site while a second pin is placed distally in line with the extension deformity of the distal radius (**a–b**). A handheld goniometer can be used to judge the degree of deformity and anticipated correction (**c**). A small hypodermic needle was placed in the radiocarpal joint for better orientation.

Perform the osteotomy

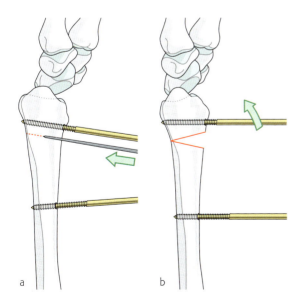

Fig 5.1-11a–b The osteotomy is performed by using an osteotome at the site of the deformity. The malunion with dorsal angulation is corrected by a dorsal open wedge osteotomy and appropriate lengthening of the radius.

5 Reduction and fixation (cont)

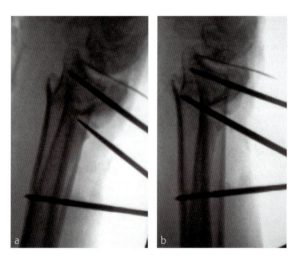

Fig 5.1-12a–b The lateral intraoperative images demonstrate the position of the Schanz pins and the intended osteotomy site (**a**). The osteotomy was performed by use of the osteotome (**b**). Interoperative imaging is used to determine the exact location of the osteotomy and to avoid damaging the median nerve and flexor tendons.

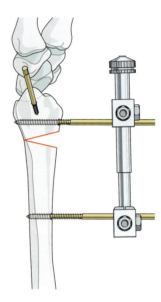

Fig 5.1-13 As an option, and as used in this case, the osteotomy and reduction can be aided with an external fixator. Attach an external fixation pin holding clamp to each Schanz pin. Then place an additional Schanz pin into the distal fragment from the radial direction. This is used to help regain the anticipated radial length and angulation of the distal fragment.

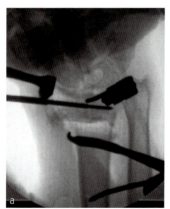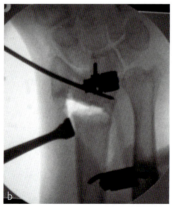

Fig 5.1-14a–b Intraoperative images show the external fixation and the osteotomy site.

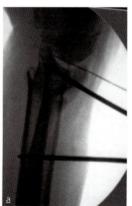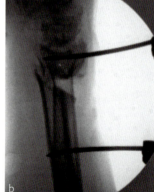

Fig 5.1-15a–b The correction following the osteotomy is seen in the lateral intraoperative images, precorrection (**a**) and after correction with a more appropriate alignment (**b**).

5 Reduction and fixation (cont)

Fixation of intermediate column

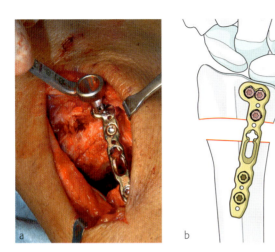

Fig 5.1-16a–b   For fixation of the distal radius, two contoured VA LCP dorsal plates 2.4 were sequentially applied, starting with the plate for the intermediate column.

Fixation of radial column

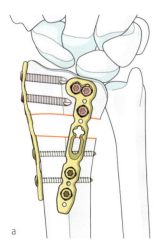 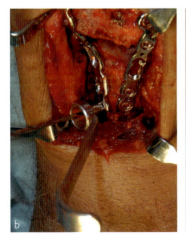 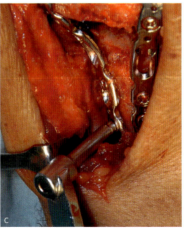

Fig 5.1-17a–c   This was followed by fixation of the radial column. Note the use of the conical drill guide to allow variable directions for the locking head screws.

The double plating fixation procedure follows the usual steps of selecting, preparing and applying the plates, stabilizing the radial column, ensuring correct plate positioning, and inserting the screws. For further information on these steps see chapter 4.5 Distal radius—dorsally displaced intraarticular fracture treated with double plating.

5 Reduction and fixation (cont)

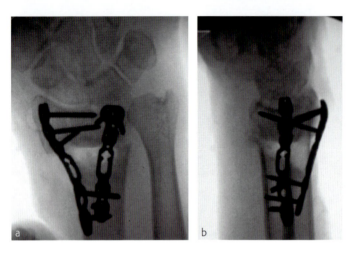

Fig 5.1-18a–b Intraoperative images following plate fixation ensured correct plate placement. Note that the defect created by the osteotomy is still clearly evident.

Bone graft

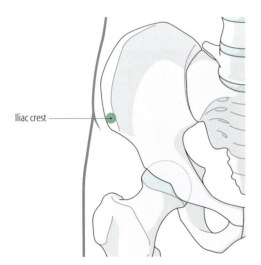

Iliac crest

Fig 5.1-19 Harvest corticocancellous graft material from the iliac crest.

Harvesting

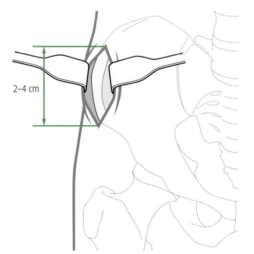

2–4 cm

Fig 5.1-20 Make a longitudinal incision over the lateral aspect of the palpable iliac crest avoiding the anterior aspect and the iliofemoral nerve. Mark out the pre-planned graft size to be harvested considering the shape and size of the defect in the distal radius. Harvest the selected graft using a sharp osteotome.

5   Reduction and fixation (cont)

Insert the bone graft

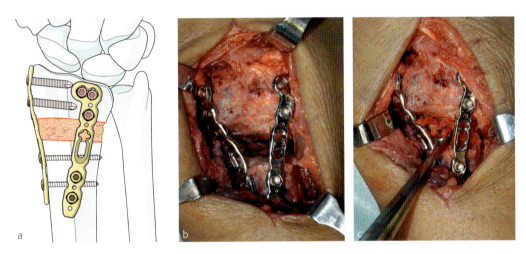

Fig 5.1-21a–c   The defect created by the osteotomy was filled with the iliac crest graft.

Complete the fixation

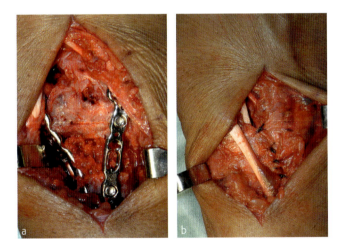

Fig 5.1-22a–b   Once the bone graft was in place, the extensor retinaculum was reapproximated and the wound irrigated and closed. The EPL tendon is left above the retinaculum.

6 Rehabilitation

Aftercare, follow-up, and functional exercises

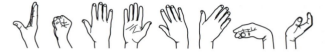

Fig 5.1-23 The patient should receive the standard postoperative rest, injury elevation, follow-up, removal of stitches, and immobilization as required. Following surgery, begin active controlled range of motion exercises. For further information, see the rehabilitation topic in chapter 4.1 Radial styloid—fracture treated with a radial column plate.

7 Outcome

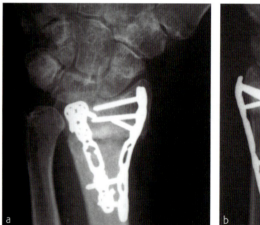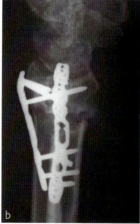

Fig 5.1-24a–b At the 4-month follow-up the postoperative x-rays showed the integration of the bone graft and the completed fixation.

7 Outcome (cont)

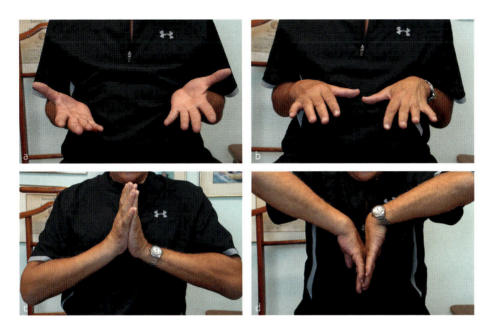

Fig 5.1-25a–d The patient showed some limitation of wrist flexion but the extension, pronation, and supination were good and the patient was without pain.

Video

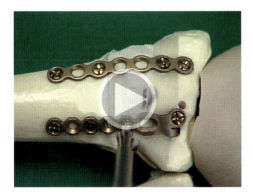

Video 5.1-1 This video demonstrates a corrective osteotomy on a distal radius with fixation with a minicondylar plate 2.0.

8 Alternative technique

Dorsal malunion treated through a palmar approach

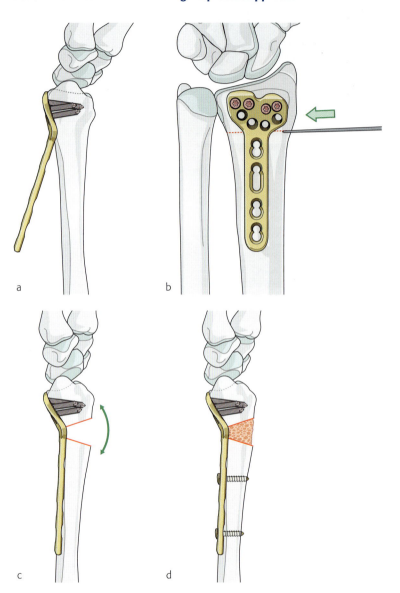

Fig 5.1-26a–d   Occasionally, plates placed on the dorsal aspect of the radius can result in tendon irritation and rupture because of the intimate contact between the tendons and the plate. As an alternative, if the fixation is performed with a plate on the palmar aspect of the radius (as shown, applying a palmar plate to assist with the osteotomy (**a–b**), correcting alignment (**c**), and eventual fixation (**d**)), then the tendons and median nerve are protected by the pronator quadratus.

With the use of angular stable implants such as an LCP locking plate, most corrective osteotomies can be performed through the palmar approach using cancellous bone graft instead of a more complex autogenous corticocancellous graft. Many osteotomies can now be performed palmarly, and instead of sculptured bone graft, which is a demanding technique, surgeons can use cancellous chopped chips.

8 Alternative technique (cont)

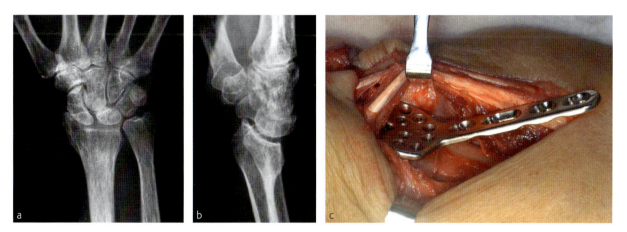

Fig 5.1-27a–c As an illustration, these x-rays show a dorsally displaced malunion on a right-handed patient (**a–b**). The intraoperative image shows that through a palmar approach the angular stable implant is applied with the proximal limb placed off the palmar cortex based on the planned angular correction (**c**).

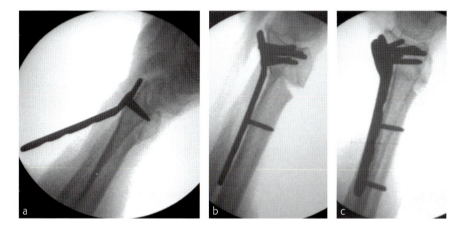

Fig 5.1-28a–c Intraoperative imaging shows the strategic placement of the implant (**a**) followed by the osteotomy and the plate then applied to the shaft to correct the deformity (**b**) with placement of cancellous bone graft to complete the fixation (**c**).

5.2 Distal radius—palmar extraarticular malunion treated with osteotomy and plate

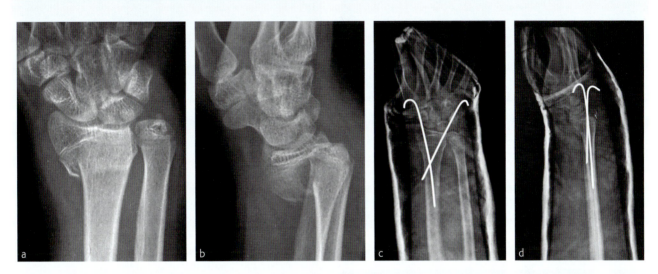

Fig 5.2-1a–d A 15-year-old male school student sustained a displaced fracture of the right distal radius in a motorcycle injury, for which he received treatment in a regional hospital with closed reduction and percutaneous K-wire fixation. The patient was initially immobilized in a short arm plaster cast, which was removed along with the K-wires 15 days after surgery. The PA and lateral x-rays show the initial fracture and K-wire fixation.

1 Case description (cont)

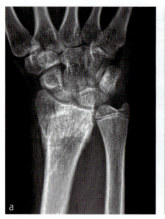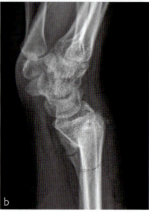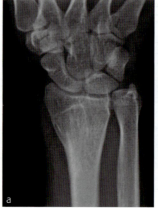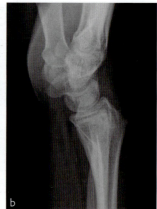

Fig 5.2-2a–b At the 5-week follow-up, new PA and lateral x-rays showed a malunited fracture of the distal radius. There was shortening of the radius by 5 mm, radial inclination of 15 degrees, and palmar angulation of 40 degrees. On the lateral view, a triangle of callus was shown on the palmar aspect of the radius. The growth plate was open in the ulna and partially closed in the radius.

Fig 5.2-3a–b The patient returned 6 months after the initial trauma having a mature symptomatic malunited fracture of the distal radius. He complained of pain, deformity, and functional limitation of the forearm and wrist. The physical examination showed reduction of wrist extension and increased flexion compared with the opposite limb. Limitation of supination of the forearm was also demonstrated, and there was pain during active and passive movement and forearm rotation. Examination of radial inclination and shortening showed there had been no improvement. The growth plate was closed in both the ulna and the radius. In the lateral view, a compensatory extension of the capitate was evident because of the flexed position of the lunate as a result of the increase in palmar angulation of the radius.

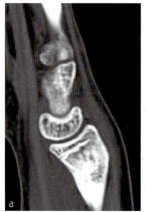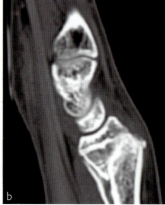

Fig 5.2-4a–b The sagittal view CT scans showed the exact plane of the malunited fracture and the apex of the deformity, both elements that help when planning an osteotomy. Additionally, an x-ray of the normal contra-lateral wrist was used for preoperative planning.

2 Indications

Palmar extraarticular radius malunion

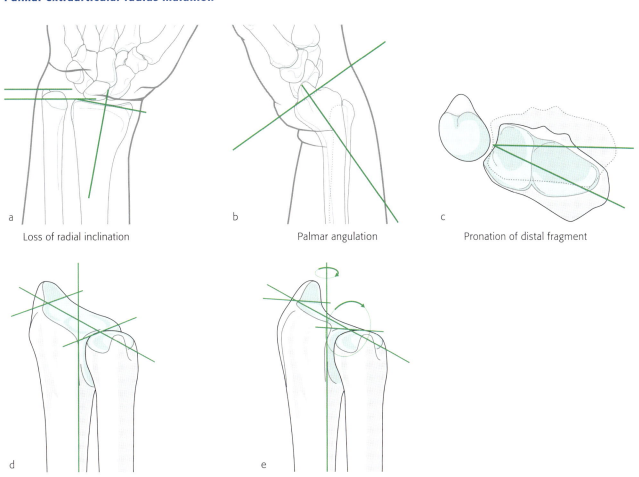

a   Loss of radial inclination

b   Palmar angulation

c   Pronation of distal fragment

d   Oblique view with normal angulation

e   Oblique view with palmar angulation

Fig 5.2-5a–e   Although less frequent than dorsally displaced malunions, malunited extraarticular fractures of the distal radius can also occur with increased palmar angulation, radial shortening, and pronation of the distal fragment, which can modify the loads transmitted in the carpus and the distal radioulnar joint (DRUJ) with increased risk of developing posttraumatic osteoarthritis.

Corrective osteotomy for malunion

As discussed in the previous chapter, consideration for a corrective osteotomy to treat distal radial malunion depends on how much deformity can be accepted and when best to operate. While there may be some contraindications, it is generally accepted that there are advantages to early operative treatment, such as decreased likelihood of deformity, or when the correction is through an immaturely healed fracture site, which is always easier.

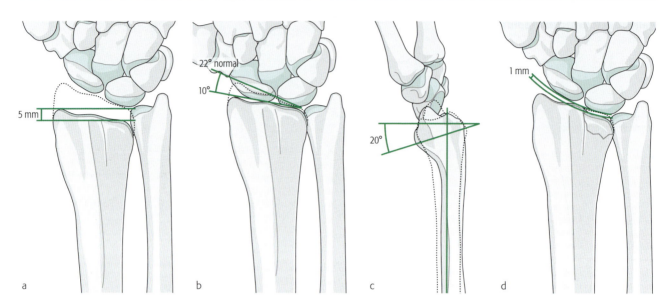

Fig 5.2-6a–d   As for the question of how much deformity can be accepted, as with dorsal malunion, there are broad guidelines on what are acceptable levels of palmar deformity. These are as follows:
a   Not greater than 5 mm of radial shortening
b   Not less than 10 degrees of radial inclination
c   Not greater than 20 degrees of palmar angulation
d   Not greater than 1 mm of step-off of the articular surface.

Regardless of these measurements, for the young patient in this case the decreased range of motion, decreased grip strength, presence of pain with motion and activity, and the unacceptable clinical appearance by the patient made for strong indicators for a corrective osteotomy.

Imaging

When dealing with malunions, the correct length of the radius in relation to the ulna should always be established preoperatively by taking x-rays of the opposite wrist.

---

3 Preoperative planning

Equipment

- Variable angle (VA) locking compression plate (LCP) distal radius set
- VA LCP volar column plate 2.4
- Autogenous bone graft or bone substitute
- Potential need for external fixator
- Image intensifier

Patient preparation and positioning

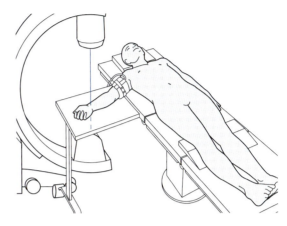

Fig 5.2-7 Position the patient supine and place the forearm on a hand table. Supinate the forearm. The position of the limb should allow complete imaging in the frontal and sagittal plane of the distal radius. A nonsterile pneumatic tourniquet is used. Prophylactic antibiotics are optional.

---

4 Surgical approach

Approach

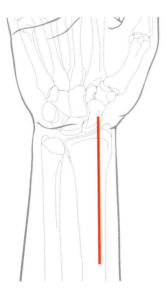

Fig 5.2-8 The surgical approach used was a modified Henry palmar approach (see Chapter 1.6 Modified Henry palmar approach to the distal radius).

5 Reduction and fixation

Plan the osteotomy

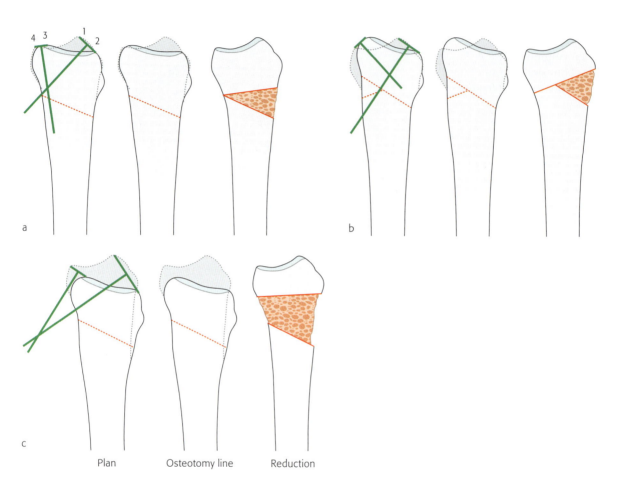

Plan   Osteotomy line   Reduction

Fig 5.2-9a–c In preparing for an osteotomy procedure three types of osteotomies can be considered:
- Incomplete (opening wedge) (**a**)
- Rocking (**b**)
- Complete (full thickness interpositional) (**c**).

By analyzing the perpendicular lines (of normal versus the malunited alignment) and where they intersected it was determined that the osteotomy once created did not need lengthening of the distal fragment, therefore an incomplete osteotomy technique was selected. Details on how to determine which osteotomy to perform are outlined in the plan of the osteotomy topic in chapter 5.1 Distal radius—dorsal extraarticular malunion treated with osteotomy and double plating.

5 Reduction and fixation (cont)

Perform the osteotomy

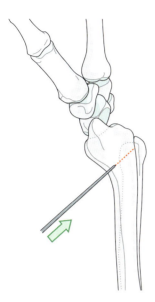

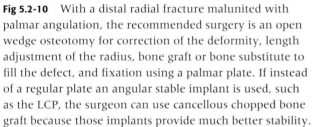

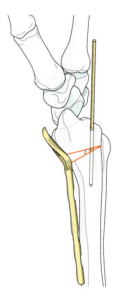

Fig 5.2-10 With a distal radial fracture malunited with palmar angulation, the recommended surgery is an open wedge osteotomy for correction of the deformity, length adjustment of the radius, bone graft or bone substitute to fill the defect, and fixation using a palmar plate. If instead of a regular plate an angular stable implant is used, such as the LCP, the surgeon can use cancellous chopped bone graft because those implants provide much better stability.

Fig 5.2-11 Through the modified Henry palmar approach, an open wedge osteotomy was performed that adjusted radial length, corrected the excessive palmar angulation, and restored the normal radial inclination. The osteotomy is performed at the site of the maximum deformity. Provide provisional fixation with a K-wire. The correction of the deformity is facilitated by utilizing the anatomical shape of the implant.

5 Reduction and fixation (cont)

Insert the first screw

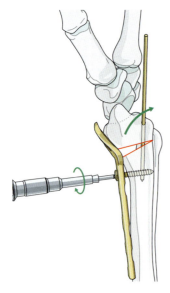

Fig 5.2-12 The first screw is placed through the implant proximal to the osteotomy. By tightening this screw an indirect reduction of the deformity will result.

Determine and correct radial inclination

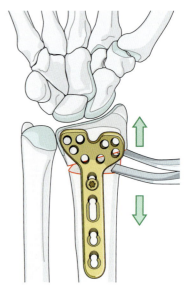

Fig 5.2-13 The deformity in the frontal plane is corrected using the laminar spreader to correct the radial inclination.

Insert additional screws

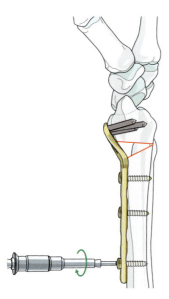

Fig 5.2-14 Additional screws proximally and distally are used to complete the fixation.

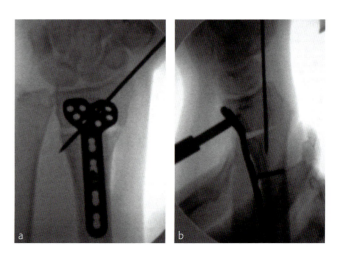

Fig 5.2-15a–b Intraoperative images show the correction obtained with the performed osteotomy in both the coronal and sagittal plane. These images also show the correct location of the plate, where care was taken not to exceed the watershed line nor to interfere with the provisional fixation maintained by the K-wire.

5 Reduction and fixation (cont)

Insert bone graft

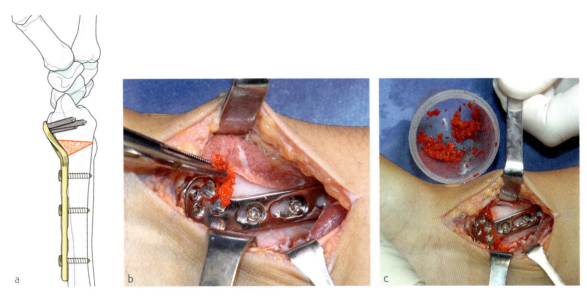

Fig 5.2-16a–c Autogenous cancellous bone graft was used to fill the space left by the osteotomy. The bone was stabilized with an LCP volar column plate 2.4.

Complete the fixation

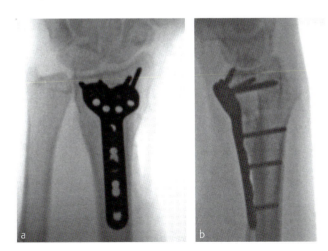
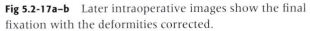
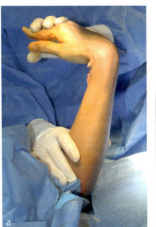
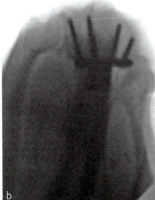

Fig 5.2-17a–b Later intraoperative images show the final fixation with the deformities corrected.

Fig 5.2-18a–b The skyline view demonstrated no protrusion of the tip of the screws on the dorsal aspect of the radius.

5 Reduction and fixation (cont)

Reduction: option

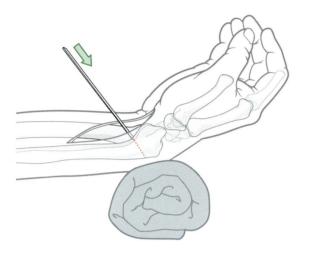

Fig 5.2-19   The osteotomy is usually performed at the site of the maximum deformity.

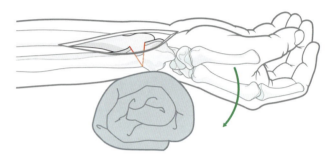

Fig 5.2-20   As an alternative, reduction can be achieved with hyperextension of the wrist using a rolled towel or bolster.

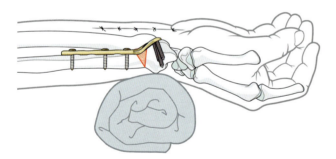

Fig 5.2-21   Fixation and bone graft of the deformity.

6 Rehabilitation

Aftercare, follow-up, and functional exercises

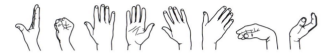

Fig 5.2-22 The patient should receive the standard postoperative rest, injury elevation, follow-up, removal of stitches, and immobilization as required. Following surgery, begin active controlled range of motion exercises. For further information, see the rehabilitation topic in chapter 4.1 Radial styloid—fracture treated with a radial column plate.

7 Outcome

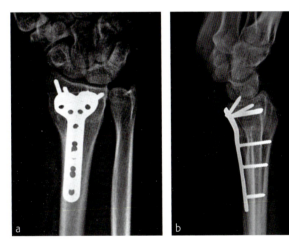

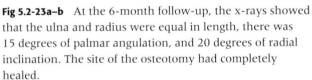

Fig 5.2-23a–b At the 6-month follow-up, the x-rays showed that the ulna and radius were equal in length, there was 15 degrees of palmar angulation, and 20 degrees of radial inclination. The site of the osteotomy had completely healed.

7 Outcome (cont)

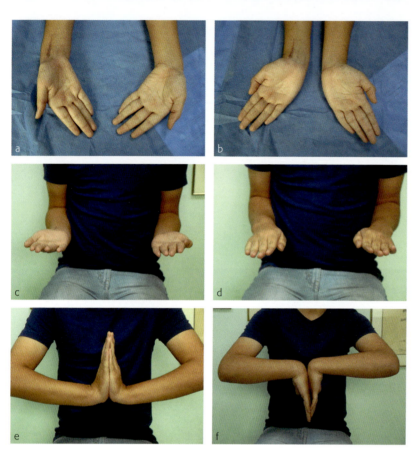

Fig 5.2-24a–f At this stage, there was good ulnar and radial deviation, and the patient could achieve excellent range of motion.

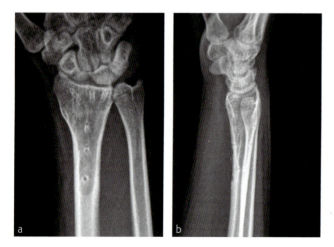

Fig 5.2-25a–b At a later follow-up, the plate was removed without problems for the patient.

5.3 Distal radius—intraarticular malunion treated with osteotomy and palmar plate

1 Case description

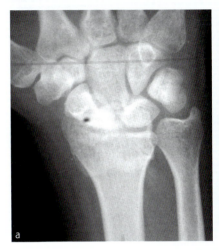 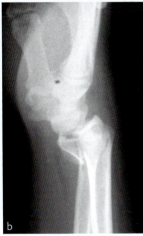

Fig 5.3-1a–b A 28-year-old salesman sustained a fall onto his outstretched hand. The PA and lateral x-rays taken immediately after the fall showed a palmar articular shearing fracture and palmar displacement with an articular step-off of 3 mm and involvement of two-thirds of the articular surface. There was articular incongruity at the lunate facet, and a distance between the palmar and dorsal rim of 9 mm, with palmar subluxation of the carpus evident. He was initially provided with nonoperative treatment of a short cast for 6 weeks.

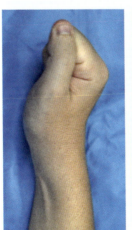 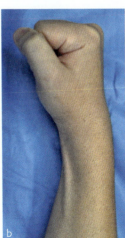 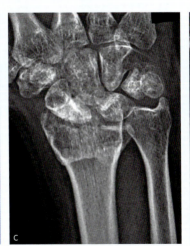 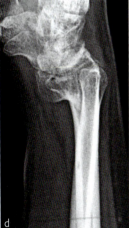

Fig 5.3-2a–d Four months after the initial trauma, he presented complaining of pain, deformity, and noticeable limitation in range of motion. The x-rays taken at that stage showed a malunited intraarticular fracture of the distal radius with palmar subluxation of the carpus and still with articular step-off of 3 mm.

399

1 Case description (cont)

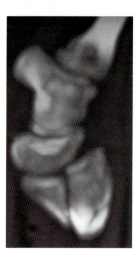

Fig 5.3-3 In the sagittal view CT scan, the palmar carpal subluxation was evident. The fracture was incompletely healed with both articular incongruity as well as fibrous union at the distal margin.

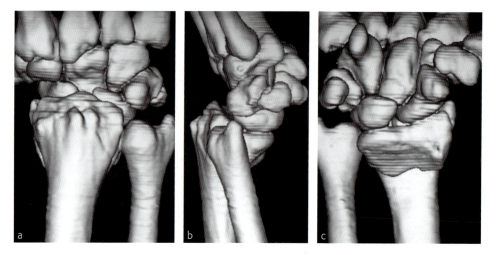

Fig 5.3-4a–c A set of 3-D CT scans offered enough information about the deformity to indicate the need for an osteotomy and fixation.

2 Indications

Intraarticular radius malunion

While extraarticular malunion of the distal radius is more common, intraarticular malunion involving the radiocarpal joint or distal radioulnar joint (DRUJ) can also occur. Articular incongruity on the joint surface ultimately leads to cartilage degeneration, and residual articular incongruity of greater than 1 mm will predictably lead to posttraumatic arthritis. For this reason, a corrective osteotomy should be considered for any distal radius malunion with joint involvement and associated incongruence.

Indications for surgery in malunited intraarticular distal radial fractures

The following are indications for surgery:
- Any step-off greater than 1 mm, as it causes articular incongruity
- Carpus subluxation, as it affects carpal kinematics and overall wrist function and is difficult to tolerate by the patient
- Malunited fractures that have a relatively simple intraarticular component.

Note that the osteotomy should be performed as early as possible since it can be made entirely through the immature callus following the planes of the deformity, thus achieving a more anatomical reduction of the articular surface.

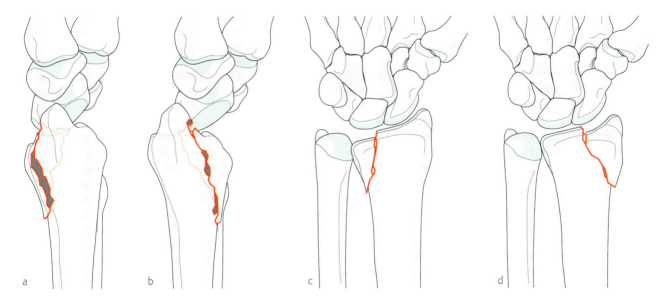

Fig 5.3-5a–d Examples of malunited intraarticular distal radial fractures amenable for corrective osteotomy include:
a Malunited palmar shearing fracture with palmar subluxation of the carpus
b Malunited dorsal shearing fracture with dorsal subluxation of the carpus
c Dorsal die punch fractures with frank incongruity between the sigmoid notch and the head of the ulna
d Malunited radial styloid fractures with frank radiocarpal incongruity.

2 Indications (cont)

Contraindications for surgery in malunited intraarticular distal radial fractures

The following are contraindications for surgery:
- Involves advanced posttraumatic arthritis
- Older patients with low demand and/or minimal symptoms
- Involves less than 1 mm articular displacement
- Involves a complex deformity with both distal radial and carpal injuries.

Imaging

In an intraarticular distal radial fracture malunion, obtaining the x-ray of the initial injury is especially helpful to both understand the articular injury and in the preoperative planning of the osteotomy. Also, a high-resolution CT with multiplanar reformatting is helpful to identify the fracture plane, which is possible upward of 8 to 12 weeks after the injury. An MRI or wrist arthroscopy may play a useful role in evaluating the amount of cartilage damage.

3 Preoperative planning

Equipment

- Variable angle (VA) locking compression plate (LCP) distal radius set
- VA LCP volar column plate 2.4
- Osteotome
- Oscillating saw
- Potential need for autogenous bone graft
- Image intensifier

Patient preparation and positioning

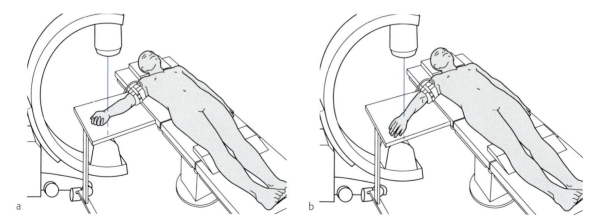

Fig 5.3-6a–b To begin, position the patient supine and place the forearm on a hand table. Supinate the forearm (**a**). The position of the limb should allow complete imaging in the frontal and sagittal plane of the distal radius. The forearm is later placed in a pronated position for the dorsal approach (**b**). A nonsterile pneumatic tourniquet is used. Prophylactic antibiotics are optional.

4 Surgical approach

Palmar and dorsal approaches

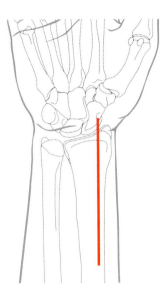

Fig 5.3-7 Two surgical approaches were used to treat this patient's injury. First, a modified Henry palmar approach was required (see Chapter 1.6 Modified Henry palmar approach to the distal radius).

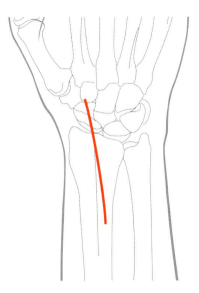

Fig 5.3-8 The second surgical approach used was a dorsal approach (see chapter 1.8 Dorsal approach to the distal radius). With this dorsal approach, only the third extensor compartment was opened. The intermediate and radial columns were approached separately using a single dorsal skin incision.

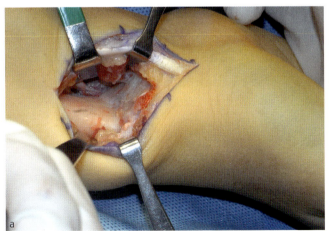

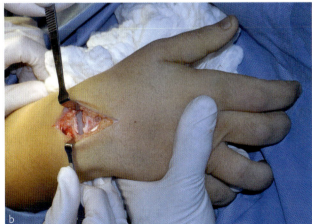

Fig 5.3-9a–b Through the modified Henry approach, the palmar aspect of the radius was exposed and the malunion became evident (**a**). The dorsal approach, followed by a dorsal capsulotomy of the joint surface, revealed the exact location of the articular step (**b**).

5 Reduction

Osteotomy

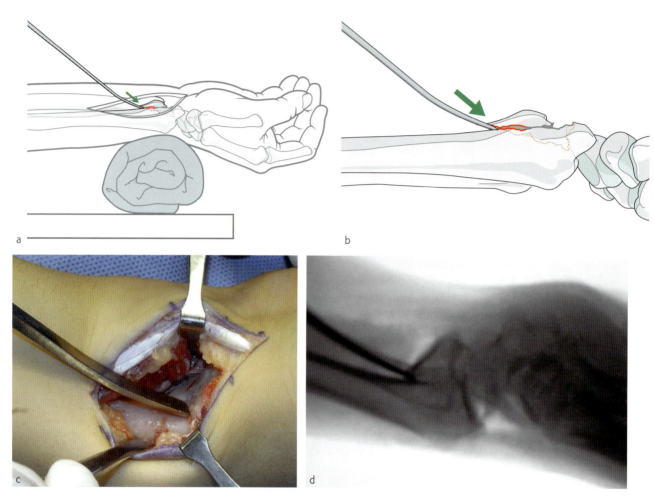

a

b

c

d

Fig 5.3-10a–d Through the palmar approach, the osteotomy was initiated using an osteotome and was guided through the plane of the malunion using the image intensifier.

5 Reduction (cont)

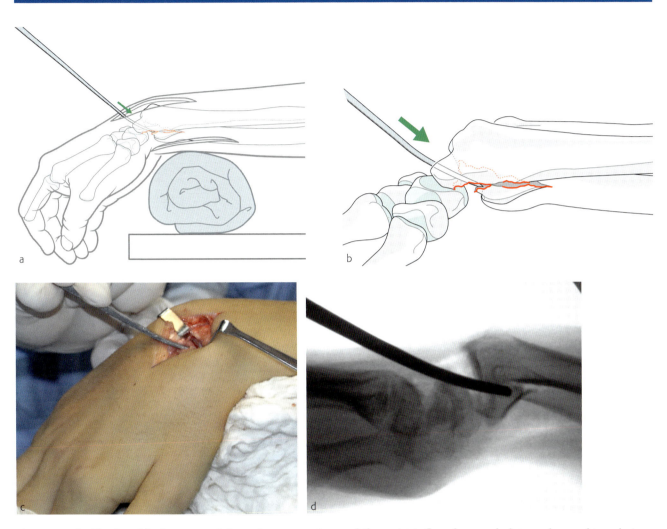

Fig 5.3-11a–d   The hand is then turned down into pronation and the wrist is flexed over a bolster or layer of towels to help determine the exact location of the step-off. The osteotome is used to implement the osteotomy from distal to proximal, and is guided by the image intensifier until the palmar and dorsal cuts meet and the palmar fragment becomes free to be reduced. It is important to leave the radiocarpal ligaments attached to the palmar fragment to avoid the risk of carpal instability. A palmar capsulotomy is prohibited, otherwise carpal instability can develop.

5 Reduction (cont)

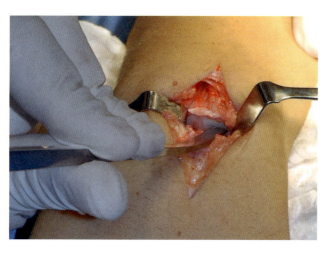

Fig 5.3-12   The dorsal view allowed a clearer view of the articular step, and allows precise placement of the osteotome to create the osteotomy.

Hyperextend the wrist

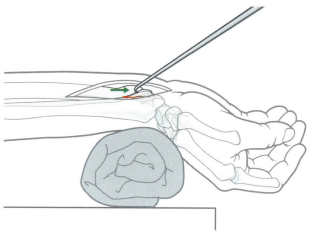

Fig 5.3-13   To assist in reduction of the osteotomy, place a rolled towel or bolster under the wrist and hyperextend it. Perfect anatomical reduction can be achieved by direct manipulation using a dental pick or a fine hook.

Alternative: reduction using plate

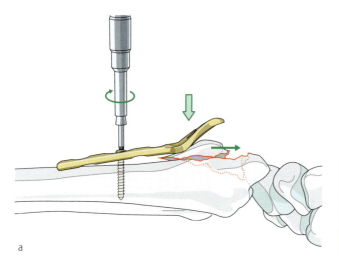

a

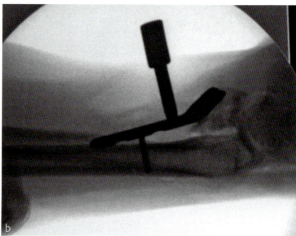

b

Fig 5.3-14a–b   The plate can be used to push the palmar fragment to achieve reduction using an appropriate screw through the oblong plate hole. The reduction must be confirmed with the use of image intensification.

Palmar plate fixation

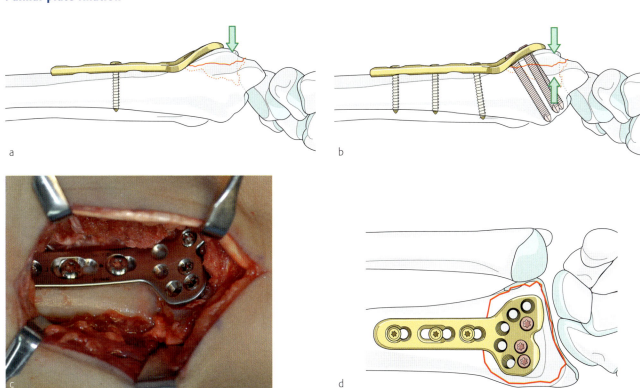

a

b

c

d

Fig 5.3-15a–d   Fixation of the distal radius should be performed with an appropriate palmar plate ensuring it buttresses the articular fragments and avoids later displacement. For this patient, stable fixation of the osteotomized palmar fragment was achieved using an LCP volar column plate 2.4, which allowed for early rehabilitation of the radiocarpal and radioulnar joints.

The fixation procedure follows the usual steps of selecting and applying the plate, inserting distal and proximal screws, and intraoperative imaging. For further information on these steps see chapter 4.6 Distal radius—multifragmentary intraarticular fracture treated with a palmar plate.

6 Fixation (cont)

Complete the fixation

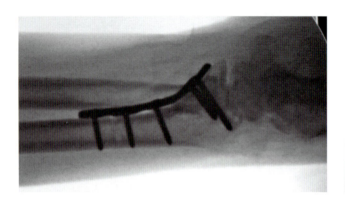

Fig 5.3-16 Final screws were inserted and the distal radius fixation completed. Intraoperative images showed correct placement of the plate.

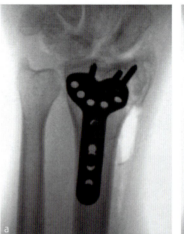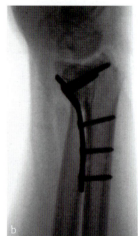

Fig 5.3-17a–b The final intraoperative images showed the anatomical reduction.

7 Rehabilitation

Aftercare, follow-up, and functional exercises

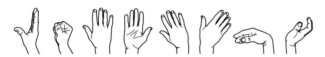

Fig 5.3-18 The patient should receive the standard postoperative rest, injury elevation, follow-up, removal of stitches, and immobilization as required. Following surgery, begin active controlled range of motion exercises. For further information see the rehabilitation topic in chapter 4.1 Radial styloid—fracture treated with a radial column plate.

8   Outcome

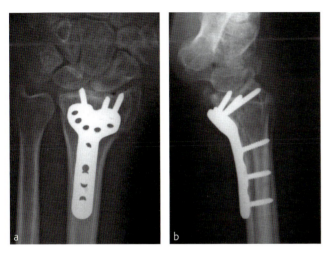

Fig 5.3-19a–b   At the 4-month follow-up, the AP and lateral x-rays showed complete healing.

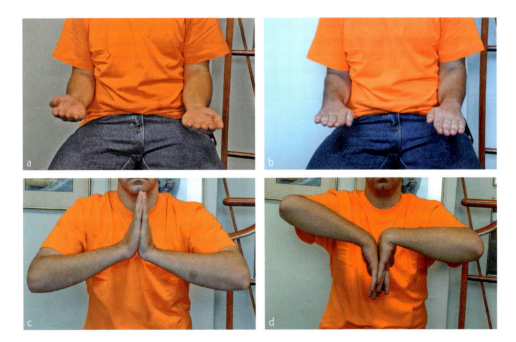

Fig 5.3-20a–d   The clinical outcome resulted in no pain and a good functional result.

9 Alternative technique: case description

Intraarticular malunion treated with osteotomy and a radial column plate and screws

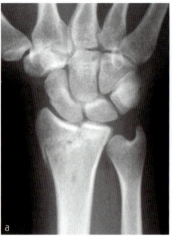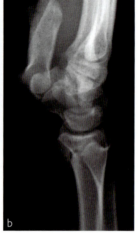

Fig 5.3-21a–b A 22-year-old female medical student suffered a fracture of the distal radius, a pelvis fracture, and other injuries in a motor vehicle accident. After initial treatment, she was seen by medical specialists 2 months after the injury, and while healing had progressed with her other injuries, she continued to have wrist pain and limitation in range of motion. The PA and lateral x-rays showed a displaced partially healed fracture of the radial styloid having an evident displacement with radiocarpal incongruity.

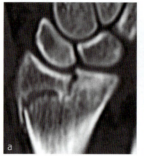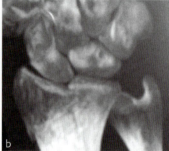

Fig 5.3-22a–b The radial CT scans demonstrated a 2 mm articular step-off and displacement on supination of the radial styloid, both of which were causing radiocarpal incongruity.

Indications

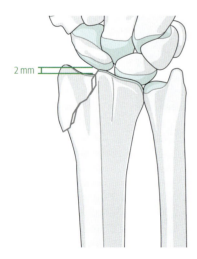

2 mm

Fig 5.3-23 Incongruency on the joint surface of the radius ultimately leads to cartilage degeneration and this is especially so when there is a malunited radial styloid with a step-off of 2 mm or more and frank radiocarpal incongruity. For this reason, a corrective osteotomy and radial column plate fixation with additional headless compression screws was considered for this patient.

9   Alternative technique: case description (cont)

Surgical approach

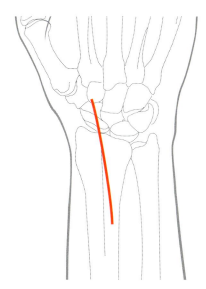

Fig 5.3-24   The surgical approach used was a dorsal approach (see chapter 1.8 Dorsal approach to the distal radius). With this dorsal approach, only the third extensor compartment was opened. The intermediate and radial columns were approached separately using a single dorsal skin incision.

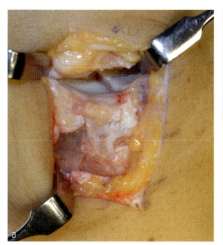
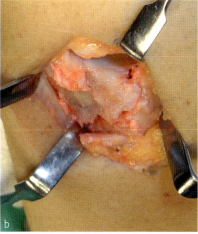

Fig 5.3-25a–b   Through a dorsal approach, the third compartment was opened in line with the extensor pollicis longus (EPL) tendon in the extensor retinaculum. The EPL tendon is freed, protected, and retracted to the radial side of the wrist. The fourth and second compartments were elevated subperiosteally, leaving both compartments intact. The fourth compartment was retracted ulnarly and the second compartment radially. The lateral column and part of the intermediate column were exposed. The dorsal capsule was incised to expose the joint, making the step-off of the joint surface clearly visible. The line of the fracture was identified using the magnifying loupes.

10 Alternative technique: reduction and fixation

Reduction

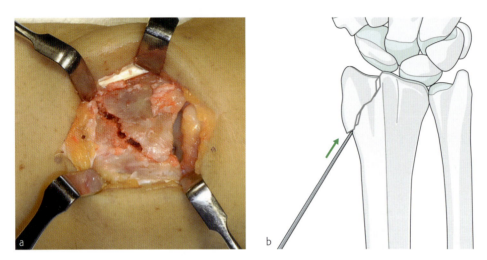

Fig 5.3-26a–b With the deformity now in clear view (**a**), using a narrow osteotome and a small curette, an osteotomy is performed through the immature callus (**b**).

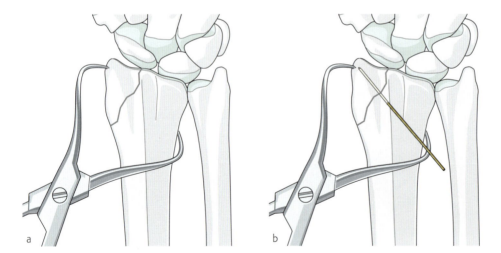

Fig 5.3-27a–b Reduce the osteotomized fragment using pointed reduction forceps (**a**). Then insert a guide wire from the radius metaphysis into the styloid fragment as perpendicular as possible to the fracture site (**b**).

10 Alternative technique: reduction and fixation (cont)

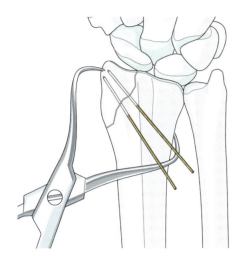

Fig 5.3-28 Pass an additional guide wire across the fracture site, gaining purchase into the cortex of the radial styloid.

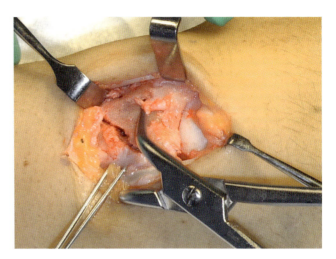

Fig 5.3-29 Following the osteotomy and temporary reduction, provisional fixation was performed using the guide wires. Reduction was checked using the image intensifier and by direct vision of the joint surface.

Fixation with radial column plate

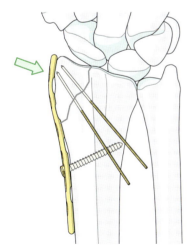

Fig 5.3-30 An LCP radial column plate 2.4 was placed over the radial column. The appropriate plate is selected according to the fracture configuration and contoured if necessary. Slide the plate underneath the first compartment and apply it onto the radial column. Insert a standard cortex screw into the oblong plate hole proximal to the malunion. Tightening this screw will reduce the radial styloid.

10 Alternative technique: reduction and fixation (cont)

Insert the additional lag screws

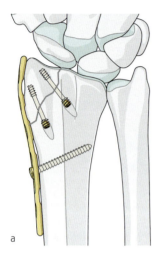 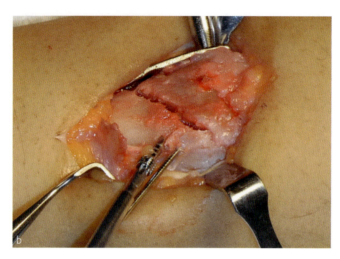

Fig 5.3-31a–b Using guide wires, two 3 mm headless compression screws are inserted exerting interfragmentary compression on the osteotomy line.

Insert proximal and distal screws

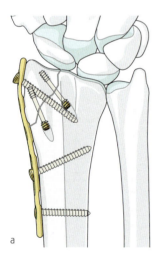 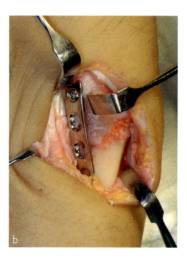

Fig 5.3-32a–b Complete the radial column plate fixation by inserting proximal and distal screws into the plate holes. The plate increases stability and allows unrestricted early mobility.

10 Alternative technique: reduction and fixation (cont)

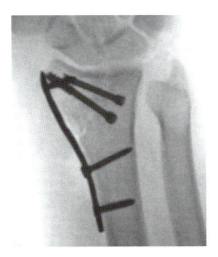

Fig 5.3-33 Intraoperative images showed the anatomical reduction and the correct placement of the plates and screws.

Complete the fixation

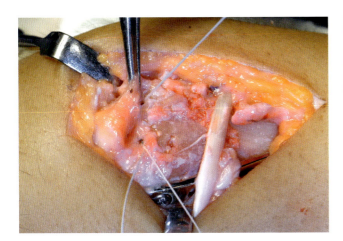

Fig 5.3-34 Two bone anchors were placed on the dorsal rim of the radius.

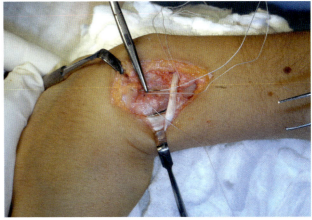

Fig 5.3-35 The dorsal capsule was sutured back onto the dorsal rim of the radius using the anchor's sutures.

10 Alternative technique: reduction and fixation (cont)

Outcome

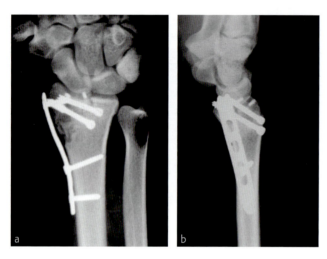

Fig 5.3-36a–b At the 3-month follow-up, the radiological images indicated good healing.

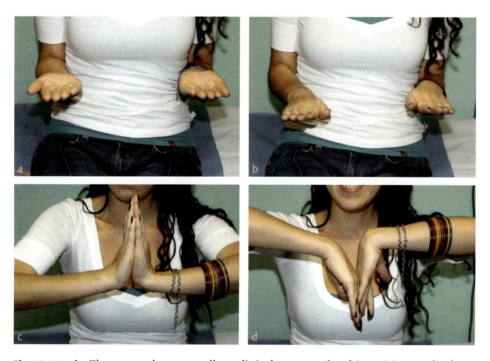

Fig 5.3-37a–d There was also an excellent clinical outcome for this aspiring medical professional.

5.4 Distal radius—extraarticular and intraarticular malunion treated with osteotomy and dorsal double plating

1 Case description

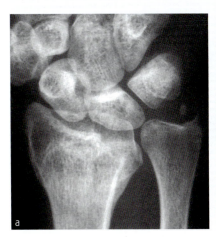 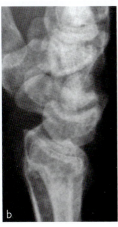

Fig 5.4-1a–b A 27-year-old house cleaner had a fall while working yet did not present for medical advice until 6 months later. She had suffered a complex fracture of her right distal radius and had limited wrist and forearm motion. She complained of persistent pain with both work-specific and normal activities of daily living. The PA and lateral x-rays revealed a combined intraarticular and extraarticular distal radial fracture malunion.

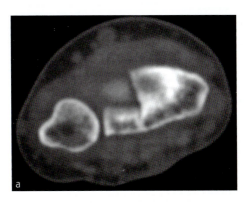 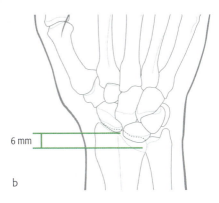

6 mm

Fig 5.4-2a–b The axial CT scan showed an impaction of the lunate facet with a 6 mm step-off and gap, and intraarticular incongruency of the distal radioulnar joint (DRUJ).

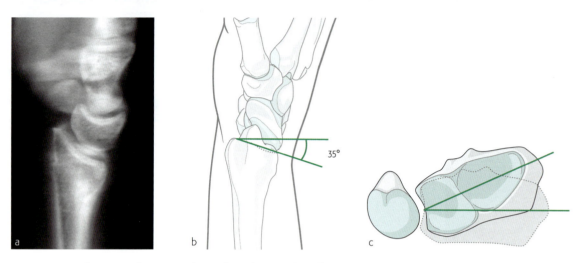

Fig 5.4-3a–c   The sagittal CT scan showed 35 degrees dorsal angulation due to the extraarticular metaphyseal deformity. Radial shortening and supination of the distal fragment were also evident.

2 Indications

Combined intraarticular and extraarticular malunion

In some instances following a distal radial fracture, a combined intraarticular and extraarticular malunion can occur, which can adversely affect both the radiocarpal and radioulnar joint functions. As discussed in the previous chapters in this section, deformity involving greater than 1 mm step-off at the articular surface, or greater than 10 degrees of dorsal angulation as a result of extraarticular malunion, are indications for treatment by osteotomy. Both these levels of deformity were greatly exceeded in this patient. Careful understanding of the component parts of the malunion is crucial to planning the type and location of the osteotomies.

Imaging

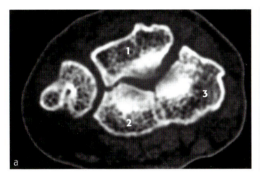
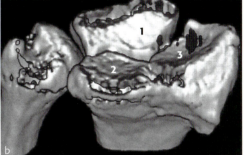
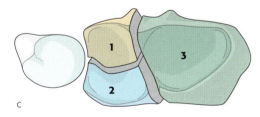

Fig 5.4-4a–c Axial 2-D CT and 3-D CT scans provide a clearer understanding of the articular incongruity and the fact that the articular malunion in this case consisted of three major components. These include both the dorsal and lunate facets and the radial styloid.

3 Preoperative planning

Equipment

- Variable angle (VA) locking compression plate (LCP) distal radius set
- VA LCP dorsal plates 2.4
- 2.0 mm cortex screw
- 1.1 mm or 1.2 mm K-wires
- Oscillating saw
- Osteotome
- Image intensifier

Patient preparation and positioning

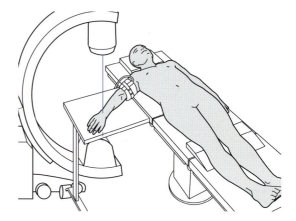

Fig 5.4-5 Position the patient supine and place the forearm on the hand table. Pronate the forearm. The position of the limb should allow complete imaging in the frontal and sagittal plane of the distal radius. A nonsterile pneumatic tourniquet is used. Prophylactic antibiotics are optional.

4 Surgical approach

Approach

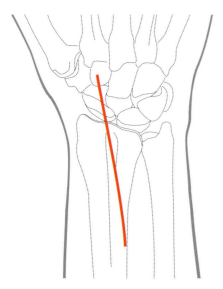

Fig 5.4-6 The surgical approach used was a dorsal approach (see chapter 1.8 Dorsal approach to the distal radius).

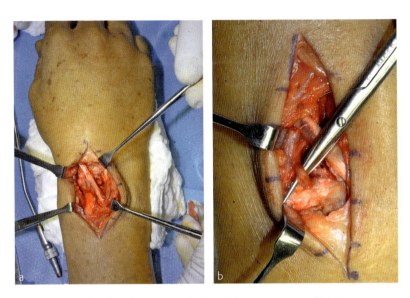

Fig 5.4-7a–b The dorsal exposure isolated the extensor pollicis longus. The posterior interosseous nerve was identified and sectioned.

5 Reduction

Plan the osteotomy

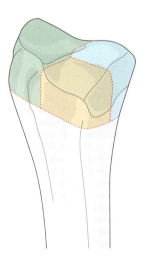

Fig 5.4-8 Osteotomy lines are planned onto the bone following the various fracture patterns. Once performed, the osteotomies separate the dorsoulnar component and the metaphysis.

5 Reduction (cont)

Perform the articular component osteotomy

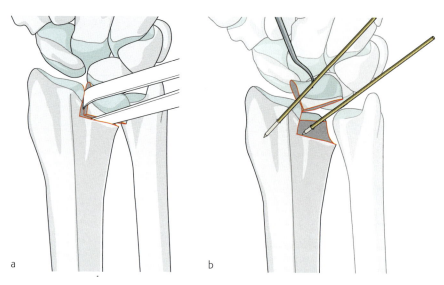

a   b

Fig 5.4-9a–b An osteotomy is first performed at the articular site. The dorsal lunate facet is osteotomized and retracted distally. This will now expose the back of the palmar lunate facet and displaced radial styloid (**a**). K-wires are introduced into the palmar lunate facet and radial styloid components to be later used as joysticks (**b**).

Perform the metaphyseal component osteotomy

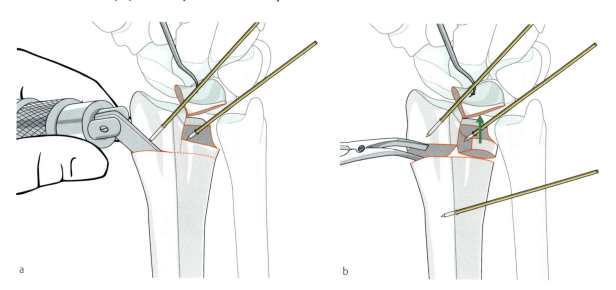

a   b

Fig 5.4-10a–b An osteotomy is then performed at the site of the metaphyseal malunion (**a**). Note that it is important to release the attachment of the brachioradialis to gain realignment for adequate length of the articular component. The osteotomy is opened using a laminar spreader and the dorsal metaphyseal deformity reduced leaving a gap in the metaphyseal area of the bone (**b**).

5   Reduction (cont)

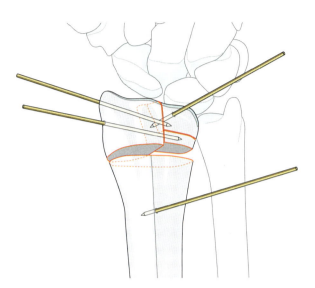

Fig 5.4-11   The K-wire is removed from the palmar lunate facet and the dorsal lunate facet is repositioned and held with a K-wire through both lunate facet fragments. The reduction of both the articular and metaphyseal deformities are temporarily held with K-wires.

Bone graft

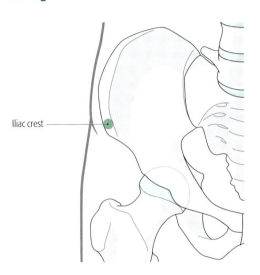

Fig 5.4-12   Harvest the corticocancellous graft material from the iliac crest.

Harvesting bone wedge

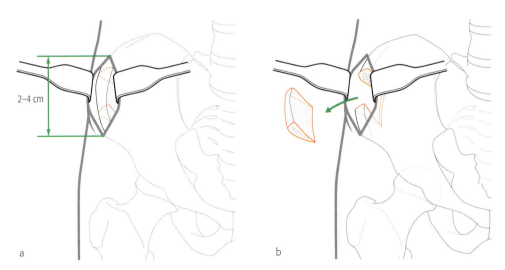

a

b

Fig 5.4-13a–b   Expose the crest over a 2–4 cm segment and mark out the preplanned graft size to be harvested (**a**). Consider the shape and size of the defect in the distal radius and how the graft will fill the defect created by the osteotomy (**b**). Harvest the selected graft using a sharp osteotome. Control bleeding with a wound pack and use a small suction drain if necessary. Close the skin and apply a pressure dressing.

5   Reduction (cont)

Insert the bone graft

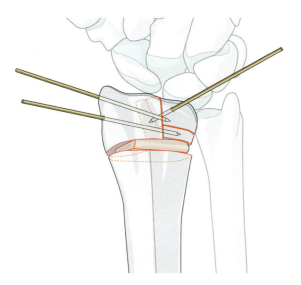

Fig 5.4-14   Once the optimal anatomical position is achieved, the parts are temporarily fixated and the iliac crest bone wedge is introduced into the metaphyseal osteotomy site.

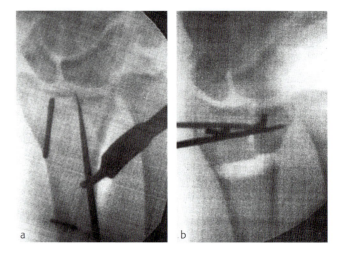

Fig 5.4-15a–b   Intraoperative images show the correction of both the intraarticular and extraarticular malunions and their temporarily stabilization with K-wires.

6   Fixation

Fixation of articular components

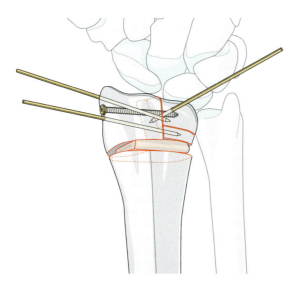

Fig 5.4-16   It may be necessary to fix the articular components with a radially inserted 2.0 mm lag screw.

6 Fixation (cont)

Fixation of intermediate column

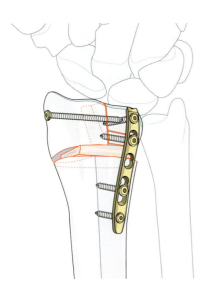

Fig 5.4-17   To fixate the metaphysis, two plates are placed on the dorsal side. First, the intermediate column must be supported by a suitable intermediate column dorsal plate. For this patient, a straight plate was used.

The fixation procedure follows the usual steps of selecting, contouring, and applying the plate, and inserting proximal and distal screws. For further information on these steps see the fixation of intermediate column topic in chapter 4.5 Distal radius—dorsally displaced intraarticular fracture treated with double plating.

Fixation of radial column

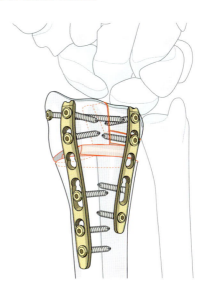

Fig 5.4-18   To complete the fixation, a straight plate was used for the radial column.

The fixation procedure follows the usual steps of selecting, contouring, and applying the plate, and inserting proximal and distal screws; however on this occasion, the plate was placed more adjacent to the intermediate column plate on the dorsal side.

7 Rehabilitation

Aftercare, follow-up, and functional exercises

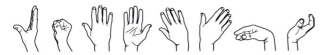

Fig 5.4-19   The patient should receive the standard postoperative rest, injury elevation, follow-up, removal of stitches, and immobilization as required. Following surgery, begin active controlled range of motion exercises. For further information, see the rehabilitation topic in chapter 4.1 Radial styloid—fracture treated with a radial column plate.

8 Outcome

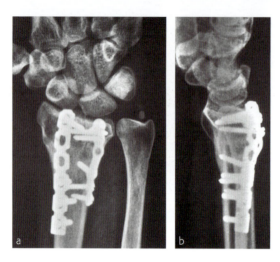

Fig 5.4-20a–b At the 1-year follow-up the osteotomies were shown to be healed.

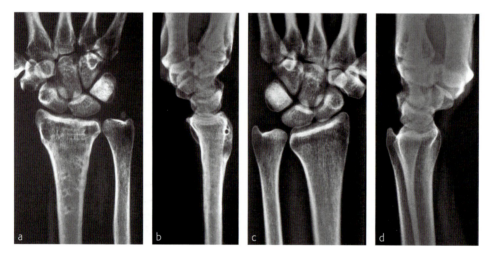

Fig 5.4-21a–d At an 11-year follow-up the implants were electively removed.

8 Outcome (cont)

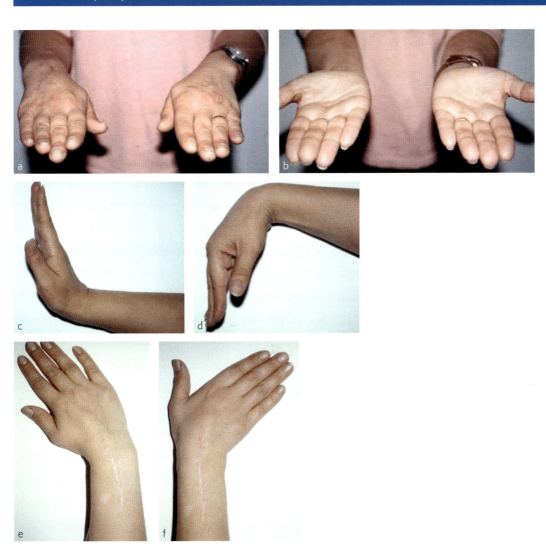

Fig 5.4-22a–f The patient had excellent function and range of motion, with no wrist arthritis.

5.5 Rheumatoid arthritis treated with radiolunate arthrodesis

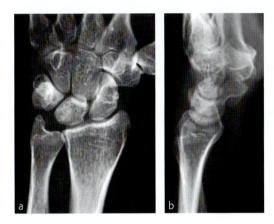

Fig 5.5-1a–b A 60-year-old female beauty therapist presented complaining of progressive pain and functional limitation in her left wrist after suffering rheumatoid arthritis for 15 years. The PA and lateral x-rays revealed joint space narrowing at the radiolunate joint and the distal radioulnar joint (DRUJ).

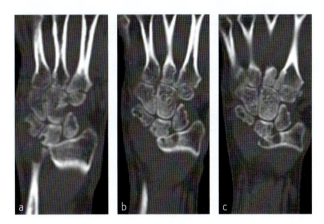

Fig 5.5-2a–c The CT scans demonstrated ongoing arthritis with radiolunate joint space narrowing, ulnar translation (displacement in an ulnar direction) of the carpus, and cystic changes at the radiolunate articulation.

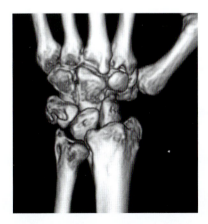

Fig 5.5-3 The 3-D CT scans further indicated the ulnar translation of the carpus.

429

Wrist dysfunction from rheumatoid arthritis

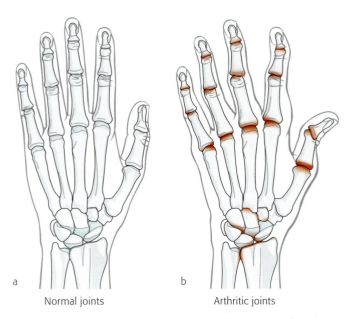

a   Normal joints   b   Arthritic joints

Fig 5.5-4a–b Rheumatoid arthritis is a well-recognized problem where the body's own immune system starts to attack the joints. Often affecting the hand and wrist, it results in inflammation, pain, and stiffness and thickening in the affected joints, and may even eventually affect the major organs. Initial treatment can include medications, steroids, and support braces or immobilization, but severe cases can be treated with surgical treatment to repair or fuse the joints.

Symptomatic wrist dysfunction of any etiology can require reconstruction, and salvage procedures are frequently the only way to offer the patient a stable pain-free wrist. A number of surgical options that ideally preserve motion and avoid complications in the long term can be considered:

- Limited wrist arthrodesis
- Proximal row carpectomy (which is contraindicated in this case because the rheumatoid arthritis affects the lunate facet of the distal radius)
- Arthroplasty (involving replacement of the wrist joint)
- Total wrist arthrodesis.

Limited wrist arthrodesis

A limited wrist arthrodesis involves the surgical fusion of a selection of bones in the wrist depending on the extent of the affected area. The ultimate goals of a limited wrist arthrodesis include eliminating pain that is related to the joints that have focal arthritis while simultaneously preserving as much motion as possible through the remaining articular surfaces. Frequently, the radiolunate or radioscaphoid joints are involved and significant pain and deformity are noted. In some cases (as will be seen in the alternative techniques later in this chapter) the partial or full removal of an affected carpal is necessary in an attempt to preserve functional motion.

2 Indications (cont)

Radiolunate arthrodesis

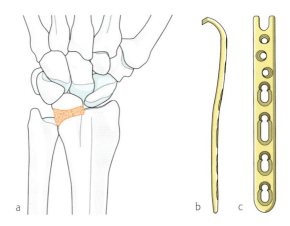

Fig 5.5-5a–c A radiolunate arthrodesis is a limited wrist arthrodesis procedure indicated when there is palmar or ulnar translation of the carpus or localized radiolunate arthritis (**a**), commonly seen in patients with rheumatoid arthritis but also noted in those with die punch fractures within the lunate fossa. For this patient, a locking compression plate (LCP) distal ulna (hook) plate was placed into the dorsal rim of the lunate at one end and to the radius at the other, fusing the segments together (**b–c**).

Imaging

X-rays and CT scans and laboratory testing may support an initial diagnosis of rheumatoid arthritis. They may also help to exclude other diseases with similar symptoms.

3 Preoperative planning

Equipment

- LCP distal ulna plate 2.0
- 1.4 mm to 1.6 mm K-wires
- Bone nibbler/rongeur
- Image intensifier

Patient preparation and positioning

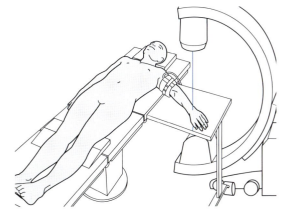

Fig 5.5-6 Position the patient supine and place the forearm on the hand table. Pronate the forearm. The position of the limb should allow complete imaging in the frontal and sagittal plane of the distal radius. A nonsterile pneumatic tourniquet is used. Prophylactic antibiotics are optional.

431

4 Surgical approach

Approach

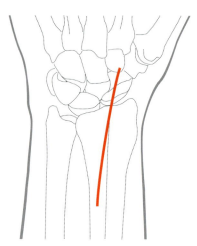

Fig 5.5-7 The surgical approach used was a dorsal approach (see chapter 1.8 Dorsal approach to the distal radius). The incision was through the third extensor compartment.

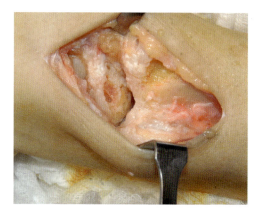

Fig 5.5-8 The dorsal capsule of the left wrist was opened in a T-fashion, exposing the radiolunate joint. Note the absence of hyaline cartilage on the lunate.

5 Reduction

Bone graft

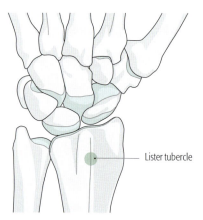

Lister tubercle

Fig 5.5-9 Harvest graft material from the distal radius for later insertion into the affected wrist joints. A good and safe place is proximal and slightly radial to Lister tubercle. When harvesting, retract the tendons of the second compartment radially and the extensor pollicis longus in an ulnar direction.

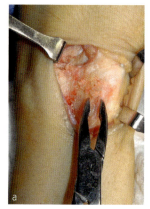
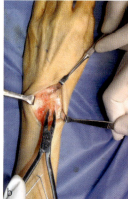

Fig 5.5-10a–b Through the existing dorsal approach, and with the extensor tendons retracted radially and ulnarly, the Lister tubercle was used as a source of autogenous bone graft.

5 Reduction (cont)

Reduce the lunate and insert the graft

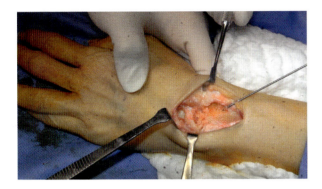

Fig 5.5-11 After decortication of the articular surfaces of both the lunate and lunate fossa, and placing the autogenous bone graft between the joint surfaces, the lunate is reduced and provisionally held with a K-wire.

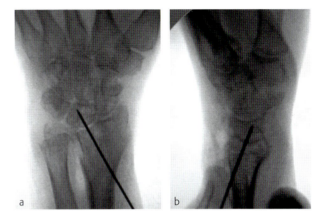

Fig 5.5-12a–b The PA and lateral intraoperative images show the placement of the K-wire. The lunate is reduced in neutral position.

6 Fixation

Select and apply the plate

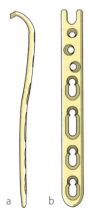

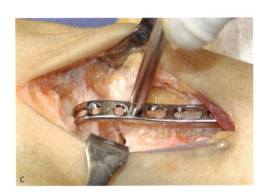

Fig 5.5-13a–c Insert the hook plate. The plate adapts well to the radiolunate articulation. The hooks are placed into the dorsal rim of the lunate. Once applied, the hook plate will be well seated and avoids the lunocapitate joint. Take great care that the hooks of the hook plate do not force the lunate into extension. A temporary radiolunate K-wire can prevent this.

6 Fixation (cont)

Insert screws

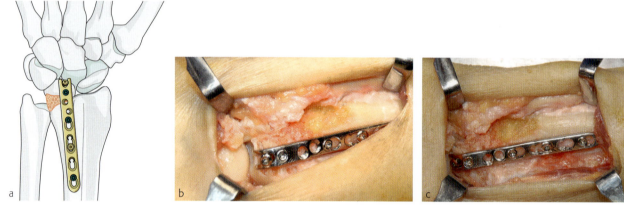

Fig 5.5-14a–c   Angular stable screws are used to fix the plate to both the lunate and radius metaphysis. The most distal screw is directed proximally into the distal radius and placed under compression.

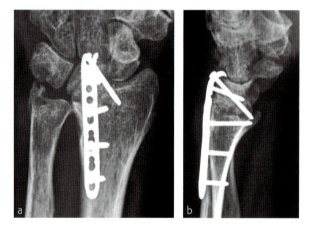

Fig 5.5-15a–b   One locking screw was inserted into the lunate and a lag screw was also placed through the lunate and was threaded on the palmar cortex of the radius.

7 Rehabilitation

Aftercare, follow-up, and functional exercises

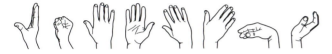

Fig 5.5-16 The patient should receive the standard postoperative rest, injury elevation, follow-up, removal of stitches, and immobilization as required. Following surgery, begin active controlled range of motion exercises. For further information, see the rehabilitation topic in chapter 4.1 Radial styloid—fracture treated with a radial column plate.

8 Outcome

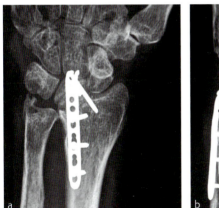
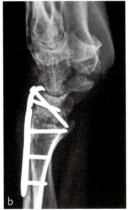
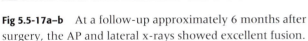

Fig 5.5-17a–b At a follow-up approximately 6 months after surgery, the AP and lateral x-rays showed excellent fusion.

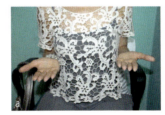
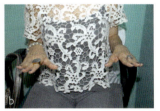
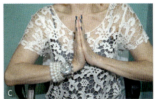
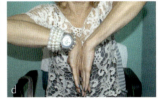

Fig 5.5-18a–d Full forearm rotation was achieved but with some limitation of wrist flexion and extension. However, the patient was completely pain free.

9   Alternative technique 1

Radioscapholunate arthrodesis

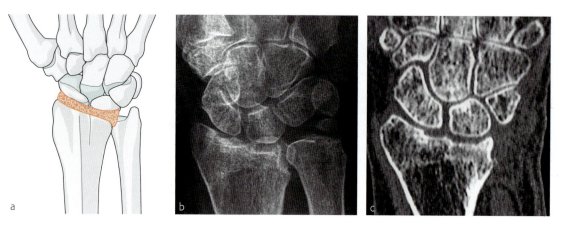

Fig 5.5-19a–c   A radioscapholunate arthrodesis is a limited wrist arthrodesis procedure indicated for patients with degenerative joint disease throughout the radiocarpal joint (**a**). It involves the entire joint surface. The x-ray and CT scans show radiocarpal osteoarthritis on a right hand following a malunited intraarticular distal radial fracture (**b–c**). Note that the cartilage of the midcarpal joint was not damaged, which is a prerequisite to indicate this technique.

Fixation and outcome

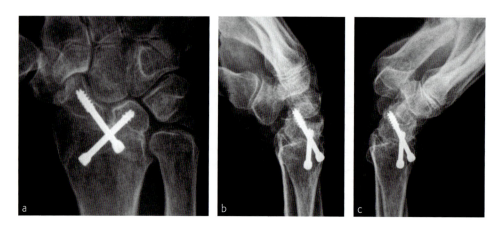

Fig 5.5-20a–c   The radioscapholunate arthrodesis involved the placement of two 3.0 mm headless compression screws coming from the radius, one into the scaphoid and one into the lunate. At the 5-year follow-up, PA and lateral x-rays showed excellent fusion, and the patient showed painless functional wrist motion. Clinical motion (flexion and extension) can be seen in the lateral x-rays.

10 Alternative technique 2

Radioscapholunate arthrodesis with resection of the distal half of the scaphoid

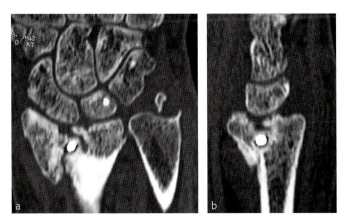

Fig 5.5-21a–b   The CT scans of this patient demonstrate arthritic involvement of both the radiolunate and radioscaphoid joint as sequelae of a malunited distal radial fracture initially treated by closed reduction and percutaneous fixation. The cartilage of the midcarpal joint was not damaged. Note the palmar subluxation of the carpus in the lateral view and a gap of 4–5 mm in the distal radial articular surface. Further treatment with a radioscapholunate arthrodesis was required.

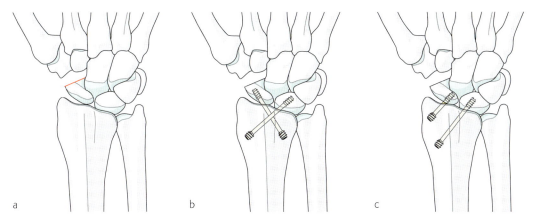

Fig 5.5-22a–c   When the radiocarpal joint undergoes a fusion procedure, the wrist's range of motion is considerably reduced, often as much as 50%. For this reason, removal of the distal half of the scaphoid is sometimes recommended to improve motion through the midcarpal joint (**a**). Fixation can involve screws inserted in a cross formation (**b**) or coming parallel from the radial styloid (**c**).

10 Alternative technique 2

Fixation and outcome

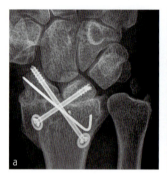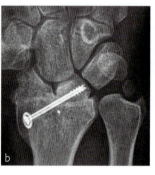

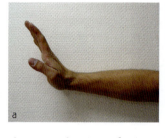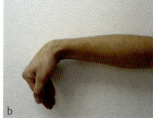

Fig 5.5-24a–b   A good range of motion was achieved by the 7-year follow-up.

Fig 5.5-23a–b   Treatment involved removal of the distal half of the scaphoid along with insertion of two 3.5 mm screws with washers and a K-wire. The PA view x-ray shows total healing of the fusion 4 months after surgery (**a**). Note that the normal relationship between the scaphoid and lunate was preserved in order to maintain the congruency of the midcarpal joint. Solid fusion is shown at 6 months following surgery (**b**). The screw from the radius into the scaphoid was removed at that time because of tendon irritation.

5.6 Kienbock's disease treated with total wrist arthrodesis

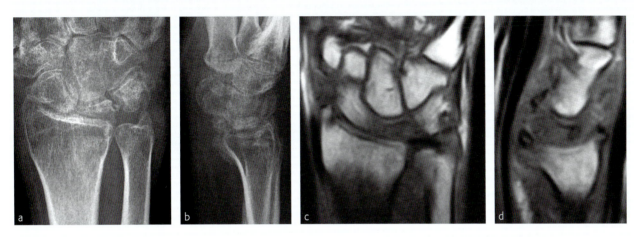

Fig 5.6-1a–d   A 47-year-old right-hand dominant taxi driver experienced a mildly painful wrist for 3 years until he suffered a torsional injury lifting a heavy object (car wheel). His wrist pain became extreme. The PA and lateral x-rays showed Kienbock´s disease stage IIIB with severe lunate collapse and osteoporosis (**a–b**). The MRIs confirmed the diagnosis, with loss of vascularization and collapse of the lunate being evident (**c–d**).

The clinical examination revealed noticeable swelling of the wrist and limited motion. He had only 10 degrees of wrist extension and 5 degrees of flexion, with only 10 degrees of ulnar deviation and absence of radial deviation. Grip strength in the affected hand had fallen markedly to just 15.5 kg (average grip strength for the normal population at the same age was 52 kg).

2 Indications

Kienbock's disease (avascular necrosis of the lunate)

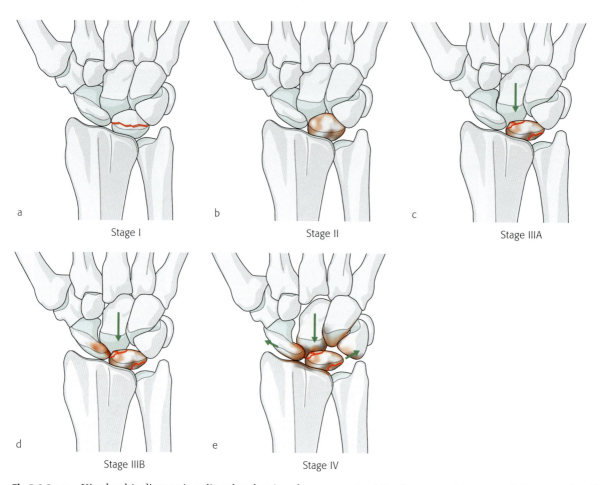

a   Stage I   b   Stage II   c   Stage IIIA

d   Stage IIIB   e   Stage IV

Fig 5.6-2a–e Kienbock's disease is a disorder that involves necrosis of the lunate and its potential eventual collapse. It results from an interruption of blood supply to the lunate caused by any number of factors, but typically involving an initial trauma to the wrist. The extent of collapse and fragmentation of the lunate can be used to help classify the disorder, as follows:

- Stage I: Normal lunate fracture
- Stage II: Sclerosis of the lunate without collapse
- Stage IIIA: Lunate collapse and fragmentation in addition to proximal migration of the capitate
- Stage IIIB: Lunate collapse and fragmentation in addition to proximal migration of the capitate plus fixed flexion deformity of the scaphoid
- Stage IV: Degeneration around the lunate with radiocarpal and midcarpal arthritic changes.

Symptomatic wrist dysfunction of any etiology can require reconstruction, and salvage procedures are frequently the only way to offer the patient a stable pain-free wrist. A number of surgical options that ideally preserve motion and avoid complications in the long term can be considered:

- Limited wrist arthrodesis
- Proximal row carpectomy
- Arthroplasty
- Total wrist arthrodesis.

2 Indications (cont)

Total wrist arthrodesis

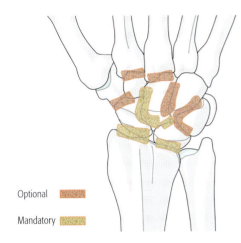

Optional ▨

Mandatory ▨

Fig 5.6-3 A total wrist arthrodesis involves the total fusion of the radiocarpal and midcarpal joints. This is a salvage procedure where the patient has lost functional wrist motion or suffers persistent and unrelenting pain and extensive intercarpal arthritis. The ultimate goal is a pain-free and stable wrist with restoration of functional grip strength.

Choice of implant

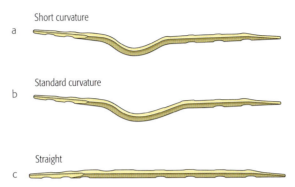

a   Short curvature

b   Standard curvature

c   Straight

Fig 5.6-4a–c A wrist fusion plate with short or standard curvature (or in some indications no bend at all) is the implant of choice. The precontoured curved plates reduce the need for intraoperative bending to follow the natural contours of the wrist. The plate also places the hand in an optimal position. The design of the curved wrist fusion plates places the radius in 10 degrees extension, which is ideal as the goal is to achieve the arthrodesis with the wrist in 10 degrees of extension and 15 degrees of ulnar deviation. For this patient, the short curved plate was selected.

3 Preoperative planning

Equipment

- Locking compression plate (LCP) wrist fusion set
- Wrist fusion plate 2.7/3.5
- Bone nibbler/rongeur
- Osteotome
- Image intensifier

Patient preparation and positioning

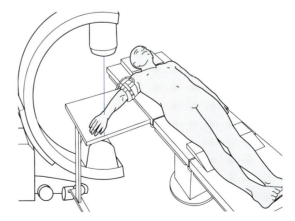

Fig 5.6-5 Position the patient supine and place the forearm on the hand table. Pronate the forearm. The position of the limb should allow complete imaging in the frontal and sagittal plane of the distal radius. A nonsterile pneumatic tourniquet is used. Prophylactic antibiotics are optional.

4 Surgical approach

Approach

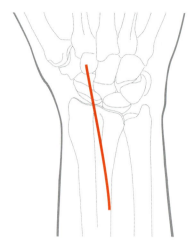

Fig 5.6-6 The surgical approach used was a dorsal approach (see chapter 1.8 Dorsal approach to the distal radius). With this dorsal approach, there was a straight longitudinal incision between the third and fourth extensor compartments.

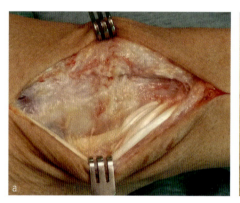

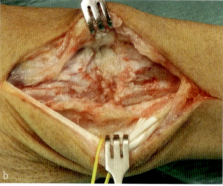

Fig 5.6-7a–b A straight dorsal longitudinal incision was made (**a**). The dorsal side of the wrist after longitudinal capsular opening (**b**).

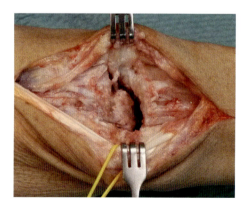

Fig 5.6-8 Chondral debridement of the radiocarpal and midcarpal joints was undertaken until reaching bleeding surfaces.

5 Reduction

Bone graft

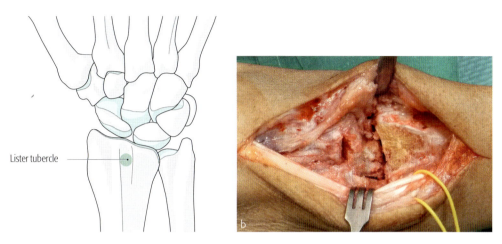

Fig 5.6-9a–b Harvest graft material from the distal radius for later insertion into the affected wrist joints. On this occasion, Lister tubercle and the dorsal half of the distal radius were removed for use as bone graft material.

Insert the bone graft

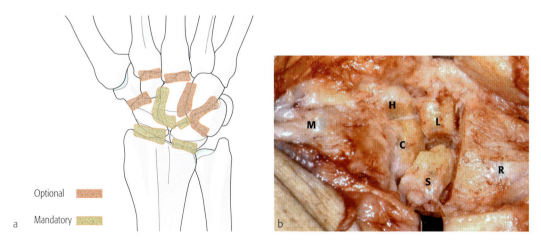

Joints to fuse (below):
R: Radius
L: Lunate
S: Scaphoid
C: Capitate
H: Hamate
M: Third metacarpal

Fig 5.6-10a–b Expose and prepare the joint surfaces to be included in the fusion. Then distribute the cancellous bone graft throughout the radiocarpal and midcarpal joints to enhance the fusion procedure.

6 Fixation

Select and apply the plate

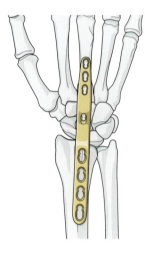

Fig 5.6-11 Insert the wrist fusion plate through the approach and position the plate directly over the third metacarpal distally and the radius proximally.

Measure screw depth

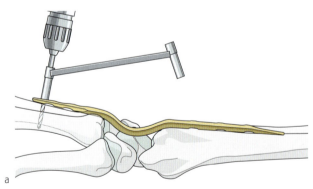

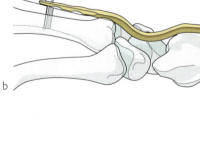

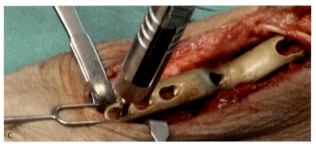

Fig 5.6-12a–c Place the drill guide in the first (most distal) hole and drill with a 2.0 mm drill bit to the desired length. Remove the drill and drill guide and measure for screw length.

6   Fixation (cont)

Insert distal screws

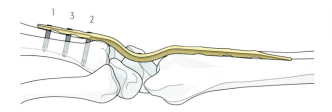

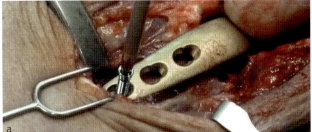

Fig 5.6-13   In this procedure, 2.7 mm compression or locking screws are used for the distal end of the plate, going into the capitate or metacarpals. Larger 3.5 mm compression or locking screws are used for the radius. Insert the 2.7 mm distal screws first (with recommended sequence of screw insertion shown).

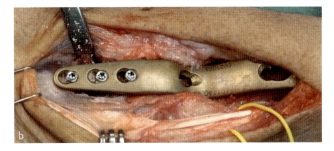

Fig 5.6-14a–b   Intraoperative images show the 2.7 mm locking screws being placed into the third metacarpal.

Measure and insert screw into the capitate

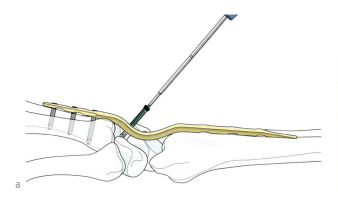

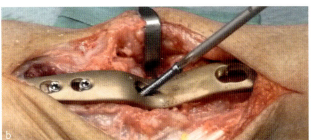

Fig 5.6-15a–b   Determine screw length and insert a 2.7 mm locking screw through the central plate hole into the capitate.

6   Fixation

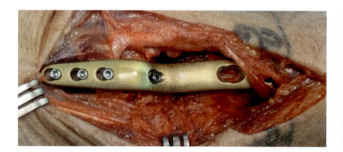

Fig 5.6-16   The distal fixation into the third metacarpal and capitate is shown.

Align plate and measure proximal screw depth

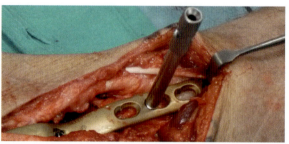

Fig 5.6-17   Align the plate over the radius. Place the drill guide in the third most proximal hole and drill with a 2.5 mm drill bit to the desired length. This will become screw number 5. Remove the drill and drill guide and measure for screw length. Verify with image intensification.

Insert proximal screws

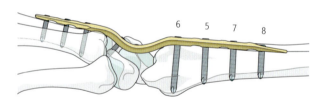

Fig 5.6-18   The 3.5 mm compression or locking screws are now used for insertion into the radius (with recommended sequence of screw insertion shown). The fifth screw can be applied as a compression screw in order to apply the plate toward the dorsal cortex of the radius.

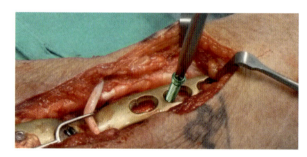

Fig 5.6-19   The intraoperative image shows a 3.5 mm locking screw being placed into the radius.

6 Fixation (cont)

Complete the fixation

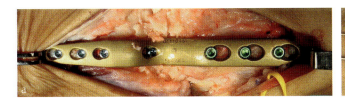
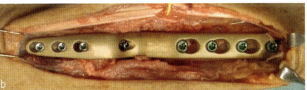

Fig 5.6-20a–b   Local bone graft from the earlier debridement was inserted into the area to complete the fixation.

7 Rehabilitation

Aftercare, follow-up, and functional exercises

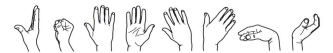

Fig 5.6-21   The patient should receive the standard postoperative rest, injury elevation, follow-up, removal of stitches, and immobilization as required. Following surgery, begin active controlled range of motion exercises. For further information, see the rehabilitation topic in chapter 4.1 Radial styloid—fracture treated with a radial column plate.

8 Outcome

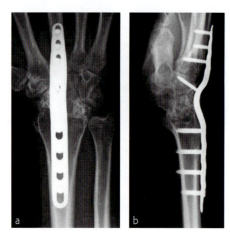

Fig 5.6-22a–b At the 13-week follow-up, the x-rays showed the total wrist arthrodesis was complete with full integration of the bone graft.

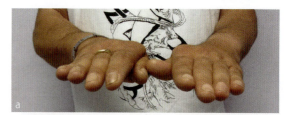

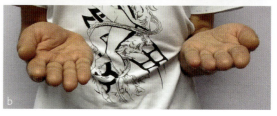

Fig 5.6-23a–b After a period of 6 months following wrist fusion surgery, the patient returned to his job as a taxi driver. At the 5-year follow-up, he noted occasional discomfort with strenuous activity, but generally good range of motion (**a–b**), and grip strength that had improved to 46.5 kg. He had a patient satisfaction rating of 9 (VAS: 0-10).

Video

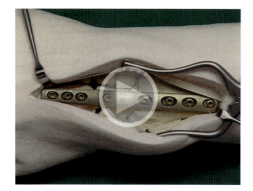

Video 5.6-1 This video demonstrates a wrist arthrodesis with a wrist fusion plate.

5.7 Malunited fracture with associated ulnar abutment syndrome treated with an ulnar shortening osteotomy

1 Case description

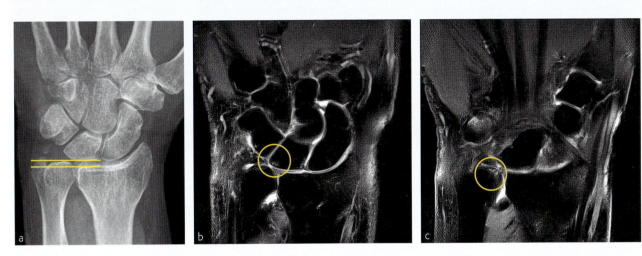

Fig 5.7-1a–c A 64-year-old man sustained a closed fracture of his nondominant left distal radius after a fall. The fracture was managed nonoperatively in a short arm cast for 6 weeks and healed with a minor loss of radial length.

Following nonoperative treatment, new PA x-rays showed positive ulnar variance of 2 mm and an avulsion of the tip of the ulnar styloid (**a**). Forearm rotation became increasingly painful and limited his ability to fully pronate. New MRI scans revealed edematous changes in the ulnar corner of the lunate and the opposing part of the ulnar head (**b–c**), which were the result of ongoing impact between the ulna and the lunate.

Radioulnar length discrepancy and ulnar abutment syndrome

A minor degree of radioulnar length discrepancy is not uncommon after a healed distal radial fracture, however, enduring symptoms are unusual. In this case, relative lengthening of the ulna (as a consequence of radial shortening) has resulted in reduced forearm rotation (due to distal radioulnar joint [DRUJ] subluxation), and ulnar sided wrist pain. Patients complain that ulnar sided wrist pain is worse in full pronation and flexion. There is often a reduced range of total forearm rotation compared with the normal side. For this patient, initial management with rest, splint immobilization, and steroid injections had failed to resolve the symptoms, so an ulnar shortening osteotomy was recommended.

Ulnar abutment (or ulnar impaction) syndrome is caused by excessive impact between the ulna and its closest carpals, typically the lunate, and often as a result of positive ulnar variance. The condition can range from simple wear patterns, to triangular fibrocartilage complex perforation, to advanced cases with ulnocarpal osteoarthritis.

Ulnar variance

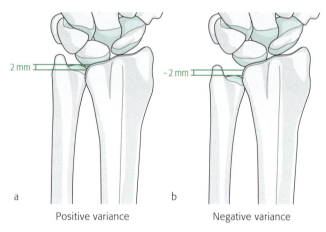

Positive variance   Negative variance

Fig 5.7-2a–b Variation in relative length of the distal articular surfaces of the ulna and radius is described as ulnar variance. When the articular surface of the ulna is more distal compared with the articular surface of the radius there is positive ulnar variance (**a**), and a more proximal ulnar length results in negative ulnar variance (**b**). Variance of 2 mm or greater typically requires operative treatment. The variance can be assessed in a variety of ways radiologically but it is mandatory to obtain a comparison x-ray of the uninjured side to judge the relevance of the radiological measurements.

Imaging

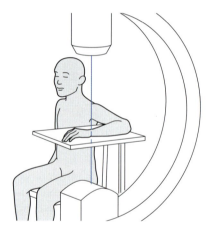

Fig 5.7-3 Plain x-rays in a standardized position should be taken. For best results, seat the patient and place the affected arm with 90 degrees of abduction at the shoulder, flexed 90 degrees at the elbow, with the arm lying in neutral forearm rotation.

2   Indications (cont)

Achieving shortening

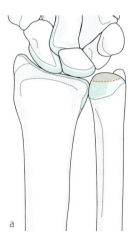
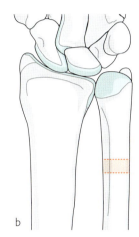
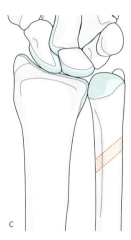

a   b   c

Fig 5.7-4a–c   When treating radioulnar length discrepancies through ulnar shortening, the procedure can be achieved by:
- Removing a portion of bone from the ulnar head (wafer resection) via open or arthroscopic surgery
- Or by shortening the bone through a distal diaphyseal osteotomy (ulnar shortening osteotomy).

A wafer resection does not address subluxation of the DRUJ and is indicated in primary ulnocarpal abutment rather than secondary abutment created by radial shortening. A wafer resection removes the terminal portion of the ulnar head but accurate resection of a preplanned amount is difficult to achieve. However, the DRUJ is not disturbed (**a**).

An ulnar shortening osteotomy can be performed precisely and allows an exact resection, producing an accurate amount of shortening (**b**). In appropriate cases, the DRUJ can be realigned. A straight plate is used to stabilize the osteotomy. Alternatively, an oblique osteotomy creates a larger surface area for bone union and also stabilizes rotation of the fragments, preventing a rotational malunion (**c**). An oblique osteotomy also has advantages in applying internal fixation. A straight plate is again used to stabilize the osteotomy but with a lag screw being passed perpendicularly across the osteotomy site. An oblique osteotomy was chosen for this patient.

Choice of implant

A locking compression plate (LCP) ulna osteotomy system 2.7 and a straight plate can be used to create an exact preplanned amount of shortening and to produce stable fixation.

3 **Preoperative planning**

Equipment

- LCP ulna osteotomy set
- LCP ulna osteotomy plate 2.7
- 1.4 mm to 1.6 mm K-wires
- Oscillating saw
- Image intensifier

Patient preparation and positioning

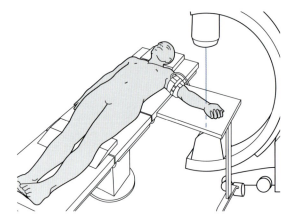

Fig 5.7-5   Position the patient supine and place the forearm on a hand table. Supinate the forearm. The position of the limb should allow complete imaging in the frontal and sagittal plane of the distal ulna and radius. A nonsterile pneumatic tourniquet is used. Prophylactic antibiotics are optional.

4 Surgical approach

Approach

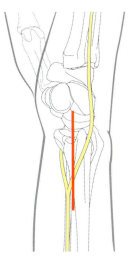

Fig 5.7-6 The surgical approach used was an ulnar approach (see chapter 1.10 Ulnar approach to the distal ulna).

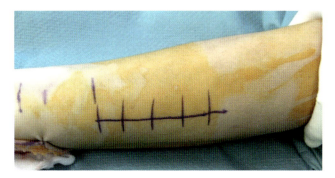

Fig 5.7-7 The approach was made via a longitudinal incision over the distal subcutaneous border of the ulna.

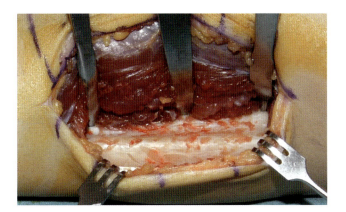

Fig 5.7-8 The flexor carpi ulnaris (FCU) is retracted toward the radial side. This protects the ulnar neurovascular bundle and reveals the flat surface of the distal ulnar diaphysis.

5   Reduction

Insert the shortening guide

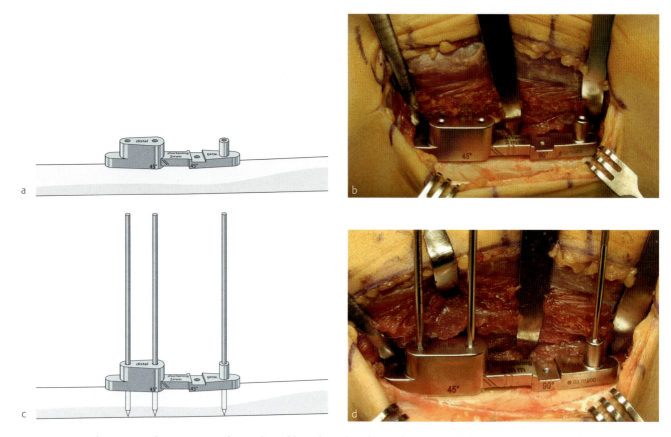

Fig 5.7-9a–d   The correct shortening guide is selected based on the planned amount of shortening (2 mm in this case). The shortening block is placed on the flattest part of the distal ulna (**a–b**). The guide is attached to the distal ulna using K-wires that must penetrate both cortices (**c–d**). Intraoperative x-rays are taken to ensure correct alignment.

5 Reduction (cont)

Select the cutting block and angle and perform the osteotomy

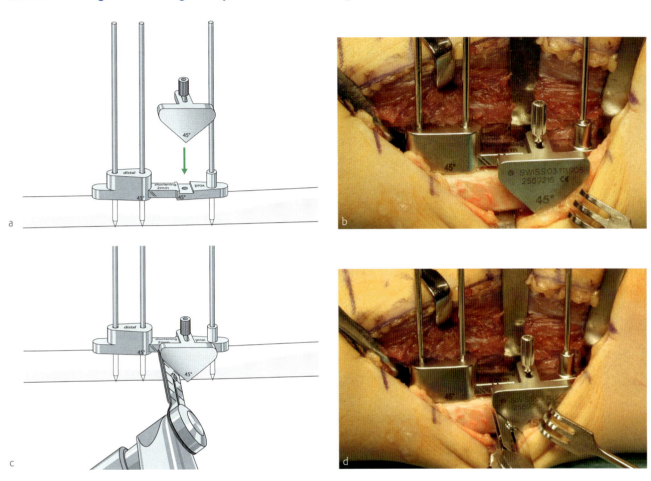

Fig 5.7-10a–d   The appropriate cutting block is selected (in this case, an oblique osteotomy had been planned) and applied to the shortening guide (**a–b**). The preplanned osteotomy is made using parallel saw blades of the preselected size (2 mm) (**c–d**). The saw blades must cut the far cortex fully to enable a neat apposition of the osteotomy surfaces.

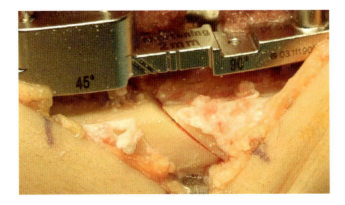

Fig 5.7-11   The slice of resected bone was excised and the guide block was then removed.

6   Fixation

Select and insert the plate

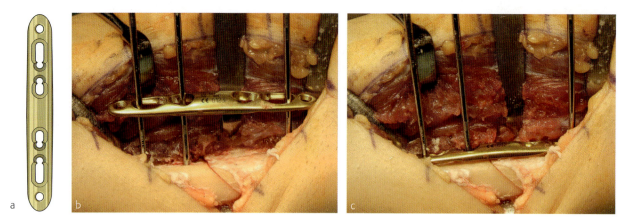

Fig 5.7-12a–c   The plate is selected and introduced over the K-wires and pushed down onto the surface of the bone (**a–b**). Rotational alignment is maintained by virtue of the K-wires (**c**).

Insert screws

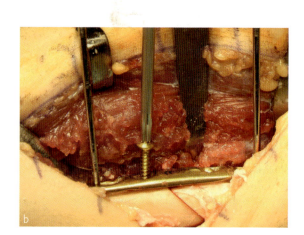

Fig 5.7-13a–b   The implant must be stabilized by sequentially removing each K-wire and replacing it with a cortex screw.

6 Fixation (cont)

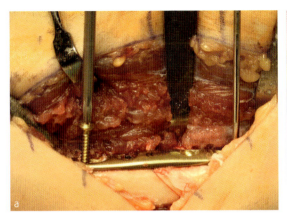
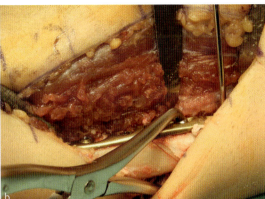

Fig 5.7-14a–b Two distal screws were inserted first, which secured the alignment of the plate onto the bone surface (**a**). Before removing the proximal K-wire, a plate reduction clamp was applied to temporarily stabilize the position of the implant on the proximal part of the osteotomy (**b**).

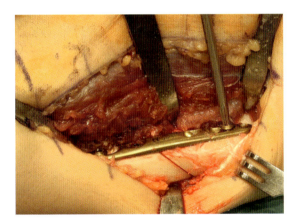

Fig 5.7-15 The proximal screw was inserted and tightened and the osteotomy gap closes into compression. It is critical to compress into the axilla of the oblique osteotomy for stability.

6 Fixation (cont)

Insert lag screw

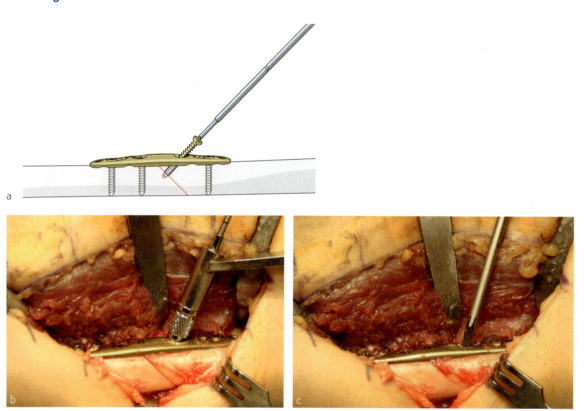

Fig 5.7-16a–c A cortex screw is inserted through the plate as a lag screw to further compress the osteotomy and improve its stability.

Insert locking screws

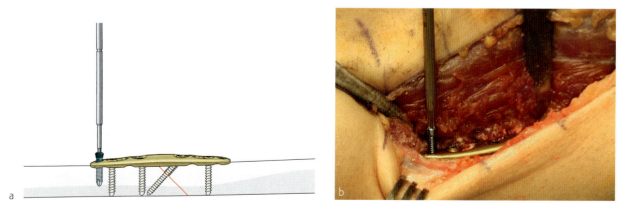

Fig 5.7-17a–b Locking screws are inserted at each end of the implant once full compression has been achieved.

6 Fixation (cont)

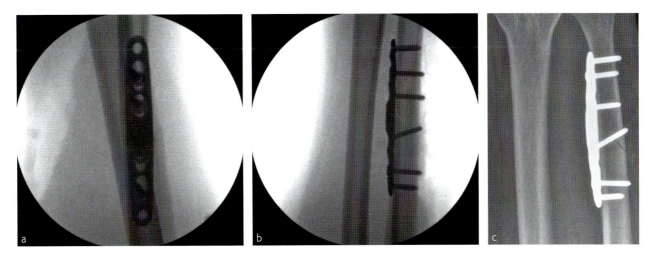

Fig 5.7-18a–c Intraoperative images confirmed the correct placement of the implant and correct length of the lag screw. Verification of the amount of ulnar shortening achieved should be performed.

Distal radioulnar joint assessment

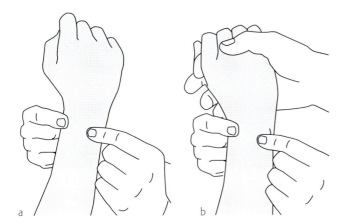

Fig 5.7-19a–b After fixation, the DRUJ should be assessed for both forearm rotation and stability. The methods for determining if DRUJ instability exists are shown in the fixation topic in chapter 4.1 Radial styloid—fracture treated with a radial column plate.

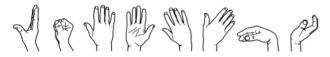

7 Rehabilitation

Aftercare, follow-up, and functional exercises

Fig 5.7-20   The patient should receive the standard postoperative rest, injury elevation, follow-up, removal of stitches, and immobilization as required. Following surgery, begin active controlled range of motion exercises. For further information, see the rehabilitation topic in chapter 4.1 Radial styloid—fracture treated with a radial column plate.

8 Outcome

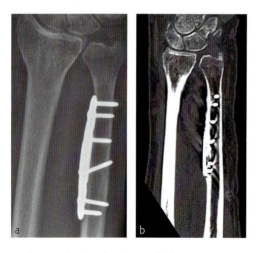

Fig 5.7-21a–b   At the 6-month follow-up, the x-ray and CT scan images confirmed radiological union.

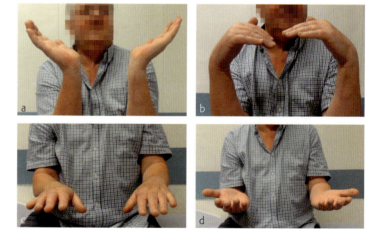

Fig 5.7-22a–d   The patient had obtained excellent range of motion, and with the ulna/lunate abutment resolved, was pain free.

8 Outcome (cont)

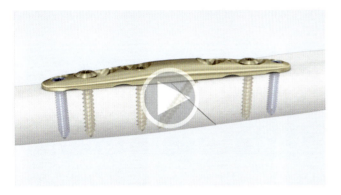

Video 5.7-1   This video demonstrates an ulnar shaft treated with an oblique shortening osteotomy using the LCP ulna osteotomy system 2.7.

9 Alternative technique 1

Ulnar shortening using a standard dynamic compression plate

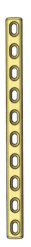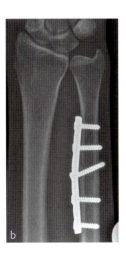

Fig 5.7-23a–b   A standard dynamic compression plate (DCP) or limited contact LC-DCP 3.5 can be used instead of the ulnar shortening system. The osteotomy is created freehand, either transverse or (as shown here) obliquely. The implant must be prebent to produce compression on the far cortex and an oblique osteotomy must be planned so that compression can occur into the axilla.

10 Alternative technique 2

Metaphyseal ulnar shortening using a distal ulna plate

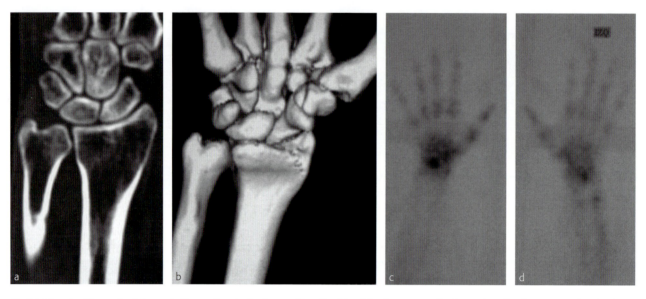

Fig 5.7-24a–d   The principle and alternative techniques described in this chapter so far have involved osteotomies in the diaphysis, where cortical bone is thick and cancellous surface area is limited. Consequently, healing can be slow. Yet, the distal ulnar metaphysis has a large cancellous surface area with thin cortical bone, and so a more distally placed osteotomy should heal more quickly as a result.

A 39-year-old machine operator with long standing pain at the ulnar side of the left wrist had undergone unsuccessful nonoperative treatment. The 2-D and 3-D CT scans showed the incongruity of the distal ulnar joint (**a–b**). Bone scans showed increased uptake of technetium nucleotide (and therefore abnormalities) around the DRUJ (**c–d**).

10 Alternative technique 2 (cont)

Select the plate

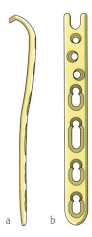

Fig 5.7-25a–b As selected for this patient, the distal ulna (hook) plate, with its locking screws on both sides of the osteotomy (which is created freehand in either a transverse or oblique fashion), provides excellent stability for this more distally placed procedure.

Determine the level of variance

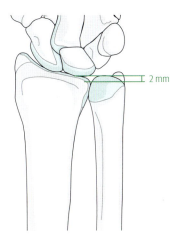

Fig 5.7-26 The first step is to assess and determine the level of variance. For this patient there was 2 mm of positive ulnar variance.

Apply the plate

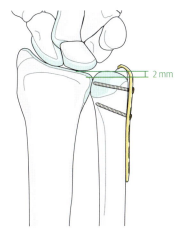

Fig 5.7-27 The plate is applied with the hook over the ulnar styloid, and temporary fixation is made with two screws into the ulnar head.

Perform the osteotomy

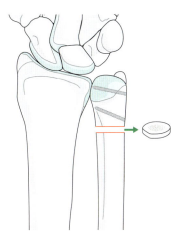

Fig 5.7-28 The plate and screws are removed and a 2 mm wafer of bone is resected from the distal ulnar metaphysis.

10 Alternative technique 2 (cont)

Reapply the plate

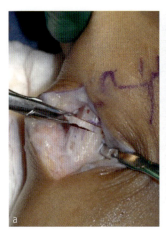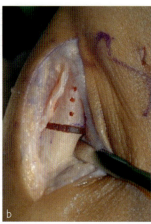

Fig 5.7-29a–b Intraoperative images show the 2 mm wafer being created and removed, revealing the site of the osteotomy.

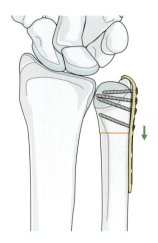

Fig 5.7-30 The plate and distal screws are reapplied.

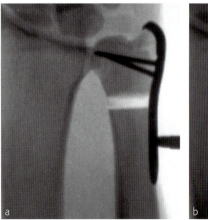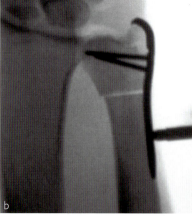

Fig 5.7-31a–b Using a drill guide as a handle, the plate can be moved proximally and the osteotomy site and ulna, reduced.

10 Alternative technique 2 (cont)

Insert proximal screws

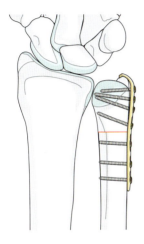

Fig 5.7-32 The proximal screws are placed, with axial compression applied through the plate.

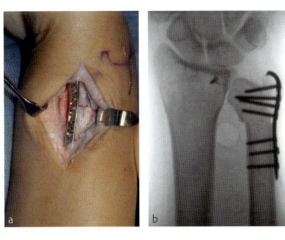

Fig 5.7-33a–b The ulna plate and screws are now secured with the osteotomy site placed under compression.

Option: oblique osteotomy

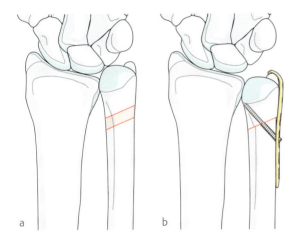

Fig 5.7-34a–b As a further option, the procedure can be performed with an oblique osteotomy (**a**), allowing for the placement of a lag screw to provide additional support (**b**).

Outcome

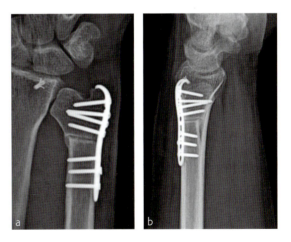

Fig 5.7-35a–b By the 3-month follow-up after surgery, complete union had been achieved.

10 Alternative technique 2 (cont)

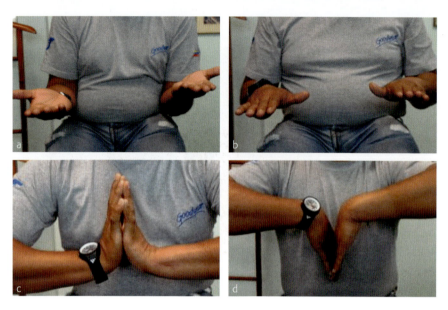

Fig 5.7-36a–d The patient had achieved a fully functional recovery without pain.

5.8 Long-standing nonunion treated with resection of the distal ulna and double plating of the radius

1 Case description

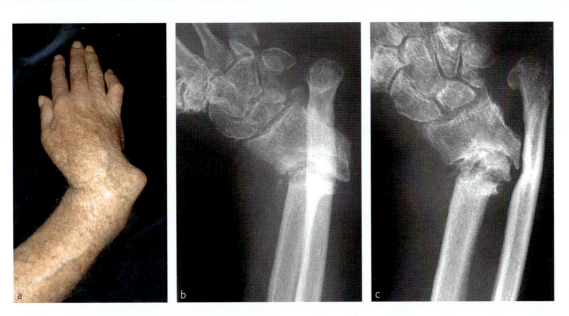

Fig 5.8-1a–c A 67-year-old retired man had a long-standing extraarticular nonunion of his right distal radius, with obvious deformity. Clinical images and x-rays demonstrated shortening, angulation, and the suggestion of synovial pseudarthrosis. The patient was previously told nothing could be done, yet ongoing instability, deformity, and pain forced him to continue to seek medical advice.

Nonunion of the distal radius

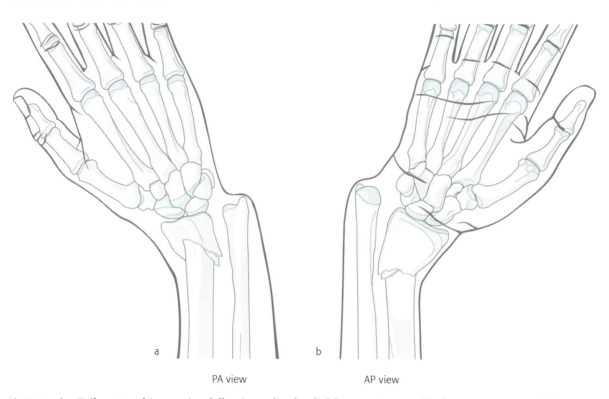

PA view   AP view

Fig 5.8-2a–b Failure to achieve union following a distal radial fracture is exceedingly uncommon. Failed internal fixation, infection, or Charcot arthropathy are among the most likely causes. If untreated, due to its proximity to the radiocarpal joint, there is a potential for the nonunion to develop into a mobile pseudarthrosis adding to the complexity of any reconstruction. Furthermore, the limited size of the distal metaphyseal and articular component as well as the likelihood of associated disuse osteoporosis presents a definite challenge to achieving stable internal fixation and ultimate union.

Distal ulna resection

While preservation of the distal radioulnar joint (DRUJ) is helpful for both motion and stability, with long-standing nonunions such as with this low-demand patient, length discrepancy and posttraumatic DRUJ arthrosis may require resection of the distal ulna, which can provide local bone graft material.

2 Indications (cont)

Choice of implant

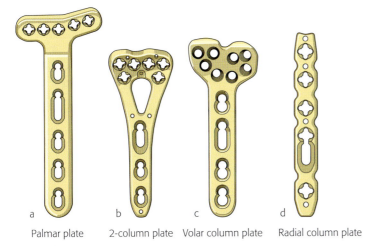

a	b	c	d
Palmar plate	2-column plate	Volar column plate	Radial column plate

Fig 5.8-3a–d Given a nonunion to such an extent along a patient's distal radial shaft, longer angular stable plates and plates with larger multiple-hole heads and variable angle (VA) locking screw options should be considered to help with stability. For added stability, insertion of a radial column plate is also recommended.

3 Preoperative planning

Equipment

- A palmar locking plate with longer shaft
- Radial column plate 2.4
- 1.4 mm to 1.6 mm K-wires
- Small external distractor
- Autogenous bone graft or bone substitute
- Oscillating saw
- Image intensifier

Patient preparation and positioning

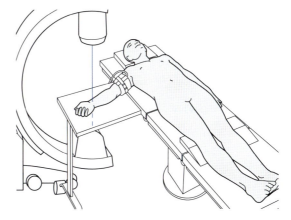

Fig 5.8-4 Position the patient supine and place the forearm on a hand table. Supinate the forearm. The position of the limb should allow complete imaging in the frontal and sagittal plane of the distal radius. A nonsterile pneumatic tourniquet is used. Prophylactic antibiotics are optional.

4 Surgical approach

Approaches

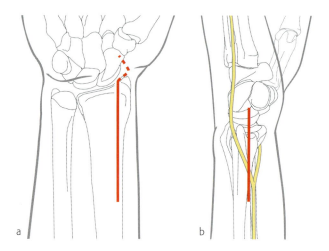

Fig 5.8-5a–b The initial surgical approach used was a modified Henry palmar approach (see Chapter 1.6 Modified Henry palmar approach to the distal radius). This was followed by an ulnar approach to the ulna (see chapter 1.10 Ulnar approach to the distal ulna).

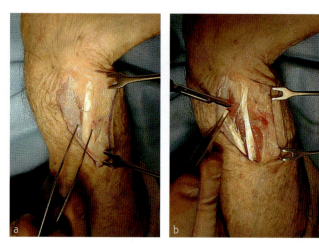

Fig 5.8-6a–b The distal radius was approached through the modified Henry palmar incision. The flexor carpi radialis (FCR) tendon was identified (**a**). The contracted FCR tendon was sectioned followed by the tendon of the brachioradialis (**b**).

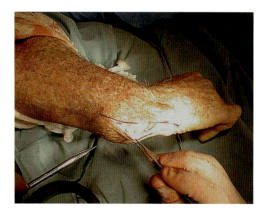

Fig 5.8-7 The second incision was then performed based along the ulna. This allowed the ulna to be osteotomized.

4 Surgical approach (cont)

Ulnar osteotomy

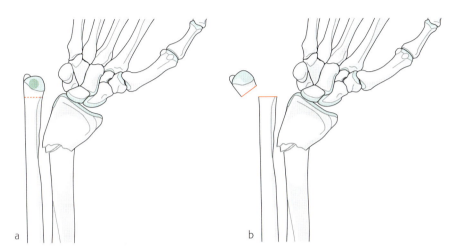

Fig 5.8-8a–b   Measure and remove a section of ulna to create equal length along the radius and ulna. The resected bone material is then able to be used for bone graft material later on.

5 Reduction

Insert external fixation pins

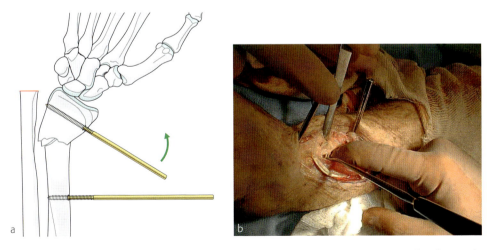

Fig 5.8-9a–b   Two small threaded external distractor pins/K-wires are inserted to be used as joysticks, with one pin in the distal radial metaphysis and one in the proximal shaft.

5 Reduction (cont)

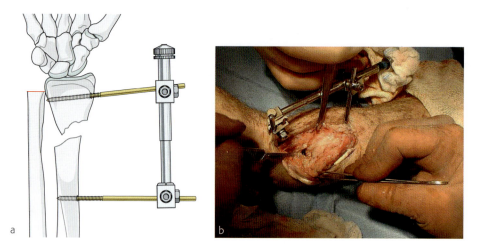

Fig 5.8-10a–b The nonunion is then realigned and the position secured with the small distractor (**a**). Debridement of the nonunion required removal of the synovial membrane (**b**).

Insert the bone graft

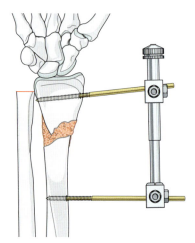

Fig 5.8-11 Once realigned, prepare and insert the bone graft obtained from the ulnar osteotomy.

6 Fixation

Palmar plate fixation

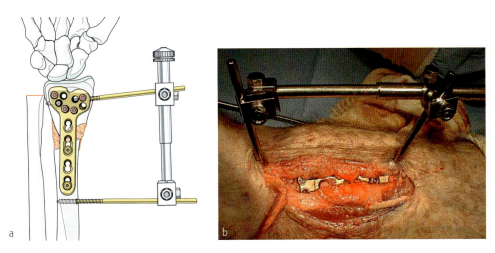

Fig 5.8-12a–b   Fixation of the distal radius should be performed with an appropriate palmar plate. The usual steps involve selecting an appropriate plate based on the configuration of the nonunion, inserting distal screws, inserting proximal screws, and intraoperative imaging.

Radial column plate fixation

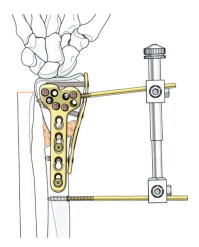

Fig 5.8-13   This is followed by insertion of a radial column plate for further stability. The steps involve selecting, contouring, and applying the plate, stabilizing the radial column, and inserting proximal and distal screws.

7 Rehabilitation

Aftercare, follow-up, and functional exercises

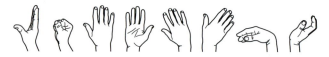

Fig 5.8-14 The patient should receive the standard postoperative rest, injury elevation, follow-up, removal of stitches, and immobilization as required. Following surgery, begin active controlled range of motion exercises. For further information, see the rehabilitation topic in chapter 4.1 Radial styloid—fracture treated with a radial column plate.

8 Outcome

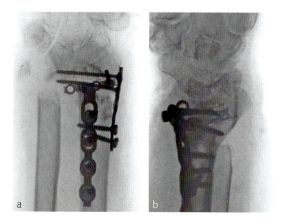

Fig 5.8-15a–b At the 6-month follow-up, x-rays showed union of the distal radius with restoration of a more normal alignment.

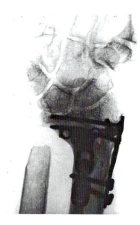

Fig 5.8-16 The x-ray at 3 years postoperatively showed complete healing.

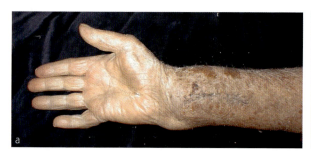

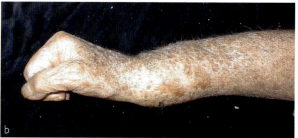

Fig 5.8-17a–b The result was that the patient had a stable and well-aligned forearm and wrist. Despite many previous years of dysfunction, his hand function had now returned with good strength and normal sensation.

5.9 Chronic intercarpal arthritis treated with scaphoid resection and 4-corner fusion

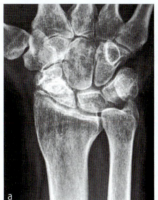 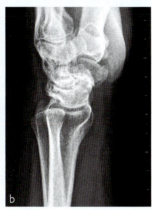

Fig 5.9-1a–b A 42-year-old male jewelry shop owner and designer fell on his outstretched wrist but did not seek treatment until 1 year later, when he had persistent pain and limitation of wrist mobility. The x-rays showed evidence of osteoarthritic changes in the radioscaphoid joint and a scaphoid fracture nonunion.

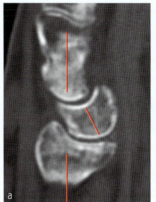 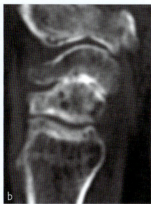

Fig 5.9-2a–b The sagittal CT scans showed carpal collapse, deformity, and shortening of the scaphoid, while osteoarthritic changes were also evident.

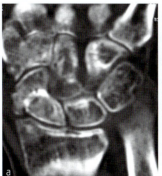 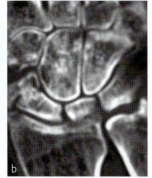

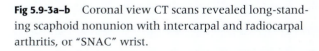

Fig 5.9-3a–b Coronal view CT scans revealed long-standing scaphoid nonunion with intercarpal and radiocarpal arthritis, or "SNAC" wrist.

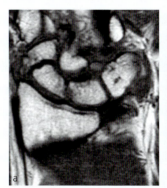 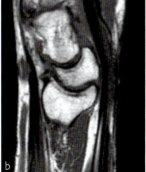

Fig 5.9-4a–b The MRI showed cartilage loss at the radioscaphoid joint. Treatment involving four-corner fusion was offered as a salvage procedure.

475

2   Indications

Intercarpal osteoarthritis and the SLAC/SNAC wrist

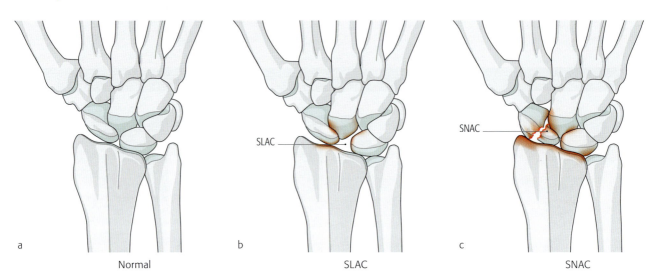

a   Normal   b   SLAC   c   SNAC

Fig 5.9-5a–c   It has already been shown in this publication that scaphoid fractures and surrounding ligament damage are common, and due to a wide variety of factors, can fail to heal. The result can be especially problematic when the scaphoid injury is not initially diagnosed or when the patient fails to seek immediate medical treatment. Potential results from such situations include necrosis and nonunion, but it can also lead to conditions such as scapholunate advanced collapse (SLAC) and scaphoid nonunion advanced collapse (SNAC), which are forms of osteoarthritis greatly affecting wrist function. Typically, both conditions result in loss of wrist mobility, swelling in the intercarpal joints, distortion of the shape of the scaphoid, change to joint kinematics, and pain. For many patients, surgical salvage procedures provide an effective treatment option.

2   Indications (cont)

Classification of scaphoid nonunion advanced collapse

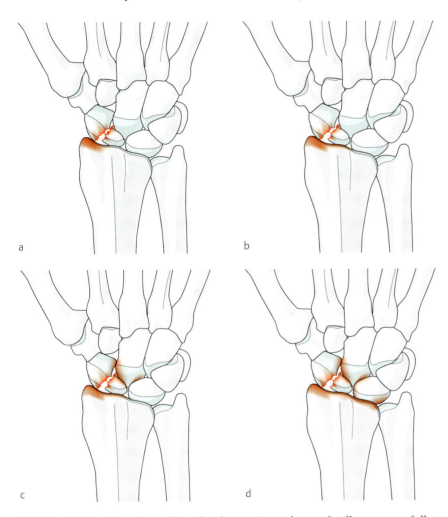

Fig 5.9-6a–d   The four stages of scaphoid nonunion advanced collapse are as follows:

a   Stage I: Arthritis at the radial styloid

b   Stage II: Arthritis of the scaphoid fossa

c   Stage III: Arthritis of the capitolunate/midcarpal joint

d   Stage IV: Diffuse arthritis of the carpus.

Symptomatic wrist dysfunction of any etiology can require reconstruction and salvage procedures are frequently the only way to offer the patient a stable pain-free wrist. A number of surgical options that ideally preserve motion and avoid complications in the long term can be considered:

- Limited wrist arthrodesis
- Proximal row carpectomy
- Arthroplasty
- Total wrist arthrodesis.

2   Indications (cont)

Limited wrist arthrodesis with four-corner fusion

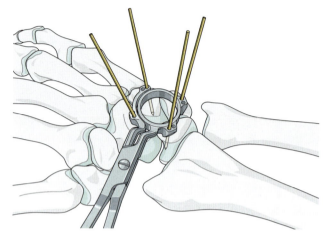

Fig 5.9-7   Four-corner fusion is a limited wrist arthrodesis treatment provided to those with advanced degenerative changes in the wrist where the carpals are fused (eg, the lunate, capitate, triquetrum, and hamate bones). As it involves only partial fusion, it preserves limited motion while allowing pain reduction from the affected joints. The "four corners" of the carpal bones are attached by an intercarpal fusion plate, while the scaphoid is partially or fully resected.

Choice of implant

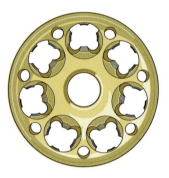

Fig 5.9-8   Four-corner fusion is performed with an intercarpal fusion plate (dorsal circular plate or spider plate). It allows variable angle (VA) screw insertion and can be adapted to the specific anatomy of the patient.

3 Preoperative planning

Equipment list

- VA locking intercarpal fusion system
- Intercarpal fusion plate
- 1.1 mm or 1.2 mm K-wires
- 1.4 mm to 1.6 mm K-wires
- Bone nibbler/rongeur
- Osteotome
- Image intensifier

Patient positioning

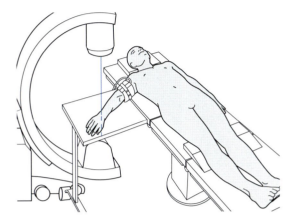

Fig 5.9-9 Position the patient supine and place the forearm on the hand table. Pronate the forearm. The position of the limb should allow complete imaging in the frontal and sagittal plane of the distal radius. A nonsterile pneumatic tourniquet is used. Prophylactic antibiotics are optional.

4 Surgical approach

Approach

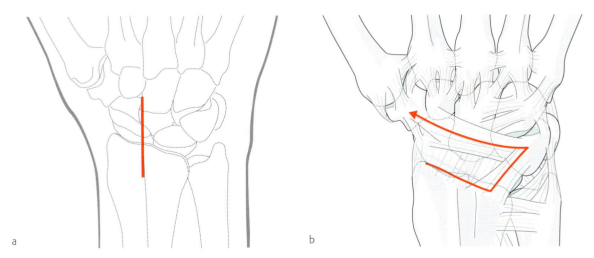

a   b

Fig 5.9-10a–b Due to the specific nature of the injury, the surgical approach used was a dorsal approach to the carpus (see chapter 1.3 Combined approach to the lunate and perilunate injuries, however in this case, only the dorsal approach was required). This approach involves a radially based capsular ligamentous flap to be elevated and a capsulotomy incision.

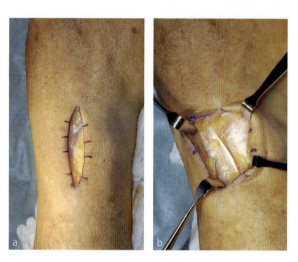

Fig 5.9-11a–b   The approach was made over the third compartment by incising the extensor retinaculum over the extensor pollicis longus (EPL) tendon. The EPL tendon was released and retracted radially, together with the extensor tendons of the second compartment.

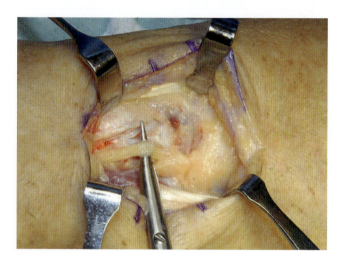

Fig 5.9-12   The posterior interosseous nerve was identified and resected to partially denervate this area of the wrist to help limit postoperative pain.

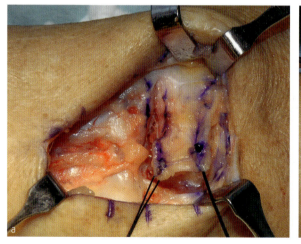
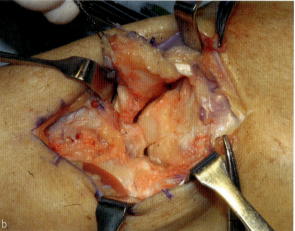

Fig 5.9-13a–b   Intraoperative photos show the radially based capsular ligamentous flap preserving the radiolunotriquetal ligament (**a**). The capsular flap was elevated by sharp dissection in an ulnar to radial direction (**b**).

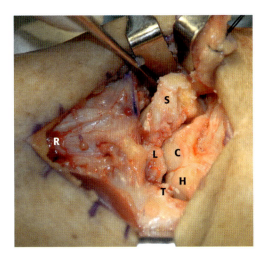

Fig 5.9-14 The carpal bones were then exposed and identified (S=scaphoid, C=capitate, H=hamate, T=triquetrum, L=lunate; with R=radius).

Excise the scaphoid

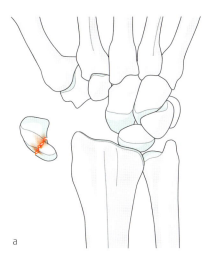
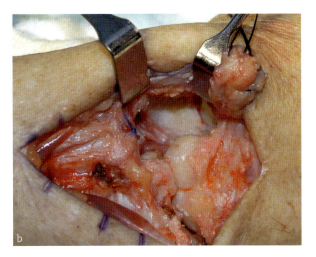

Fig 5.9-15a–b Because of the chronic nonunion and surrounding arthritic changes the first part of this procedure was to completely remove the scaphoid. Particular care must be taken to preserve the palmar radioscaphocapitate ligament. In some instances, the excised scaphoid can provide some autogenous bone graft material.

5 Reduction

Reduce rotational deformity and provisionally fix the carpal bones

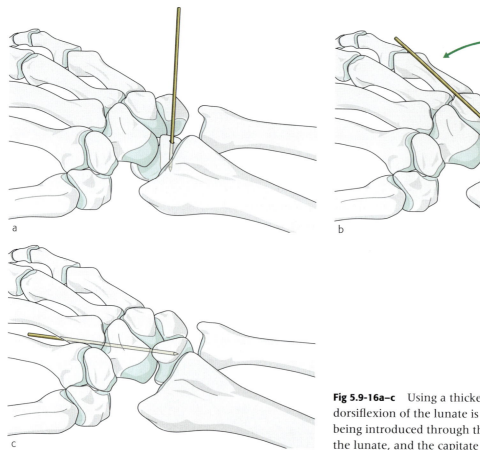

Fig 5.9-16a–c Using a thicker joystick K-wire, the dorsiflexion of the lunate is corrected and stabilized by being introduced through the capitate to align the radius, the lunate, and the capitate in neutral position.

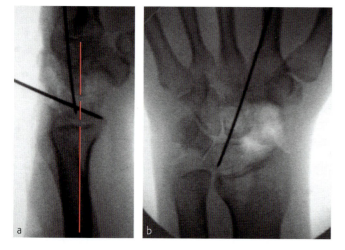

Fig 5.9-17a–b Intraoperative images show the K-wire in place.

5 Reduction (cont)

Debride the midcarpal joint

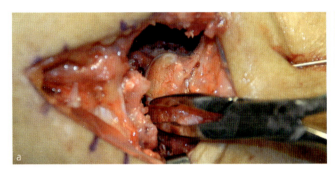 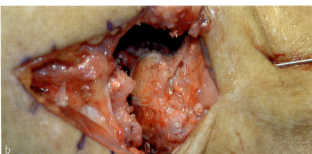

Fig 5.9-18a–b   Using a small rongeur and osteotome, the cartilage of the midcarpal joint is removed to expose the subchondral bone (debride the midcarpal joint) (**a**). Make sure that sclerotic and dense subchondral bone is removed down to cancellous bone (**b**). Preparation of the joint surfaces between the capitate/hamate and lunate/triquetrum is optional or may be carried out after provisional fixation. Excessive removal of bone should be avoided otherwise the shape of the carpus will be modified.

6 Fixation

Select fixation method and plate

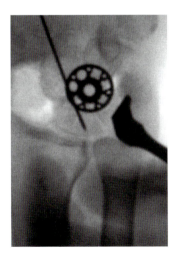

Fig 5.9-19   To achieve fusion of the midcarpal joint, the VA locking intercarpal fusion system was used (shown with the plate inserted), which is a variable angle locking technology for midcarpal limited arthrodesis. Appropriate plate size is chosen using the image intensifier and it can also be used to verify correct alignment of the carpal bones.

6 Fixation (cont)

Position reaming guide

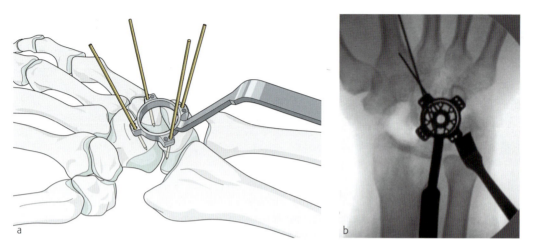

Fig 5.9-20a–b To begin, choose the reaming guide according to the selected plate and fix it temporarily with at least one 1.1 mm/1.2 mm K-wire per carpal bone over the center of the four-bone junction (**a**). If necessary, remove the palmar lunocapitate K-wire to avoid later interference with the reamer (**b**).

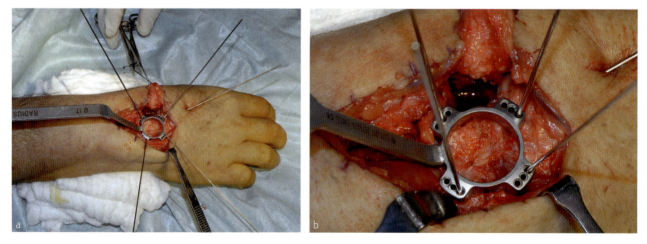

Fig 5.9-21a–b The handle of the reaming guide should be in line with the radial shaft (**a**). The reaming guide was temporarily fixed with K-wires over the center of the four-bone junction (**b**).

6 Fixation (cont)

Optional instrument: reduction reaming guide

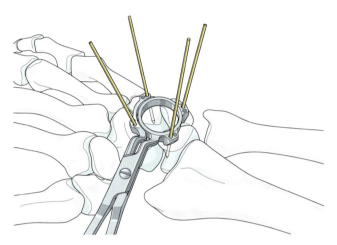

Fig 5.9-22 Use the reduction reaming guide if reduction of the carpal bones is required. This particular reaming guide has offset feet to allow it to sit comfortably on the carpus. If this guide is used, its handle must be located on the radial side of the carpus when, as in this case, a right wrist is being treated and on the ulnar side of the carpus when a left wrist is being treated.

Ream plate recess

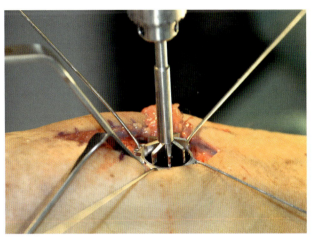

Fig 5.9-23 Choose the reamer corresponding to the (reduction) reaming guide. Ream through the reaming guide to the first laser marking line.

Apply the plate

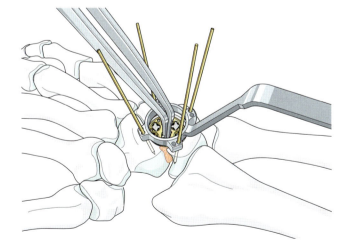

Fig 5.9-24 Use the plate holder to pick up the appropriately sized plate. Position the plate through the reduction reaming guide.

6 Fixation (cont)

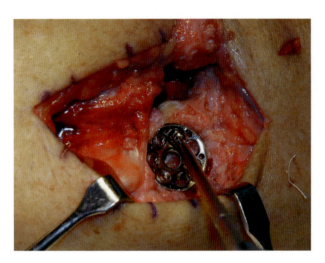

Fig 5.9-25 The plate was inserted as shown. Check for sufficient reaming depth by trial placement of the plate, ensuring that the plate edge does not project beyond the bone at any point. It is critically important to ensure the plate edge does not project beyond the proximal margin of the reamed defect otherwise wrist extension will be blocked by implant impingement.

Fix plate with locking screws

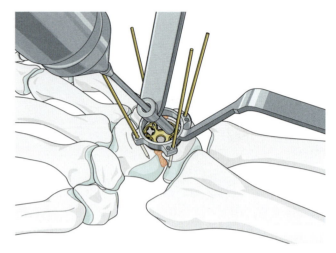

Fig 5.9-26 Start plate fixation with the placement of VA locking screws in the lunate. Use the variable angle part of the drill guide 1.8 (see marking "VARIABLE ANGLE") and fully insert it into the locking hole. Drill the hole with the 1.8 mm drill bit at the desired angle.

Measure screw length using the depth gauge

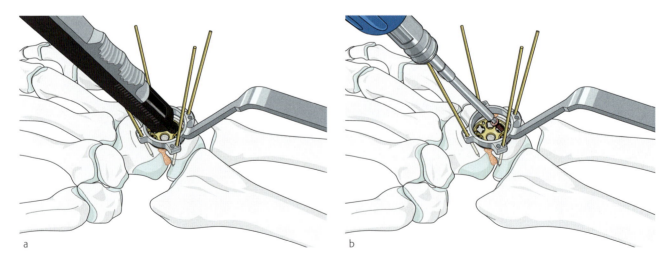

a

b

Fig 5.9-27a–b Insert locking screws using the T8 screwdriver shaft with stardrive attached to the handle with quick coupling. At least two screws should be placed in the lunate.

6   Fixation (cont)

Bone graft

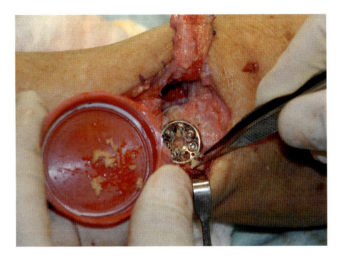

Fig 5.9-28   Fill the space between the four bones with autogenous bone graft taken from the excised scaphoid, or from the iliac crest or Lister tubercle. As an alternative, bone graft can be placed before the plate is inserted.

7   Rehabilitation

Aftercare, follow-up, and functional exercises

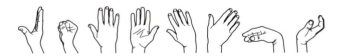

Fig 5.9-29   The patient should receive the standard postoperative rest, injury elevation, follow-up, removal of stitches, and immobilization as required. Following surgery, begin active controlled range of motion exercises. For further information, see the rehabilitation topic in chapter 4.1 Radial styloid—fracture treated with a radial column plate.

8 Outcome

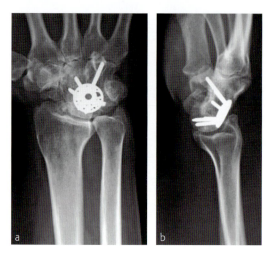

Fig 5.9-30a–b The 3-month follow-up x-rays showed that fusion was achieved.

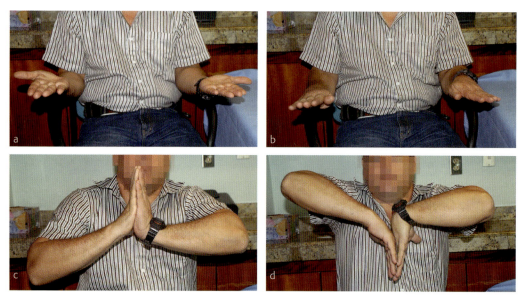

Fig 5.9-31a–d At the 1-year follow-up there was complete resolution of pain and a functional range of motion but with some limitation of flexion and extension.

8 Outcome

Video

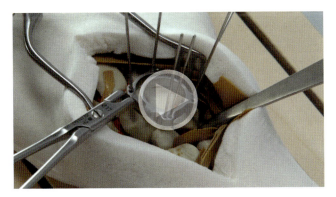

Video 5.9-1   This video demonstrates a midcarpal wrist fusion using the VA locking intercarpal fusion system.

Appendix

Further reading

Carpal injuries

Adkison JW, Chapman MW. Treatment of acute lunate and perilunate dislocations. *Clin Orthop Relat Res.* 1982;199–207.

Bain GI, McLean JM, Turner PC, et al. Translunate fracture with associated perilunate injury: 3 case reports with introduction of the translunate arc concept. *J Hand Surg Am.* 2008;33:1770–1776.

Blazar PE, Murray P. Treatment of perilunate dislocations by combined dorsal and palmar approaches. *Tech Hand Up Extrem Surg.* 2001;5:2–7.

Capo JT, Corti SJ, Shamian B, et al. Treatment of dorsal perilunate dislocations and fracture-dislocations using a standardized protocol. *Hand NY.* 2012;7:380–387.

Fenton RL. The naviculo-capitate fracture syndrome. *J Bone Joint Surg Am.* 1956;38-A:681–684.

Forli A, Courvoisier A, Wimsey S, et al. Perilunate dislocations and transscaphoid perilunate fracture-dislocations: a retrospective study with minimum ten-year follow-up. *J Hand Surg Am.* 2010;35:62–68.

Gilula LA, Destouet JM, Weeks PM, et al. Roentgenographic diagnosis of the painful wrist. *Clin Orthop Relat Res.* 1984;52–64.

Graham TJ. The inferior arc injury: an addition to the family of complex carpal fracture-dislocation patterns. *Am J Orthop (Belle Mead NJ).* 2003;32:10–19.

Green DP. The effect of avascular necrosis on Russe bone grafting for scaphoid nonunion. *J Hand Surg Am.* 1985;10:597–605.

Haddad FS, Goddard NJ. Acute percutaneous scaphoid fixation: a pilot study. *J Bone Joint Surg.* 1998;80:95–99.

Herbert TJ, Fisher WE. Management of the fractured scaphoid using a new bone screw. *J Bone Joint Surg.* 1984;66(1):114–123.

Herzberg G. Acute dorsal trans-scaphoid perilunate dislocations: Open reduction and internal fixation. *Tech Hand Up Extrem Surg.* 2000;4:2–13.

Herzberg G, Comtet JJ, Linscheid RL, et al. Perilunate dislocations and fracture-dislocations: a multicenter study. *J Hand Surg Am.* 1993;18:768–779.

Herzberg G, Forissier D. Acute dorsal trans-scaphoid perilunate fracture-dislocations: medium-term results. *J Hand Surg.* 2002;27:498–502.

Hildebrand KA, Ross DC, Patterson SD, et al. Dorsal perilunate dislocations and fracture-dislocations: questionnaire, clinical, and radiographic evaluation. *J Hand Surg Am.* 2000;25:1069–1079.

Inoue G, Kuwahata Y. Management of acute perilunate dislocations without fracture of the scaphoid. *J Hand Surg.* 1997;22:647–652.

Inoue G, Shionoya K. Herbert screw fixation by limited access for acute fractures of the scaphoid. *J Bone Joint Surg.* 1997;79:418–421.

Inoue G, Shionoya K, Kuwahata Y. Herbert screw fixation for scaphoid nonunions. An analysis of factors influencing outcome. *Clin Orthop Relat Res.* 1997 Oct;343:99–106.

Jiranek WA, Ruby LK, Millender LB, et al. Long-term results after Russe bone-grafting: the effect of malunion of the scaphoid. *J Bone Joint Surg Am.* 1992;74:1217–1228.

Johnson RP. The acutely injured wrist and its residuals. *Clin Orthop Relat Res.* 1980;33–44.

Jones DB Jr, Bürger H, Bishop AT, et al. Treatment of scaphoid waist nonunions with an avascular proximal pole and carpal collapse. A comparison of two vascularized bone grafts. *J Bone Joint Surg Am.* 2008;90:2616–2625.

Jupiter JB, Nunez FA Jr, Nunez F, et al. Current perspective on complex wrist fracture-dislocation. *Instr Course Lect.* 2018;67:155–174.

Kardashian G, Christoforou DC, Lee SK. Perilunate dislocations. *Bull NYU Hosp Jt Dis.* 2011;69:87–96.

Knoll VD, Allan C, Trumble TE. Trans-scaphoid perilunate fracture dislocations: results of screw fixation of the scaphoid and lunotriquetral repair with a dorsal approach. *J Hand Surg Am.* 2005; 30:1145–1152.

Komurcu M, Kurklu M, Ozturan KE, et al. Early and delayed treatment of dorsal transscaphoid perilunate fracture-dislocations. *J Orthop Trauma.* 2008;22:535–540.

Kremer T, Wendt M, Riedel K, et al. Open reduction for perilunate injuries—clinical outcome and patient satisfaction. *J Hand Surg Am.* 2010;35:1599–1606.

Krief E, Appy-Fedida B, Rotari V, et al. Results of perilunate dislocations and perilunate fracture dislocations with a minimum 15-year follow-up. *J Hand Surg Am.* 2015;40:2191–2197.

Mack GR, Bosse MJ, Gelberman RH, et al. The natural history of scaphoid non-union. *J Bone Joint Surg Am.* 1984;66:504–509.

Mayfield JK, Johnson RP, Kilcoyne RK. Carpal dislocations: pathomechanics and progressive perilunar instability. *J Hand Surg Am.* 1980;5:226–241.

Merrell GA, Wolfe SW, Slade JF III. Treatment of scaphoid nonunions: quantitative meta-analysis of the literature. *J Hand Surg Am.* 2002;27:685–691.

Minami A, Kaneda K. Repair and/or reconstruction of scapholunate interosseous ligament in lunate and perilunate dislocations. *J Hand Surg Am.* 1993;18:1099–1106.

Nakamura R, Horii E, Watanabe K, et al. Proximal row carpectomy versus limited wrist arthrodesis for advanced Kienbock's disease. *J Hand Surg.* 1998;23:741–745.

Nunez FA Jr, Luo TD, Jupiter JB, et al. Scaphocapitate syndrome with associated trans-scaphoid, trans-hamate perilunate dislocation. *Hand.* 2016;12(2):27-31.

Robbins RR, Carter PR. Iliac crest bone grafting and Herbert screw fixation of nonunions of the scaphoid with avascular proximal poles. *J Hand Surg Am.* 1995;20:818–831.

Russe O. Fractures of the carpal navicular. *J Bone Joint Surg Am.* 1960;42:759–768.

Scalcione LR, Gimber LH, Ho AM, et al. Spectrum of carpal dislocations and fracture-dislocations: imaging and management. *Am J Roentgenol.* 2014;203:541–550.

Schuind F, Haentjens P, Van Innis F, et al. Prognostic factors in the treatment of carpal scaphoid nonunions. *J Hand Surg Am.* 1999;24:761–776.

Sheetz KK, Bishop AT, Berger RA. The arterial blood supply of the distal radius and ulna and its potential use in vascularized pedicled bone grafts. *J Hand Surg Am.* 1995;20:902–914.

Sotereanos DG, Mitsionis GJ, Giannakopoulos PN, et al. Perilunate dislocation and fracture dislocation: a critical analysis of the volar-dorsal approach. *J Hand Surg Am.* 1997;22:49–56.

Souer JS, Rutgers M, Andermahr J, et al. Perilunate fracture-dislocations of the wrist: comparison of temporary screw versus K-wire fixation. *J Hand Surg Am.* 2007;32:318–325.

Straw RG, Davis TR, Dias JJ. Scaphoid nonunion: treatment with a pedicled vascularized bone graft based on the 1,2 intercompartmental supraretinacular branch of the radial artery. *J Hand Surg.* 2002;27:413–416.

Teisen H, Hjarbaek J. Classification of fresh fractures of the lunate. *J Hand Surg.* 1988;13:458–462.

Trumble T. Fractures and dislocations of the carpus. In: Trumble T, ed. *Principles of Hand Surgery and Therapy.* Philadelphia: Saunders;2000:90–125.

Trumble T, Verheyden J. Treatment of isolated perilunate and lunate dislocations with combined dorsal and volar approach and intraosseous cerclage wire. *J Hand Surg Am.* 2004;29:412–417.

Wozasek GE, Moser KD. Percutaneous screw fixation for fractures of the scaphoid. *J Bone Joint Surg.* 1991;73;138–142.

Zaidemberg C, Siebert JW, Angrigiani C. A new vascularized bone graft for scaphoid nonunion. *J Hand Surg Am.* 1991;16:474–478.

Carpal instability

Allieu Y, Brahin B, Ascencio G. Carpal instabilities: radiological and clinico-pathological classification. *Ann Radiol.* 1982;25:275–287.

Berger RA. The ligaments of the wrist: a current overview of anatomy with considerations of their potential functions. *Hand Clin.* 1997;13:63–82.

Brunelli GA, Brunelli GA. Carpal instability with scapho-lunate dissociation treated using the flexor carpi radialis and scapho-trapezoid ligament repair: foundations, technique and results of preliminary series. *Rev Chir Orthop Reparatrice Appar Mot.* 2003;89:152–157.

Cooney WP, Bussey R, Dobyns JH, et al. Difficult wrist fractures: perilunate fracture-dislocations of the wrist. *Clin Orthop Rel Res.* 1987;214:136–147.

Fenton RL. The naviculo-capitate fracture syndrome. *J Bone Joint Surg Am.* 1956;38:681–684.

Garcia-Elias M, Lluch AL, Stanley JK. Three-ligament tenodesis for the treatment of scapholunate dissociation: indications and surgical technique. *J Hand Surg Am.* 2006;31:125–134.

Geissler WB, Freeland AE, Savoie FH, et al. Intracarpal soft-tissue lesions associated with an intra-articular fracture of the distal end of the radius. *J Bone Joint Surg Am.* 1996;78:357–365.

Goldfarb CA, Stern PJ, Kiefhaber TR. Palmar midcarpal instability: the results of treatment with 4-corner arthrodesis. *J Hand Surg Am.* 2004;29:258–263.

Johnson RP. The evolution of carpal nomenclature: a short review. *J Hand Surg Am.* 1990;15:834–838.

Larsen CF, Amadio PC, Gilula LA, et al. Analysis of carpal instability, I: description of the scheme. *J Hand Surg Am.* 1995;20:757–764.

Lichtman DM, Bruckner JD, Culp RW, et al. Palmar midcarpal instability: results of surgical reconstruction. *J Hand Surg Am.* 1993;18:307–315.

Lichtman DM, Wroten ES. Understanding midcarpal instability. *J Hand Surg Am.* 2006;31:491–498.

Linscheid RL, Dobyns JH. Treatment of scapholunate dissociation. *Hand Clin.* 1992;8:645–652.

Linscheid RL, Dobyns JH, Beabout JW, et al. Traumatic instability of the wrist: diagnosis, classification, and pathomechanics. *J Bone Joint Surg Am.* 1972;54:1612–1632.

Mayfield JK, Johnson RP, Kilcoyne RK. Carpal dislocations: pathomechanics and progressive perilunar instability. *J Hand Surg Am.* 1980;5:226–241.

Minami A, Kaneda K. Repair and/or reconstruction of scapholunate interosseous ligament in lunate and perilunate dislocations. *J Hand Surg Am.* 1993 Nov;18(6):1099–1106.

Mitsuyasu H, Patterson RM, Shah MA, et al. The role of the dorsal intercarpal ligament in dynamic and static scapholunate instability. *J Hand Surg Am.* 2004;29:279–288.

Rettig ME, Raskin KB. Long-term assessment of proximal row carpectomy for chronic perilunate dislocations. *J Hand Surg Am.* 1999;24:1231–1236.

Rikli DA, Honigmann P, Babst R, et al. Intra-articular pressure measurement in the radioulnocarpal joint using a novel sensor: in vitro and in vivo results. *J Hand Surg Am.* 2007;32:67–75.

Ritt MJPF, Linscheid RL, Cooney WP, et al. The lunotriquetral joint: kinematic effects of sequential ligament sectioning, ligament repair, and arthrodesis. *J Hand Surg Am.* 1998;23:432–445.

Saffar P. Classification of carpal instabilities. In: Büchler U, ed. *Wrist Instability.* London: Martin Dunitz;1996:29–34.

Shin AY, Weinstein LP, Berger RA, et al. Treatment of isolated injuries of the lunotriquetral ligament: a comparison of arthrodesis, ligament reconstruction and ligament repair. *J Bone Joint Surg.* 2001;83:1023–1028.

Siegel JM, Ruby LK. A critical look at intercarpal arthrodesis: review of the literature. *J Hand Surg Am.* 1996; 21:717–723.

Taleisnik J. *The Wrist*. New York: Churchill Livingstone;1985.

Viegas SF. Ligamentous repair following acute scapholunate dissociation. In: Gelberman RH, ed. *Master Techniques in Orthopedic Surgery: The Wrist.* New York: Raven Press;1994:135–146.

Walsh JJ, Berger RA, Cooney WP. Current status of scapholunate interosseous ligament injuries. *J Am Acad Orthop Surg.* 2002;10:32–42.

Watson HK, Ashmead D IV, Makhlouf MV. Examination of the scaphoid. *J Hand Surg Am.* 1988;13:657–660.

Watson HK, Weinzweig J, Zeppieri J. The natural progression of scaphoid instability. *Hand Clin.* 1997;13:39–49.

Zdravkovic V, Sennwald GR. A new radiographic method of measuring carpal collapse. *J Bone Joint Surg.* 1997; 79:167–169.

Distal radial injuries

Cohen MD, Jupiter JB. Fractures of the distal radius. In: Browner BD, ed. *Skeletal Trauma: Basic Science, Management, and Reconstruction.* 4th ed. Philadelphia: WB Saunders, 2009:1405–1458.

Dumontier C, Meyer zu Rexkendorf G, Sautet A, et al. Radiocarpal dislocations: classification and proposal for treatment. A review of twenty-seven cases. *J Bone Joint Surg Am.* 2001;83:212–218.

Fernandez DL. Correction of post-traumatic wrist deformity in adults by osteotomy, bone-grafting, and internal fixation. *J Bone Joint Surg Am.* 1982;64:1164–1178.

Fernandez DL. Fractures of the distal radius: operative treatment. *Instr Course Lect.* 1993;42:73–88.

Fernandez DL, Ring D, Jupiter JB. Surgical management of delayed union and nonunion of distal radius fractures. *J Hand Surg Am.* 2001;26A:201–209.

Gong HS, Cho HE, Kim J, et al. Surgical treatment of acute distal radioulnar joint instability associated with distal radius fractures. *J Hand Surg Eur.* 2015; 40:783–789.

Hanel DP, Lu TS, Weil WM. Bridge plating of distal radius fractures: the Harborview method. *Clin Orthop Relat Res.* 2006;445:91–99.

Jakob M, Rikli DA, Regazzoni P. Fractures of the distal radius treated by internal fixation and early function. A prospective study of 73 consecutive patients. *J Bone Joint Surg.* 2000;82:340–344.

Jupiter JB, Ring D. A comparison of early and late reconstruction of malunited fractures of the distal end of the radius. *J Bone Joint Surg Am.* 1996;78:739–748.

Karnezis IA, Panagiotopoulos E, Tyllianakis, et al. Correlation between radiological parameters and patient-rated wrist dysfunction following fractures of the distal radius. *Injury.* 2005;36:1435–1439.

Krämer S, Meyer H, O'Loughlin PF, et al. The incidence of ulnocarpal complaints after distal radial fracture in relation to the fracture of the ulnar styloid. *J Hand Surg Eur.* 2013;38:710–717.

Lafontaine M, Hardy D, Delince PH. Stability assessment of distal radius fractures. *Injury.* 1989;20:208–210.

Leslie BM, Medoff RJ. Fracture specific fixation of distal radius fractures. *Tech Orthop.* 2000;15:336–352.

Lozano-Calderón SA, Doornberg J, Ring D. Fractures of the dorsal articular margin of the distal part of the radius with dorsal radiocarpal subluxation. *J Bone Joint Surg Am.* 2006;88:1486–1493.

MacKenney PJ, McQueen MM, Elton R. Prediction of instability in distal radius fractures. *J Bone Joint Surg Am.* 2006;88:1944–1951.

Melone CP Jr. Articular fractures of the distal radius. *Orthop Clin North Am*. 1984;15:217–236.

Nunez FA Jr, Zhongyu L, Campbell D, et al. Distal ulna hook plate: angular stable implant for fixation of distal ulna. *J Wrist Surg*. 2013 Feb;2(1):87–92.

Orbay JL, Fernandez DL. Volar fixed-angle plate fixation for unstable distal radius fractures in the elderly patient. *J Hand Surg Am*. 2004;29:96–102.

Rikli DA, Regazzoni P. Fractures of the distal end of the radius treated by internal fixation and early function. A preliminary report of 20 cases. *J Bone Joint Surg*. 1996;78(4):588–592.

Ring D, Prommersberger KJ, González del Pino J, et al. Corrective osteotomy for intra-articular malunion of the distal part of the radius. *J Bone Joint Surg Am*. 2005;87:1503–1509.

Souer JS, Ring D, Matschke S, et al. Effect of an unrepaired fracture of the ulnar styloid base on outcome after plate-andscrew fixation of a distal radial fracture. *J Bone Joint Surg Am*. 2009; 91:830–838.

Taleisnik J, Watson HK. Midcarpal instability caused by malunited fractures of the distal radius. *J Hand Surg Am*. 1984;9:350–357.

Zenke Y, Sakai A, Oshige T, et al. The effect of an associated ulnar styloid fracture on the outcome after fixation of a fracture of the distal radius. *J Bone Joint Surg*. 2009; 91:102–107.

Distal radioulnar joint injuries

Adams BD, Berger RA. An anatomic reconstruction of the distal radioulnar ligaments for posttraumatic distal radioulnar joint instability. *J Hand Surg Am*. 2002;27:243–251.

Allan CH, Joshi A, Lichtman DM. Kienböck's disease: diagnosis and treatment. *J Am Acad Orthop Surg*. 2001;9:128–136.

Bednar MS, Arnoczky SP, et al. The microvasculature of the triangular fibrocartilage complex: its clinical significance. *J Hand Surg Am*. 1991;16:1101–1105.

Bilos ZJ, Chamberland D. Distal ulnar head shortening for treatment of triangular fibrocartilage complex tears with ulna positive variance. *J Hand Surg Am*. 1991;16:1115–1119.

Breen TF, Jupiter JB. Extensor carpi ulnaris and flexor carpi ulnaris tenodesis of the unstable distal ulna. *J Hand Surg Am*. 1989;14:612–617.

Chen NC, Wolfe SW. Ulna shortening osteotomy using a compression device. *J Hand Surg Am*. 2003;28:88–93.

Chun S, Palmer AK. The ulnar impaction syndrome: follow-up of ulnar shortening osteotomy. *J Hand Surg Am*. 1993;18:46–53.

Constantine KJ, Tomaino MM, Herndon JH, et al. Comparison of ulnar shortening osteotomy and the wafer resection procedure as treatment for ulnar impaction syndrome. *J Hand Surg Am*. 2000;25:55–60.

Darrow JC Jr, Linscheid RL, Dobyns JH, et al. Distal ulnar recession for disorders of the distal radioulnar joint. *J Hand Surg Am*. 1985;10:482-491.

Ekenstam F, Hagert CG. Anatomical studies on the geometry and stability of the distal radioulnar joint. *Scand J Plast Reconstr Surg*. 1985;19:17–25.

Friedman SL, Palmer AK. The ulnar impaction syndrome. *Hand Clin*. 1991;7:295–310.

Geissler WB, Fernandez DL, Lamey DM. Distal radioulnar joint injuries associated with fractures of the distal radius. *Clin Orthop Relat Res*. 1996 Jun;327:135–146.

Hulsizer D, Weiss AP, Akelman E. Ulnar-shortening osteotomy after failed arthroscopic débridement of the triangular fibrocartilage complex. *J Hand Surg Am*. 1997;22:694–698.

Kapandji IA. The Kapandji-Sauve procedure. *J Hand Surg*. 1992;17:125–126.

Nunez FA Jr, Barnwell J, Li Z, et al. Metaphyseal ulnar shortening osteotomy for the treatment of ulnocarpal abutment syndrome using distal ulna hook plate: Case series. *J Hand Surg Am*. 2012;37A:1574–1579.

Palmer AK, Werner FW. Biomechanics of the distal radioulnar joint. *Clin Orthop Relat Res*. 1984;187:26–35.

Malunion of distal radial fractures

Amadio PC, Botte MJ. Treatment of malunion of the distal radius. *Hand Clin*. 1987;3:541–561.

Fernandez DL. Correction of post-traumatic wrist deformity in adults by osteotomy, bone-grafting, and internal fixation. *J Bone Joint Surg*. 1982;64A:1164–1178 and 2000;120:23–26.

Fernandez DL. Malunion of the distal radius: current approach to management. *Instr Course Lect*. 1993;42:99–113.

Fernandez DL, Jupiter B. *Fractures of the Distal Radius: A Practical Approach to Management*. New York: Springer;1996.

González del Pino J, Nagy L, González E, et al. Complex intra-articular osteotomy for malunion of the distal radius. Indications and surgical technique. *Rev Orthop Traumatol*. 2000;44:406–417.

Jenkins NH, Mintowt-Czyz WJ. Mal-union and dysfunction in Colles' fracture. *J Hand Surg*. 1988;13B:291–293.

Jupiter JB, Fernandez DL. Complications following distal radial fractures. *Instr Course Lect*. 2002;51:203–219.

Jupiter JB, Ring D. A comparison of early and late reconstruction of malunited fractures of the distal end of the radius. *J Bone Joint Surg Am*. 1996;78A:739–748.

Knirk JL, Jupiter JB. Intra-articular fractures of the distal end of the radius in young adults. *J Bone Joint Surg Am*. 1986;68A:647–659.

Lozano-Calderon SA, Brouwer KM, Doornberg JN, et al. Long-term outcomes of corrective osteotomy for the treatment of distal radius malunion. *J Hand Surg Am*. 2010;35E:370–380.

Prommersberger KJ, Van Schoonhoven J, Lanz UB. Outcome after corrective osteotomy for malunited fractures of the distal end of the radius. *J Hand Surg*. 2002;27B:55–60.

Rikli DA, Regazzoni P. Fractures of the distal end of the radius treated by internal fixation and early function. A preliminary report of 20 cases. *J Bone Joint Surg*. 1996;78(4):588–592.

Ring D, Roberge C, Morgan T, et al. Osteotomy for malunited fractures of the distal radius: a comparison of structural and nonstructural autogenous bone grafts. *J Hand Surg Am*. 2002;27A:216–222.

Ring D, Prommersberger KJ, Gonzalez del Pino J, et al. Corrective osteotomy for intra-articular malunion of the distal part of the radius. *J Bone Joint Surg Am*. 2005;87A:1503–1509.

Arthrodesis of the wrist

Bain GI, Watts AC. The outcome of scaphoid excision and fourcorner arthrodesis for advanced carpal collapse at a minimum of ten years. *J Hand Surg Am*. 2010; 35(5):719–725.

Bolano LE, Green DP. Wrist arthrodesis in post-traumatic arthritis: A comparison of two methods. *J Hand Surg Am*. 1993;18:786–791.

Borisch BN, Haussmann P. Radio-lunate arthrodesis in the rheumatoid wrist: a retrospective clinical and radiological long-term follow-up. *J Hand Surg*. 2002;27:61–72.

Chamay A, Della Santa D, Vilaseca A. Radiolunate arthrodesis factor of stability for the rheumatoid wrist. *Ann Chir Main*. 1983;2:5–17.

Cohen MS, Kozin SH. Degenerative arthritis of the wrist: proximal row carpectomy versus scaphoid excision and four-corner arthrodesis. *J Hand Surg Am*. 2001;26:94–104.

Cooney WP, Linscheid RL, Dobyns JH. Scaphoid fractures: problems associated with nonunion and avascular necrosis. *Orthop Clin North Am*. 1984;15:381–391.

Friedman S, Palmer A. The ulnar impaction syndrome. *Hand Clin*. 1991;7:295-310.

Garcia-Elias M, Cooney WP, An KN, et al. Wrist kinematics after limited intercarpal arthrodesis. *J Hand Surg Am*. 1989;14:791–799.

González del Pino J, Campbell D, Fischer T, et al. Variable angle locking intercarpal fusion system for four-corner arthrodesis: Indications and surgical technique. *J Wrist Surg*. 2012 Aug;1(1):73–78.

Hastings H. Arthrodesis of the osteoarthritic wrist. In: Gelberman RH, ed. *Master Techniques in Orthopaedic Surgery. The Wrist*. New York: Raven Press;1994:345–350.

Hastings H, Weiss APC, Quenzer D, et al. Arthrodesis of the wrist for post-traumatic disorders. *J Bone Joint Surg Am*. 1996;78:897–902.

Krakauer JD, Bishop AT, Cooney WP. Surgical treatment of scapholunate advanced collapse. *J Hand Surg Am*. 1994;19:751–759.

Krimmer H, Wiemer P, Kalb K. Comparative outcome assessment of the wrist joint—mediocarpal partial arthrodesis and total arthrodesis. *Handchir Mikrochir Plast Chir*. 2000;32:369–374.

Mulford JS, Ceulemans LJ, Nam D, et al. Proximal row carpectomy vs four corner fusion for scapholunate (SLAC) or scaphoid nonunion advanced collapse (SNAC) wrists: a systematic review of outcomes. *J Hand Surg Eur*. 2009;34(2):256–263.

Nagy L, Büchler U. Long-term results of radioscapholunate fusion following fractures of the distal radius. *J Hand Surg*. 1997;22:705–710.

Ozyurekoglu T, Turker T. Results of a method of 4-corner arthrodesis using headless compression screws. *J Hand Surg Am*. 2012;37(3):486–492.

Palmer AK, Dobyns JH, Linscheid RL. Management of post-traumatic instability of the wrist secondary to ligament rupture. *J Hand Surg Am*. 1978;3:507–532.

Shin AY. Four-corner arthrodesis. *J Am Soc Surg Hand*. 2001;1:93–111.

Shin EK, Jupiter JB. Radioscapholunate arthrodesis for advanced degenerative radiocarpal osteoarthritis. *Tech Hand Up Extrem Surg*. 2007;11:180–183.

Strauch RJ. Scapholunate advanced collapse and scaphoid nonunion advanced collapse arthritis—update on evaluation and treatment. *J Hand Surg Am*. 2011; 36(4):729–735.

Watson HK, Ballet FL. The SLAC wrist: scapholunate advanced collapse pattern of degenerative arthritis. *J Hand Surg Am*. 1984;9:358–365.

Weiss APC, Hastings H. Wrist arthrodesis for traumatic conditions: a study of plate and local bone graft application. *J Hand Surg Am*. 1995;20:50–56.

Wyrick JD, Stern PJ, Kiefhaber TR. Motion-preserving procedures in the treatment of scapholunate advanced collapse wrist: proximal row carpectomy versus four-corner arthrodesis. *J Hand Surg Am*. 1995;20:965–970.

AO/OTA Fracture and Dislocation Classification

Distal radius and ulna
Hand and carpus

For further educational material about the classification and access to the complete Fracture and Dislocation Classification Compendium, please use the QR code.

Distal radius and ulna

2R3/2U3

Location: Radius/Ulna, **distal end segment** 2R3/2U3

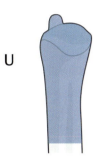

U

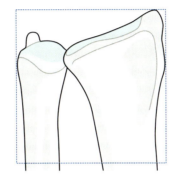

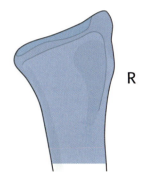

R

Types:

Radius, distal end segment,
extraarticular fracture
2R3A

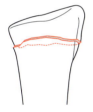

Radius, distal end segment,
partial articular fracture
2R3B

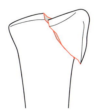

Radius, distal end segment,
complete articular fracture
2R3C

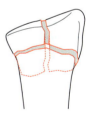

Ulna, distal end segment,
extraarticular fracture
2U3A

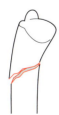

Ulna, distal end segment,
partial articular fracture
2U3B

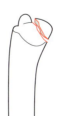

Ulna, distal end segment,
complete articular fracture
2U3C

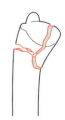

2R3A

Type: Radius, distal end segment, **extraarticular fracture** 2R3A

Group:
Radius, distal end segment, extraarticular,
radial styloid avulsion fracture
2R3A1

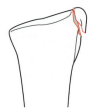

Group: Radius, distal end segment, extraarticular, **simple fracture** 2R3A2

Subgroups:

| Transverse, no displacement/tilt (may be shortened) 2R3A2.1 | Dorsal displacement/tilt (Colles) 2R3A2.2 | Volar displacement/tilt (Smith's) 2R3A2.3 |

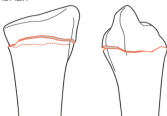 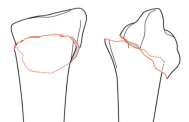 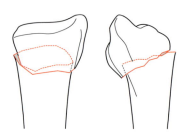

Group: Radius, distal end segment, extraarticular, **wedge or multifragmentary fracture** 2R3A3

Subgroups:

| Intact wedge fracture 2R3A3.1 | Fragmentary wedge fracture 2R3A3.2 | Multifragmentary fracture 2R3A3.3 |

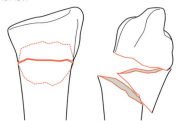 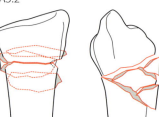 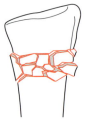 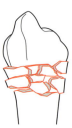

2U3A

Type: Ulna, distal end segment, **extraarticular fracture** 2U3A

Group: Ulna, distal end segment, extraarticular, **styloid process fracture** 2U3A1

Subgroups:

Tip of styloid fracture
2U3A1.1

Base of styloid fracture
2U3A1.2

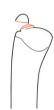

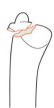

Group: Ulna, distal end segment, extraarticular, **simple fracture** 2U3A2

Subgroups:

Spiral fracture
2U3A2.1

Oblique fracture (≥30°)
2U3A2.2

Transverse fracture (<30°)
2U3A2.3

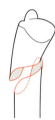

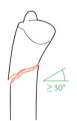

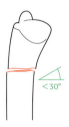

Group: Ulna, distal end segment, extraarticular, **multifragmentary fracture** 2U3A3

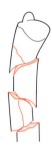

2R3B

Type: Radius, distal end segment, **partial articular fracture** 2R3B

Group: Radius, distal end segment, partial articular, **sagittal fracture** 2R3B1

Subgroups:
Involving scaphoid fossa
2R3B1.1

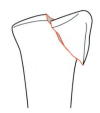

Involving lunate fossa
2R3B1.3

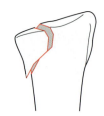

Group: Radius, distal end segment, partial articular, **dorsal rim (Barton's) fracture** 2R3B2

Subgroups:
Simple fracture
2R3B2.1

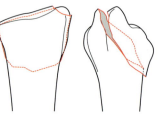

Fragmentary fracture
2R3B2.2

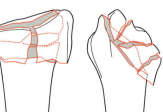

With dorsal dislocation
2R3B2.3

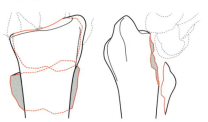

Group: Radius, distal end segment, partial articular, **volar rim (reverse Barton's, Goyrand-Smith's II) fracture** 2R3B3

Subgroups:
Simple fracture
2R3B3.1

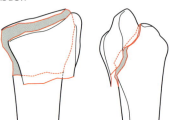

Fragmentary fracture
2R3B3.3

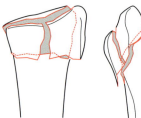

2R3C

Type: Radius, distal end segment, **complete articular fracture** 2R3C

Group: Radius, distal end segment, complete, **simple articular and metaphyseal fracture** 2R3C1

Subgroups:
Dorsomedial articular fracture 2R3C1.1*	**Sagittal articular fracture** 2R3C1.2*	**Frontal/coronal articular fracture** 2R3C1.3*

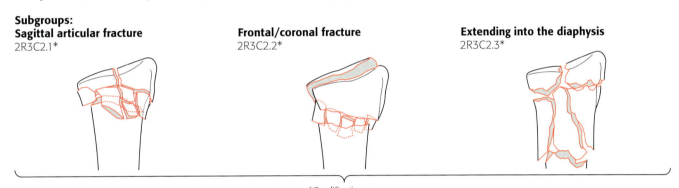

*Qualifications:
t DRUJ stable
u DRUJ unstable

Group: Radius, distal end segment, complete, simple articular, **metaphyseal multifragmentary fracture** 2R3C2

Subgroups:
Sagittal articular fracture 2R3C2.1*	**Frontal/coronal fracture** 2R3C2.2*	**Extending into the diaphysis** 2R3C2.3*

*Qualifications:
t DRUJ stable
u DRUJ unstable

Group: Radius, distal end segment, complete, **articular multifragmentary fracture, simple or multifragmentary metaphyseal fracture** 2R3C3

Subgroups:
Simple metaphyseal fracture 2R3C3.1*	Metaphyseal multifragmentary fracture 2R3C3.2*	Extending into the diaphysis 2R3C3.3*

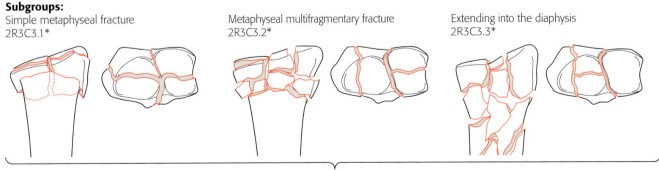

*Qualifications:
t DRUJ stable
u DRUJ unstable

Qualifications *are optional and applied to the fracture code where the asterisk is located as a lower-case letter within rounded brackets. More than one qualification can be applied for a given fracture classification, separated by a comma. For a more detailed explanation, see the compendium introduction.*

Hand and carpus

Anatomical region: Hand and carpus 7

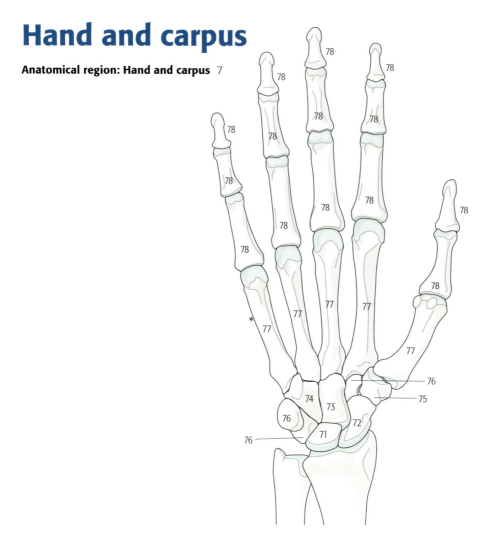

Bones:
Hand and carpus, **Lunate** 71
Hand and carpus, **Scaphoid** 72
Hand and carpus, **Capitate** 73
Hand and carpus, **Hamate** 74
Hand and carpus, **Trapezium** 75
Hand and carpus, **Other carpal bones** 76
Hand and carpus, **Metacarpal** 77
Hand and carpus, **Phalanx** 78
Hand and carpus, **Crushed, multiple fractures** 79

Qualifications are optional and applied to the fracture code where the asterisk is located as a lower-case letter within rounded brackets. More than one qualification can be applied for a given fracture classification, separated by a comma. For a more detailed explanation, see the compendium introduction.

Lunate 71

Bone: Hand and carpus, **lunate** 71

Types:

Hand and carpus, lunate,
avulsion fracture
71A

Hand and carpus, lunate,
simple fracture
71B

Hand and carpus, lunate,
multifragmentary fracture
71C

Scaphoid 72

Bone: Hand and carpus, **scaphoid** 72

Types:

Hand and carpus, scaphoid,
avulsion fracture
72A

Hand and carpus, scaphoid,
simple fracture
72B*

Hand and carpus, scaphoid,
multifragmentary fracture
72C*

*Qualifications:
a Proximal pole
b Waist
c Distal pole

Capitate 73

Bone: Hand and carpus, **capitate** 73

Types:

Hand and carpus, capitate,
avulsion fracture
73A

Hand and carpus, capitate,
simple fracture
73B

Hand and carpus, capitate,
multifragmentary fracture
73C

Hamate 74

Bone: Hand and carpus, **hamate** 74

Types:

Hand and carpus, hamate,
hook fracture
74A

Hand and carpus, hamate,
simple fracture
74B

Hand and carpus, hamate,
multifragmentary fracture
74C

Trapezium 75

Bone: Hand and carpus, **trapezium** 75

Types:

Hand and carpus, trapezium,
avulsion fracture
75A

Hand and carpus, trapezium,
simple fracture
75B

Hand and carpus, trapezium,
multifragmentary fracture
75C

Other 76._.

Bone: Hand and carpus, **other** 76.__.

| **Pisiform** | **Triquetrum** | **Trapezoid** |
| 76.1. | 76.2. | 76.3. |

→ The bone identifier (between two dots .__.) is added to the code after the anatomical region.

76.1

Hand and carpus, **pisiform** 76.1.

Type:

Hand and carpus, other, pisiform, **avulsion fracture**
76.1.A

Hand and carpus, other, pisiform, **simple fracture**
76.1.B

Hand and carpus, other, pisiform, **multifragmentary fracture**
76.1.C

76.2

Hand and carpus, **triquetrum** 76.2.

Type:

Hand and carpus, other, triquetrum, **avulsion fracture**
76.2.A

Hand and carpus, other, triquetrum, **simple fracture**
76.2.B

Hand and carpus, other, triquetrum, **multifragmentary fracture**
76.2.C

76.3

Hand and carpus, **trapezoid** 76.3.

Type:

Hand and carpus, other, trapezoid, **avulsion fracture**
76.3.A

Hand and carpus, other, trapezoid, **simple fracture**
76.3.B

Hand and carpus, other, trapezoid, **multifragmentary fracture**
76.3.C

Metacarpals 77.__.

Bone: Hand and carpus, **metacarpal** 77.__.

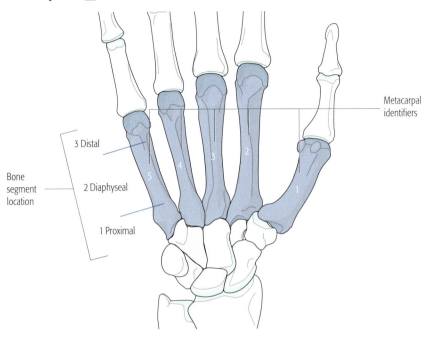

Metacarpal identifiers

3 Distal

Bone segment location

2 Diaphyseal

1 Proximal

→ The metacarpal bones are identified as follows: Thumb = 1, index = 2, long or middle = 3, ring = 4, and little = 5.
→ The metacarpal identifier is added (between two dots .__.) after the bone code.
→ The bone segment location is then added.
→ Example: Hand, 3rd metacarpal, proximal end segment = 77.3.1

Location: Hand and carpus, metacarpal, **proximal end segment** 77.__.1
→ Example code for the 3rd metacarpal is indicated with an underline 77.3.1

Types:

Hand and carpus, metacarpal, proximal end segment, **extraarticular fracture**	Hand and carpus, metacarpal, proximal end segment, **partial articular fracture**	Hand and carpus, metacarpal, proximal end segment, **complete articular**
77.3.1A	77.3.1B	77.3.1C

Location: Hand and carpus, metacarpal, **diaphyseal fracture** 77.__.2
→ Example code for the 3rd metacarpal is indicated with an underline 77.3.2
Types:

Hand and carpus, metacarpal, diaphyseal, **simple fracture**	Hand and carpus, metacarpal, diaphyseal, **wedge fracture**	Hand and carpus, metacarpal, diaphyseal, **multifragmentary fracture**
77. 3.2A	77. 3.2B	77. 3.2C

Location: Hand and carpus, metacarpal, **distal end segment** 77.__.3
→ Example code for the 3rd metacarpal is indicated with an underline 77.3.3
Types:

Hand and carpus, metacarpal, distal end segment, **extraarticular fracture**	Hand and carpus, metacarpal, distal end segment, **partial articular fracture**	Hand and carpus, metacarpal, distal end segment, **complete articular fracture**
77. 3.3A	77. 3.3B	77. 3.3C

Phalanx 78.__.__.

Bone: Hand and carpus, **phalanx** 78.__.__.

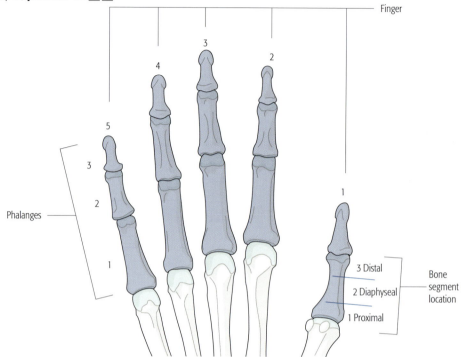

→ The fingers and phalanges are identified as follows:
Fingers: Thumb = 1, index = 2, long or middle = 3, ring = 4, and little = 5.
Phalanges: Proximal phalanx = 1, middle phalanx = 2, and distal phalanx = 3.
The finger identifier plus phalanx identifier are added (between dots .__.__.) after the bone code.
→ Example: Proximal thumb phalanx is 78.1.1.
→ The location is then added.
→ **Anatomical region+bone.Finger.Phalanx.Bone segment location**
→ Example: Proximal thumb phalanx proximal end segment is 78.1.1.1

Location: Hand and carpus, phalanx, **proximal end segment** 78.1.1.1
→ Example code for proximal thumb phalanx is indicated with an underline 78.1.1.1

Types:

Hand and carpus, phalanx, proximal end segment, **extraarticular fracture** 78.1.1.1A	Hand and carpus, phalanx, proximal end segment, **partial articular fracture** 78.1.1.1B	Hand and carpus, phalanx, proximal end segment, **complete articular fracture** 78.1.1.1C

Location: Hand and carpus, phalanx **diaphyseal fracture** 78.1.1.2
→ Example code for proximal thumb phalanx is indicated with an underline 78.1.1.2

Types:

Hand and carpus, phalanx, diaphyseal, **simple fracture** 78.1.1.2A	Hand and carpus, phalanx, diaphyseal, **wedge fracture** 78.1.1.2B	Hand and carpus, phalanx, diaphyseal, **multifragmentary fracture** 78.1.1.2C

Location: Hand and carpus, phalanx, **distal end segment** 78.1.1.3
→ Example code for proximal thumb phalanx is indicated with an underline 78.1.1.3

Types:

Hand and carpus, phalanx, distal end segment, **extraarticular fracture** 78.1.1.3A	Hand and carpus, phalanx, distal end segment, **partial articular fracture** 78.1.1.3B	Hand and carpus, phalanx, distal end segment, **complete articular fracture** 78.1.1.3C

Crushed, multiple fractures 79

Hand and carpus, **crush, multiple fractures hand** 79

Qualifications are optional and applied to the fracture code where the asterisk is located as a lower-case letter within rounded brackets. More than one qualification can be applied for a given fracture classification, separated by a comma. For a more detailed explanation, see the compendium introduction.

509

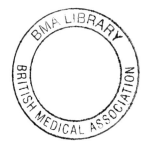